Inhibition

4/2001

Inhibition

History and Meaning in the Sciences of Mind and Brain

Roger Smith

UNIVERSITY OF CALIFORNIA PRESS
Berkeley Los Angeles

University of California Press
Berkeley and Los Angeles, California

Published by arrangement with Free Association Books, London.

Library of Congress Cataloging-in-Publication Data
Smith, Roger, 1945–
Inhibition: history and meaning in the sciences of mind and brain/ Roger Smith.
p. cm.
Includes bibliographical references and index.
ISBN 0-520-07580-3 (cloth: alk. paper)
1. Neurophysiology—History. 2. Psychology—History. 3. Inhibition. I. Title.
QP353.S65 1992
612.8—dc20 91-37839
CIP

Printed in the United States of America

The paper used in this publication meets the minimum requirements of American National Standard for Information Sciences—Permanence of Paper for Printed Library Materials, ANSI Z39.48-1984 ∞

Contents

Preface

Even avid dictionary browsers may be surprised by a book that appears to be about just one word. This book, like a dictionary, ties meaning to historical usage, but it also goes much further. It is common enough to praise the richness of language. It is less usual to unravel this quality to account for knowledge and meaning in historical context. It is even less usual to do this for scientific language, especially since most people expect scientific words to have precise and technical reference. I argue that scientific knowledge is, through its language, embedded in the meanings and evaluations of a wider Western culture. This is a history of scientific concepts of control, signified by the word "inhibition," that aims to show that the meaning of scientific knowledge about human beings is profoundly informed by—and, in turn, informs—evaluations of being human. The historical subject is what is claimed about human nature.

"Inhibition" is central to reflection on how order is possible at the social and the individual level: how social values instruct a person's action, how we exercise—or fail to exercise—our will, how the mind regulates the body, and how the brain controls the automatic physiological functions. As I will explore at length, it is a word denoting mental and physical control, and it has both scientific and lay usage. In writing about the word's meaning, I in fact discuss a wide area of both the human and the natural sciences.

The history of inhibition, conceived as a history of scientific knowledge, concerns major topics in nineteenth-century and early-twentieth-century physiology and psychology. I go into some detail, working from published primary sources. There are two reasons for this. The first, straightforwardly, is that little systematic historical work relevant to inhibition has been undertaken. Where historians or, more often, natural scientists have been before me, I use their work critically but gratefully. I owe a special debt to those scholars who have made it possible for me to incorporate the Russian and Soviet context into the account.

The second reason is more contentious. While many, but by no means all, historians have become sympathetic to arguments about the social construction of scientific knowledge, most scientists remain dismissive. It is common for scientists and commentators on science to draw a distinction between "hard" science and its "soft" imitations (such as sociology or psychology), implying that any social elements that might enter into the latter do not enter into the former. It is therefore essential to my argument to show that the indubitably "hard" science of experimental physiology (whose exponents win Nobel Prizes) shares a vocabulary, and hence a world of evaluative meaning, with the surrounding culture. Thus, the historical detail about scientific papers, especially in chapters 3 and 4, cannot be omitted. I have tried, however, to make accessible the technical writing I do touch on.

The book's primary purpose is historical. It is not subservient to either the modern natural sciences or the modern social sciences. It assumes that history creates irreducible knowledge, that is, knowledge in its own right, and that such knowledge is—and is increasingly recognized to be—an essential part of rational knowledge about being human. In writing history, I seek to know about the constitution and the reconstitution of the human subject. One way to attempt this is through describing the meanings represented in language. As it happens, those meanings discussed here will often be familiar, as we have very much taken over and perpetuated earlier usages. Thus, though historical, this history concerns ourselves.

My main debt is to the authors cited. Kurt Danziger, Christopher Lawrence, and Robert M. Young, along with the readers for the University of California Press, have helped me shape the argument. I am grateful to Horst Gundlach for advice about and help in obtaining German-language sources, and Gesine Leo has kindly revised my translations from the German. Thanks to Anne Stubbins and Susan Waddington, and especially warm gratitude to Sonja Bradshaw, for help with typing. Elizabeth Knoll and Michelle Nordon at the University of

California Press and Ann Scott and Robert M. Young at Free Association Books are my valued editors.

Bringing *Inhibition* to fruition has been a long journey. I first aired the topic at a conference organized jointly by the British Society for the History of Science and the British Sociological Association, "New Perspectives in the History and Sociology of Scientific Knowledge," at Bath in 1980. Some ideas were discussed subsequently in a paper to Cheiron: The European Society for the History of the Behavioural and Social Sciences, Heidelberg 1983, at a seminar of the Division of the History and Philosophy of Science at the University of Leeds, and at the discussion group in history of science, Lancaster University. Financial support, making possible access to sources, has come in the form of a Research Grant in the History of Science from the Royal Society.

I have sought to write in a way that combines scholarship, accessibility, an openness to ideas, and an international outlook. Though I am conscious that I do not always succeed in this, I would like to dedicate the book to my colleagues and friends in Cheiron-Europe who, at a time of immense change, have made possible a shared world.

Lancaster
July 1991

Abbreviations

C.R.A.S.	*Comptes rendus hebdomadaires des séances de l'Académie des Sciences.*
C.R.S.B.	*Comptes rendus des séances de la Société de Biologie*; or *Comptes rendus des séances et mémoires de la Société de Biologie.*
D.S.B.	*Dictionary of Scientific Biography*, ed. Charles Coulston Gillispie, 16 vols. New York: Charles Scribner's Sons, 1970–1980.
S.E.	*The Standard Edition of the Complete Psychological Works of Sigmund Freud*, trans. and ed. James Strachey, assisted by Alix Strachey and Alan Tyson, 24 vols. London: Hogarth Press, 1953–1974.
S.K.A.W.	*Sitzungsberichte der mathematisch-naturwissenschaftlichen Classe der kaiserlichen Akademie der Wissenschaft.*
S.W.	*Selected Writings of John Hughlings Jackson*, ed. James Taylor, facsimile reprint, 2 vols. London: Staples, 1958. (First publ. 1931–1932.)

CHAPTER 1

The History of Inhibition

Stop and think!

ORDER AND INHIBITION

More than a millennium and a half of Christian commentary imbued Western consciousness with a profound sense of duality between the spirit and the flesh. Each human life reenacted the drama of struggle, discipline, and sin. Catholic confessional manuals provided rules for the regulation of the flesh. A renewed seriousness in Protestant life in the eighteenth century, whether in German Pietism or in Welsh Methodism, posed the individual a stark choice between moral conduct and sin, a choice for which he or she was directly answerable to God. Theology and daily life conjoined in an acute sensibility of the threat to grace and virtue from fallen nature. Wherever one turned at the beginning of the nineteenth century, there was a sense that the mind's grasp over the body was tenuous but imperative.

This sensibility was not only theological and moralistic in content. The French Revolution revealed in an overwhelmingly terrifying manner the power of disorder latent in social existence, both to those who lived through the years of upheaval and to subsequent generations throughout the nineteenth century.[1] To conservatives—traditional rulers retained power in most of Europe for most of the nineteenth century—the Revolution and its aftermath provided exemplary justification for the control from above of the masses below. Political order and civilized values, it appeared, depended on continuing enforcement of hierarchical social arrangements between those fitted to govern and those fitted to be governed. An elaborate vocabulary of preordained or natural qualities of elites and masses, of higher and lower classes, and of mental and manual occupations informed every discussion of political life. Radical writings, proposing egalitarian, republican, and socialist conceptions of political order served only to reinforce in the minds of most educated people a fear that anarchy was threatening to break out from below. The fear took a particularly tortuous form in reactions to feminism, a movement that was to become a permanent part of political consciousness from the midcentury. One historian has thus aptly titled her collection of studies of "the woman question," *Disorderly Conduct.*[2] In parliamentary France under the Third Republic, or in Germany unified under the emperor, educated elites worried about sustaining "rational" order in the face of "irrational" mass pressures. When some liberalization did become part of political life, as with the extension of the male franchise in Britain in 1832, 1867, and 1884, it tended to be accompanied by the internalization of the traditional values of control and order in the newly empowered groups. Britain thus achieved an envied political stability, central to which was a way of thought linking control within the individual and control within the state. The Victorians repeatedly explained political success in terms of the character of Britain's peoples. English-language writers condescendingly described a contrast between themselves and the excitable Italians or Greeks, referring interchangeably to individual character and to collective order and disorder.[3]

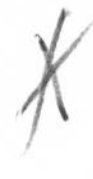

Nineteenth-century moral and political discourse unified expressions of order and disorder. Its language associated spirit and flesh, head and hand, culture and nature, male and female, and the higher classes and the masses. These were very rich linguistic resources, making it possible to characterize relationships and differentiate values in multitudinous ways and for very diverse purposes. Discourse of this quality is open-ended rather than constraining.[4] There were recurrent patterns or emphases, however, and prominent among these was a stress on the latent power of disorder to break out unless restrained by the watchful eye of the ordering power. English-language writers, at least until about 1870, did not refer to this pattern as involving inhibition, but they clearly stressed a conception of regulation equivalent to what was later described by that term.

The history of inhibition describes representations of regulation as natural phenomena. There was a gradual reformulation of religious, moral, and political "higher" powers of control in terms, initially psychological, of the mind's control over the body and, later physiological, of the brain's control over the nervous system. Language changed: speaking loosely, spirit became mind, and mind became the upper brain; flesh became body, and body became the spinal nervous system. The translated language substantially perpetuated an earlier logic of regulatory relations and a system of evaluative meaning. The most straightforward illustration is provided by writers who compared hierarchical government in society and hierarchical control in the nervous system, a comparison common even at the end of the century, long after neurophysiology had become a specialized science. As the neurologist Charles Mercier wrote, at one and the same time describing brain damage and the loss of an army commander, "But whether the immediate effect of the loss of the highest authority is an outbreak of excessive but misdirected vigour, or whether it is a general condition of diminished activity, in either case the ultimate result is a loss of efficiency on behalf of the body at large."[5]

Order was sustained most obviously by higher powers controlling lower ones. In conservative Europe, such as Imperial Germany or Tsarist Russia, rule from above accompanied a political and moral culture that embedded such hierarchical control in everyday expectations. In the more liberal systems of Britain or the United States, political and moral hierarchies were certainly also present, though newer entrepreneurial classes achieved solid economic power, and social order therefore appeared to correlate more with market relations. As other nations began to share Britain's experience of industrialization, an experience that was sometimes traumatic and always socially disruptive, the perception that order was a function of competitive economic relations became more prominent. Representation of order in terms of self-correcting relations therefore existed alongside representations of order as control from above. Vociferous and sometimes violent calls for the more equal distribution of power, for empowerment of the urban proletariat or for women's emancipation, kept order at the top of the political agenda. Conservatives and intellectuals alike worried whether disorder was implicit in such changes. Striking coal miners in the Nord, socialists agitating in Turin's factories, or crowds pouring onto the streets of Saint Petersburg dramatically reminded everyone that industrialization called into question political traditions.

These events have an economic, social, and political history. But we also wish to understand what these events meant to those who, directly or indirectly, were caught up in them. We therefore turn to look at the way people described order and disorder, using language or other forms of communication to construct meaning and significance and to give expression to their hopes and fears.

If the nineteenth century was an age of industrialization, provoking the rethinking of human relations, it was also a scientific age. Many observers, indeed, believed that science and industry were almost synonymous. What science meant in practice, including its relations with industry, was almost infinitely varied, but it always included a body of what was claimed to be reliable knowledge. Such knowledge became a powerful and widespread means for constructing sense in modern Western society. Nineteenth-century writers drew on science to interpret the events about them. Science became bound up with the search to render human life intelligible. At the same time, scientists drew on the language used to describe events about them in framing their new knowledge. A web of meaning, represented by language, constituted a common world.

This will be described for inhibition. Rather than proceed in generalities concerning either social change or the development of scientific knowledge since the early nineteenth century, I will discuss the meaning of "just" one word. Even then, I will sharpen the focus most clearly on the word's meaning in science; but, in so doing, I intend to show that the word contains meanings going far beyond the confines of scientific communities. Such claims are simple to make but complex to support.

The history of inhibition ranges across Europe and, to a lesser extent, North America from the late eighteenth century to the present. Faced by this, and faced by the need in writing history to be precise in order to be persuasive, it is necessary to attend to local developments and settings. In this study, most detailed attention is given to Britain. Negatively, this is a function of access to sources and of my restricted linguistic competencies. Positively, the case that links science to a general discourse about order can be made for this setting as well as any other. The study does, however, examine the full range of meanings associated with inhibition in the wider European world. The intention is to reconstruct the discourse of which the word was part. This introduction examines these intentions and the way they relate to other work on the history of mind and body. In chapter 2, I outline relevant notions of ordered relations in the first half of the nineteenth century. I argue in chapter 3 that these notions of order were fundamentally important to the emergent "hard" science of neurophysiology in the nineteenth century. In chapters 4 and 5, I consider the relations between brain physiology and the different branches of psychology in the late nineteenth century and the first part of the twentieth century. Finally, in conclusion, I return to the more general themes with which this study begins.

The English language is rich in psychological words that presuppose and reaffirm an individualistic sense of self. Many of these terms also convey a sense of the individual's relation to others, of emotional and moral interaction, and of the individual's place in a larger order. Such is the case for the everyday word, "inhibition."

The act of inhibition is dynamic and implies conflict, perhaps between powers within the individual, perhaps between the individual and outside forces. The relationship may refer simply to one force controlling another, or it may imply the suppression of some spontaneous or natural energy. The language often suggests that control, expressed as inhibition, whether internalized or coming from without, is a fundamental condition of social life. Significantly, three major twentieth-century scientific traditions have each worked inhibition hard as a conceptual resource: C. S. Sherrington's neurophysiology in the English-speaking world, I. P. Pavlov's theory of higher nervous activity in the Soviet world, and Sigmund Freud's psychoanalysis.

It was Freud who gave the most profound and disturbing account of such control as a precondition of social existence, though he described control as an act of unconscious repression rather than conscious inhibition. His essay, *Civilization and Its Discontents* (1930), compared the growth of the individual ego, through a power to repress the instincts, with the growth of civilization. He expected neither one nor the other to be accompanied by much happiness. "It is this battle of the giants that our nurse-maids try to appease with their lullaby about Heaven."[6] Freud rearticulated a deeply entrenched Western sensibility. Its most enduring and symbolically most prolific form has been as original sin, a heaviness of being in this world which can be assimilated but never lost: "And dust ye shall eat all the days of your life."[7] The language of Freud and the language of Genesis have now become inextricably mixed, and a popularized psychoanalysis informs everyday expression about inhibition. The inhibited person has become a stock character of popular psychology, hiding his or her real desires behind a veil of politeness, diffidence, and abstinence—and doubtless being constipated as well.

Understanding the meaning of words involves going beyond the definitions of dictionaries. Words are representations of what we hold to be the case, descriptively and evaluatively. Their history is a history of what it has been to be human. The history of even what may be thought a simple word is therefore complex. As for "inhibition," while it is embedded in a popular language describing character and conduct, it is also an extremely common term in the physiological and psychological sciences. This essay is a history of the nineteenth-century background of the latter usage. Yet it will argue that these scientific contexts share many meanings in common with the everyday world. Raymond Williams's comments on "keywords" are relevant:

> [They form a vocabulary] which is significantly not the specialized vocabulary of a specialized discipline, though it often overlaps with several of these, but a general vocabulary ranging from strong, difficult and persuasive words in everyday usage to words which, beginning in particular specialized contexts, have become quite common in descriptions of wider areas of thought and experience. This, significantly, is the vocabulary we share with others, often imperfectly, when we wish to discuss many of the central processes of our common life.[8]

A glance at the exceedingly esoteric and minutely precise world of the modern neurosciences, in which "inhibition" is a term in constant use, might suggest this is a highly implausible claim. After all, even to have any understanding of a neuroscientific paper requires an extensive training, whereas there is no difficulty about anyone using the word "inhibition" on a daily basis. Nevertheless, however remote the language of science may appear to be, we cannot simply assume that there is no connection between it and the loose expressions of popular culture. Studies in the sociology of scientific knowledge have shown how communities of scientists construct their technical vocabulary, skills, and truths on a day-to-day basis, drawing on both their own traditions and the wider culture to do so.[9] Scientific papers exhibit many features in common with other literatures, and they include terms that have both narrow technical meaning and rich metaphorical associations. Words carry social values into the heart of science.[10] All language, whether technical or nontechnical, has a rhetorical form. This is intrinsic, not just extrinsic, to what is meant when the language is used.

The history of science plays a fundamental part in understanding science's relations to the wider culture. This history will show how even the scientists' most esoteric pursuits originated in experience, in curiosity, or in concerns widely shared and how technical and popular formulations of the subject gradually separated. A study of the adaptation of language and the way occupationally separate groups adopt words for special and restricted uses uncovers the common ground of meanings embedding science in Western culture.

"Inhibition" has been a richly allusive psychological term ever since it came into common use in the nineteenth century. It also has had a seemingly neutral definition: "By inhibition we mean the arrest of the functions of a structure or organ, by the action upon it of another, while its power to execute those functions is still retained, and can be manifested as soon as the restraining power is removed."[11] This definition appears bland and unexceptional. Yet it has limited value as a guide to historical understanding since it glosses over deep and continuously debated questions concerning relations between mind and body, between the human and the physical sciences, and between values and facts.

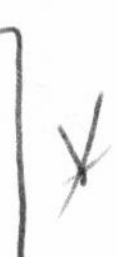

It is highly significant that nineteenth-century scientific writers used the term in *both* physiology and psychology, and this continues. Inhibition and the relation between physiology and psychology in the nineteenth century will therefore be a prominent theme in subsequent chapters. Inhibition, however, became most elaborated as an idea in neurophysiology, and the antonyms "inhibition" and "excitation" were fundamental to descriptions of the nervous system's regulatory—or, in Sherrington's term, integrative—function. Since the 1950s, inhibition has persisted as a common term in neuroscience, a discipline that its proponents consider integrates physiology and psychology.

The history of inhibition is also part of a wider history of regulation and control, concerns that are so fundamental they almost define the scope of the sciences of body, mind, and behavior. They are also central to thought about the social nature of the individual and to the very continuance of social life. The concept of regulation belongs to concerns as far apart as theodicy, the vindication of divine providence, and the history of technology. Some concrete exemplifications of this can be studied as inhibition.

A shift toward describing mental qualities as the outcome of physiological processes occurred as nineteenth-century society underwent industrialization and experienced the emotional and imaginative consequences of new technology. By the second half of the century, changes in productivity and labor were following not only from factory organization but also from new science-based chemical or electrical technologies. Regulation at the level of production in the factory, at the level of the factory machinery itself, and in relation to finance and markets was a major concern. Political economy flourished as an intellectual discipline addressing the regulation of interests in generating wealth. Discussion of order, arresting powers, equilibrium, or the balance of forces occurred equally in technological, economic, and moral contexts. When the word "inhibition" itself came into common currency, it necessarily had associations with the regulation of the economy and with technology.[12] Features from this wider world, such as the self-regulating capacities of the governor on the steam engine or of the trade cycle, may have informed the meanings of the word. In particular, the dynamics of control, through the redistribution or antagonism of forces within a closed-energy system, a physical economy, became a significant background feature of twentieth-century physiology and psychology. All this had profound implications for the ancient vision of "man a machine."[13] The story of inhibition, which represented values as natural features, is therefore one contribution to appreciating the wider meaning of order within social life.

Even "inhibition" itself, as a term referring to control, has multiple meanings. It may indicate a relationship between two forces, one power, at least for a time, arresting and thereby regulating another power. In such circumstances, the inhibitory relationship is frequently a hierarchical one, in which a higher power (such as will) controls a lower one (such as instincts). Inhibition may also indicate a competitive relationship between different but comparable forces in a limited field, the redistribution of energy in a closed system. An example would be the competition of sensations for conscious attention. But I shall not construct abstract models of different types of inhibitory relations as a contribution to specifying the logic of control systems. My purpose is a historical one, to describe the meanings that "inhibition" has had by studying the term's use in scientific knowledge.

The main lines of the story may be summarized briefly. Early-nineteenth-century writers inherited descriptions of character, beliefs in pedagogy, and moralistic attitudes that described the power of the mind over the body and that consequently addressed conduct in terms of the mind's power to regulate an individual's life. In German, the noun *Hemmung* and the verb *hemmen* (now generally translated as "inhibition" and "to inhibit") were in relatively common use. The same words also described the jostle of perceptions (*Vorstellungen*) by which one conscious element replaced another in the mind, with implications for such everyday psychological phenomena as attention. These usages continued through the nineteenth century, becoming a potent resource in medical writings, especially in medical psychology but also in neurology. The establishment of academic traditions in experimental

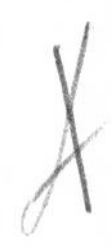

neurophysiology, which occurred in the 1820s and 1830s, went hand in hand with the construction of organizing concepts about the nervous system, notably, localization of function and the reflex. This consolidated a way of thinking about regulation in the body that extended the explanatory terms of physical science to include psychological phenomena. Inhibition was among the most productive of the concepts that made this development possible. From the late 1830s, scientists discussed inhibition as a function within the nervous system and it became the subject of considerable experimental research in its own right. The discovery of vagal (peripheral) inhibition by E. F. W. Weber (1845) and of central inhibition by I. M. Sechenov (1862) are known to scientists as major achievements. Thereafter, inhibition featured in diverse and increasingly specialized research programs in neurophysiology, gaining a special place in Sherrington's early-twentieth-century synthesis. The recognizably modern specialties of physiological psychology, experimental psychology, and neurology, each using the concept of inhibition, diverged in the second half of the nineteenth century. The new psychology continued to value inhibition as a term to describe competition between mental elements or, in the context of learning theory, the arresting action on behavior of stimuli or responses. The three sharply contrasting schools of Sherrington, Pavlov, and Freud then demand attention in understanding the transmission of the research into the twentieth century. A degree of synthesis between Western and Soviet traditions, along with a renewed commitment to the reduction of psychological explanations to physiological ones, has inspired the more recent neuroscience of the 1950s and 1960s. Both neuroscience and experimental psychology, before and after the so-called cognitive revolution around 1970, have continued to find a central place for inhibition.

A note on language is necessary, though it is not to the point to make a fetish of the particular Latin root *in + habere*. The general meaning of this root, to hold in, suggests what is of interest. "To inhibit" has a variety of cognates: to arrest, to hinder, to repress, and so forth. The same holds for the German form, *hemmen*, which was in widespread psychological use long before the parallel English, to inhibit. Thus, Grimm cited such phrases as *die Krankheit hemmt mein Vorhaben* (the illness inhibits my purpose) or *mit in der Brust gehemmtem Athem* (with inhibited breath in the breast) from the end of the eighteenth century. Schiller and Goethe frequently used the word.[14] The *Oxford English Dictionary* records that before the second half of the nineteenth century, the verb—and even more, the noun—denoted the legal restraint exercised by a higher ecclesiastical power. The word appeared occasionally in relation to temperament or bodily functions, though I have not seen a physiological meaning before 1858 (in a context described in chap. 3). Thereafter, it became common in physiology. In French, *inhibition* was introduced by the Mauritian-French-American neurologist and neurophysiologist, Charles-Édouard Brown-Séquard, around 1870, and this supplemented earlier physiological uses of *arrêter* (to arrest) and *centres modérateurs* (regulatory centers).[15] It seems likely that the French term was subsequently adopted in Italian, as *inibizione*, though the use of *inibere*, in the sense of the exercise of impeding authority, was much older.[16] In Russian, "inhibition" has commonly been translated by the word used for braking, and it has thus perhaps carried somewhat different connotations.[17]

The modern usage of the word "inhibition" and its derivatives is therefore intimately bound up with the development of scientific physiology and with the authority this discipline has acquired as knowledge of the body. By the late nineteenth century, it appeared to many writers on human physiology and psychology that inhibition was a fact of regulation that made ordered action possible. Inhibition described physical processes that sustained the life of human beings as objects in the natural world. The fact of inhibition therefore played a significant part in the nineteenth-century assimilation of humans to the laws of physical nature. It was part of the same Victorian world that so fervently examined evolutionary ideas.[18] Further, just as the development of evolutionary thought articulated issues in political economy, so the development of ideas of control in mind and brain articulated issues in moral philosophy. Scientific theories of inhibition reexpressed ways of thought already embedded in the culture. In doing so, however, they lent an authority based on the prestige of observational scientific methods. Inhibition became part of a language characterizing regulation as a natural process, thereby confirming conceptions of ordered life that people already possessed. But this return re-presented those conceptions as objective descriptions of nature.[19] The history of inhibition is a dialogue between the desire to exercise moral control and the description of natural control. This dialogue has presupposed a common discourse, that is, a world of coordinated meanings in language.[20] This book seeks to delineate this world.

The broader issues are so vast that an ordering and simplifying theme is a necessity. Thus, we turn to the detailed history of inhibition itself. Even then there will be large areas of relevant nineteenth-century culture (I have in mind literature or technology), as well as of science, that escape attention. This should require no apology: a historical interpretation may be assessed by its qualities of consistency and by its synthetic power, rather than in terms of comprehensive correspondence with a supposed historical reality. Thus, this study would be well rewarded were readers to feel that ideas about control and inhibition were "obviously" represented in writings other than those discussed here. It is exactly that familiarity and that range of usages that give significance to the subject.

Special questions arise in describing the history of scientific knowledge owing to the unique rationality and objectivity claimed for such knowledge. It is as well, therefore, to make my position clear, not by providing developed answers to philosophical questions but by indicating the subject matter of which this is a history. This subject matter is the meaning of nineteenth- and early-twentieth-century claims to knowledge about controlling relations between mind and brain and within the nervous system itself. I argue that this knowledge was intrinsically normative or evaluative, as well as empirical, in content. Thus, I presuppose—and then try to justify this presupposition through historical argument—that physiological or psychological scientific statements shared meanings with contemporary moral and social language. I suggest that there was a single discourse for scientific and ethical domains, however much that discourse was refined in specialized ways by particular occupational groups such as experimental neurophysiologists. I do not impose judgments distinguishing "science" from "nonscience," least of all by defining the former as value-free and the latter as value-laden. Quite the opposite: this is a study of science as a dimension of a shared culture.

The development of a sociology of scientific knowledge that, in its strong form, seeks causal explanations for the truth status of knowledge in social processes has transformed historical writing about science.[21] Not surprisingly, it has provoked debates, which still continue, about rationality and relativity. It is not necessary for my historical purposes, however, to enter into such issues. These purposes are hermeneutic, that is, concerned with meaning rather than causal explanation, aimed at historical interpretation rather than sociological analysis. But of course I do share with the sociological program the (relatively) weak claim that the meaning of knowledge statements has social content and therefore that the history of science is about society as well as about nature or, rather, that the categories "nature" and "society" are mutually constitutive.

What has "inhibition" meant as a term within the sciences of mind and body? To answer this question, I describe natural scientists and fellow travelers engaged in experimenting on animals, recording clinical observations, and formulating accounts of what is taken to be natural reality. Their aim was knowledge, a consistent set of representations of the natural. Clearly, knowledge, if it is to be acceptable as natural science, must satisfy correspondence conditions; that is, there must be a strict relationship between representation and what is taken to be reality. A regular and critical attention to this relationship is the very stuff of scientific practice. The relationship of scientist and his or her knowledge to its subject, however, cannot be specified in a way that excludes reference to conceptual shaping, judgment, and values. Science, simply, like any other human activity, is social. Thus, the correspondence conditions are not the sole criteria that knowledge must satisfy. A range of other conditions exist, and these conditions structure what scientists judge to be intelligible and adequate knowledge in a field. One can thus refer to the coherence conditions that must be satisfied if a claim is to be accepted as knowledge. I therefore also describe scientists integrating reasons and values, concerning what sort of thing it is they are studying, with empirical research.

That coherence as well as correspondence conditions are fundamental in establishing natural-scientific knowledge is particularly evident in the history of the sciences of human nature. No culture exists without representations of the human agents producing that culture. The history of inhibition is bound up with such representations, conceiving of humans as highly ordered and morally regulated. Theories of inhibition became a means to represent that order and regulation. The order was perceived to be in nature, as the very concept of an "organism" attests; but accounts claiming to understand that order achieved intelligible expression by drawing on meanings shared with the moral and social world.

As mentioned, there have been two major senses in which "inhibition" has helped constitute knowledge about order. In the first, the word referred to a hierarchical arrangement in which a higher power arrests or depresses a lower power. In the second, the word portrays how more or less equal powers compete for limited resources. The former was used in theories about organizational levels in the brain, the latter in psychologies describing the organization of consciousness or behavior. These usages indicated that the word denoted processes in the body or in the mind. At the same time, they indicated that the word connoted relations of power within societies: the arrest of lower by higher agents or the competition of the economic marketplace.

The connotations of words are context dependent, and "inhibition" is no exception. There has been no linear shift from general and loose to scientific and precise meaning. Twentieth-century scientists, however exacting their experimental practices, have complained periodically about the vagueness of some of their central terms like "excitation" and "inhibition."[22] This said, it is still possible to note that the late-nineteenth- and early-twentieth-century history of physiological inhibition does illustrate a common pattern in the history of scientific knowledge: the achievement of factual modes of expression through the specialization and narrowing of an independent community's linguistic practices. But just as no community, however specialized, is in fact fully independent of the wider society, so no word—least of all "inhibition"—achieves a denotative meaning freeing it from connotative evaluations. It is therefore an empirical historical matter to recover the meaning of words in context.

These matters may appear to some scientists to be remote from the history of inhibition as the history of *science*. Yet once such history moves away from reporting the serial discovery of empirical truths, all these questions follow. It cannot make sense to ask for knowledge unmediated by history and culture.

THE HISTORY OF PHYSIOLOGY AND PSYCHOLOGY

Running through the history of "inhibition," as with some other key concepts in science, such as "force" in mechanics, was an ambivalence amounting to a philosophical problem. The word referred to a causal process or to a functional relationship. Both usages were common. Sometimes scientists sought to understand inhibition as a specific physical mechanism. At other times, they used the word to describe the function of particular nerves or parts of the brain. On yet other occasions, the word characterized relations within the mind or between the brain and the mind. Language rarely drew logically refined distinctions. Instead, it provided the means for the elaboration of metaphor and the carrying over of meanings between related issues.

General accounts of biology and, to use another modern term, the biomedical sciences have stressed organization and structure-function relations as conceptual fundamentals. Biology was, in origin, a nineteenth-century science, the term "biology" being used right at the beginning of the century, and inhibition theories contributed to the general conditions of understanding in which biology became a branch of knowledge.[23] The discovery of inhibition was part of a larger endeavor to give detailed empirical content to structure-function relations, while retaining a feeling for the integrated place of those relations within the organism as a whole. The purpose of biology was to understand "organic" relations, using "organic" in the double sense of existing in an organism and of integrating a whole.

Organization and control is a central theme in the general history of biology, from Xavier Bichat's conception of life as the sum of forces resisting death to Claude Bernard's formulation of the *milieu intérieur* (internal environment) to Walter B. Cannon's principle of homeostasis to modern cybernetics and systems thinking.[24] There have been repeated attempts to portray life itself as essentially a regulatory phenomenon. Visions of social order, presupposing comparable regulatory patterns, informed these biological philosophies and, at the same time, were enriched by biological thought. Modern systems thinking, indeed, emerged as a project to provide a general mathematical theory of organized relations.[25] Cybernetics, the science of "control and communication in the animal and the machine" in Norbert Wiener's famous definition, drew on comparisons between engineering governors, early computing circuits and self-guidance systems, to interpret control as a property of action providing informative feedback on itself.[26] As Wiener recognized, the prototype of such feedback control was the purposive, regulatory power of the organism. In a well-known paper in 1943, Wiener and his collaborators pointed out how their approach to control could provide a resolution, in mechanistic explanatory terms, of the fact that biologists continued to depend on teleological descriptions (i.e., descriptions evoking purposes).[27]

A general commitment to the possibility of scientific knowledge about human beings, which is such a marked feature of modern thought, was in large measure an achievement of the nineteenth century. Experimental physiology and practical medicine greatly encouraged physical conceptions of human existence. Darwinian and other evolutionary theories drew life in general, and human life in particular, into historical continuity with nature. Karl Marx coupled social and political arrangements with natural law through the history of the material relations of production. Auguste Comte described a single method for attaining knowledge that would put the conduct of human affairs on the same footing as the control of nature. Extension of the principle of the uniformity of nature to encompass the human sphere was accompanied by struggle, indecision, and endless divergence of opinion. There was nothing inevitable about these intellectual developments, no more than for any other major historical event. Nor did new knowledge develop in a linear fashion. Much nineteenth-century thought appears in retrospect to have had an ambivalent character, pointing at one and the same time to belief that the human condition was separate from the condition of nature and to belief that integrated human and natural conditions. Language often left unresolved a choice between new or old, between a concern with human culture or human science, between a religious or a secular world view. This is not to say that such language represented apathy or confusion. Indeed, the opposite was the case: the vocabulary that sustained the possibility of compromise became a particularly valued resource and a focus for the intense emotions that accompanied cultural change.

The nineteenth-century debate on the continuity of the human with the natural sphere repeatedly employed a rhetoric for and against materialism. Calling a belief "materialism" rarely meant anything philosophically precise. It was more a way of indicating that grand issues were at stake: Christianity versus atheism, morality versus anarchy, purpose versus nihilism. Significant conflicts of social interest accompanied such debates. Nevertheless, everyone agreed that a science of physiology grounded in physical explanations, which was a prominent and challenging feature of scientific culture from the 1840s, equipped materialism as a world view with a powerful and seemingly precise resource. For many physiologists and their supporters and popularizers, this was not just *a* resource but *the* empirically authoritative program for uncovering the truth of the human condition. This was the message of individual writers and also a collective message, increasingly entrenched in educational, medical, and scientific institutions, from the Medical Surgical Academy in Saint Petersburg to the Gesellschaft der Aerzte (Society of Physicians) in Vienna to the British Association for the Advancement of Science in Belfast.

Scientific physiology had to face the ever-present question of the relation of mind and body, and its ability to do this and to contribute to the broader scientific program was dependent on creating physiological analogues for psychological events. Neurophysiological theories of reflex action and the localization of function acquired enormous significance in this context. Such topics were not neutral empirical developments in scientific knowledge. They were the vehicle for an emotive revolution in thought, laden with evaluative implications and open to seemingly endless philosophical dispute.

This was the setting in which "inhibition" proved to be an enriching term. The word evoked psychological explanation at the same time as it promoted the search for a physiological mechanism; it signaled the power of the mind over the body, yet it was part of the means by which the nervous system regulated itself; it implied purpose and value derived from mind, while it also described an order inherent in the fabric of nature. The word's very lack of precise definition sustained its richness. When the term did begin to acquire definition, in the elaborate experimental detail of late-nineteenth-century neurophysiology, this marked the point at which "inhibition" started to lose its mediating qualities for the scientific community and between that community and its public. Nevertheless, its richness has persisted in lay usage, and it has continued to attract scientific attention whenever there has been a concerted effort to synthesize an integrated physiological psychology.[28] The significance of "inhibition" to the sciences of organization and regulation has been particularly well recognized in Soviet thinking, owing to the stress Soviet historians have placed on Sechenov's contribution to making objective psychology possible.[29]

Inhibition has often appeared to be a logical necessity of biological systems: there must be a function "to provide an arrangement whereby, when the same organism has multiple response potentialities, one of these can be activated without simultaneously activating the others. If the several response systems are to be coordinated, and not independent, inhibition is required."[30] Similar points have been made in philosophical reconstructions of the history of the brain sciences. Max Neuburger identified "the significance of regulation, coordination, and other phenomena" as the distinguishing feature of the modern scientific idea of the nervous system, as opposed to the ancient theories that located a distinct controlling power in the brain.[31] He argued that knowledge of inhibition followed necessarily from unraveling the mechanism of the reflex, which he understood to be the basis of regulation. Walther Riese characterized integration as "not a fact which has to be stated empirically: it is a principle." He then attributed this principle to the work of the British neurologist, John Hughlings Jackson, and the neurophysiologist, Sherrington.[32] Nevertheless, in spite of such claims, regulation and coordination have not been the subject of major histories, except in the specific sense of their incorporation into theories of reflex action. This contrasts with the attention that has been given to localization of function and specifically cerebral localization, that is, localization of function in the higher brain or cerebral cortex.[33]

This latter theme began (we may simplify) with Albrecht von Haller's mid-eighteenth-century distinction between the properties of sensibility and irritability, and it then continued in the Bell-Magendie separation of sensory and motor nerve functions, in the distinction of levels within the central neuraxis (i.e., the brain and spinal cord), and in the post-1870 elaboration of cerebral localization of sensory-motor functions. It was significant because localization suggested physical analogues for functions that were previously considered the expression of nonphysical, mental, or vital powers. Localization thus enabled description of living and mental processes as part of the natural world. Inhibition, in its turn, is part of the history of the structural localization of control functions. Inhibition and excitation together represented the way physical structures achieved organization or action of the organism—or human being—as a whole.

However, there is more to this history in several important respects. This is because inhibition has played a complex and fascinating mediating role between mind and brain, in three ways. First, "inhibition" was a psychological and a physiological term, referring equally to the action of mind and of body or to the interaction of mind and body. Second, "inhibition" was used in the esoteric language of science and in commonplace language. And, last, "inhibition" had both factual (or descriptive) and evaluative (or prescriptive) meanings. This was an extraordinarily rich set of characteristics, as a result of which reference to inhibition flourished in circumstances where the relations between mind and body, between psychology and physiology, between science and the everyday, and between values and facts were most at issue.

Theories of inhibition have been an important means by which natural scientists have hoped to incorporate psychological volition, or mental control, into biological knowledge. In the idiom of everyday individualist and, in origin, Christian psychology, reference to the will represents belief in the real power of mental control. It has therefore been a standing challenge to biological explanation to subsume psychological volition and to substitute a biological conception of control for the traditional mental one. Thought about inhibition has often acted as a bridge in this process, naturalizing a mental value as a physical cause. It has also been an issue on which critics of mechanistic physiology have concentrated, fearing that physiology was removing the grounds for belief in mental self-control. There was no simple correspondence between these tendencies facilitating and resisting mechanistic explanation and the inside and the outside of scientific communities, even if we could define the physiological community in some precise way, which is doubtful for much of the nineteenth century, given its links with both medicine and popular writings on health and morals. We cannot describe a fear of materialism simply as existing *outside* the scientific community, as a potential source of resistance to scientific work. Rather, evaluative discussion on the way in which volition or self-regulation acts has been central *within* the history of neurophysiology and psychology. It seemed to many researchers that the idea of inhibition offered special promise as a program of research on this troubled question.

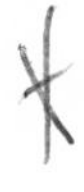

At the end of the nineteenth century, the naturalist and philosopher C. Lloyd Morgan stated that "when physiologists have solved the problem of inhibition, they will be in a position to consider that of volition."[34] He wrote after half a century of increasingly refined and specialized study of inhibition within the physiological community, and few physiologists would have made the point quite so concretely. As this community became institutionally autonomous, self-perpetuating through its own educational and career structures, and as its language became technical and tied to the minutiae of experimental practice, physiologists became less inclined to tackle the grand questions that had preoccupied earlier generations. Further, the more technical the physiological language of inhibition became, the less appropriate it was for the larger purpose. It was therefore left to more general writers like Morgan to explore topics such as volition. Yet the grand questions continued to surface at intervals, when "inhibition" again revealed its potential to act as a mediating term.

There were many reasons why volition should have been a problem area. Scientists, indeed, have often felt it to be a metaphysical desert in which no precise knowledge could bloom. Reference to volition connotes a mental value that expresses an emotional preference, a commitment of belief, or a moral principle. Thus, any attempt to construct a science of volition confronts the general problem of the relation between facts and values. This in its turn connects with the still current debate concerning causes and intentions in the explanation of human action. As a consequence, the actual historical use of a language of inhibition was to mediate values in the world of facts. As Michael J. Clark has observed, "As naturalistic accounts of the nature and origin of the mental and moral faculties became increasingly *de rigueur*, so the 'objective' physiological process of inhibition came progressively to be identified with, and substituted for, the 'subjective' psychological processes of attention, volition and moral feeling."[35] Sometimes this naturalizing step was overt and moralistic, as in tracts intended to help people cultivate their power of self-control. Sometimes, a fortiori in the specialist neurophysiology of the late nineteenth century, the evaluative connotations of the language of inhibition were highly attenuated. Most late-nineteenth-century neurophysiologists believed that "inhibition" was a word belonging to entirely factual discourse. In other writings, including some coming from the new academic psychology at the turn of the century, the evaluative expressive possibilities of the word remained nearer the surface.

Existing historical knowledge of mind and brain resembles a patchwork, with each patch executed to a different pattern and showing little indication of where it might be sewn into a whole. Earlier historians of science—to whom this history is much indebted—would not have seen it in these terms. They would have agreed that the patchwork was incomplete, but they would have had no intrinsic difficulty in seeing how it should fit together with expanding research and greater resources for the history of science. They believed that the pattern of the whole would emerge by itself, since this pattern would represent science's discovery of the objective reality or truth of psychological and physiological processes. Having rejected the sufficiency of their epistemological presuppositions, however, other ways to shape the history of knowledge are needed.

The American physiological psychologist Franklin Fearing published his standard history of reflex action in 1930. He assigned a clear role to both theory and discovery:

> The reflex arc concept has come to play a role in modern psychological and physiological theorizing which is comparable with the part played by the fundamental explanatory principles of physics and chemistry. . . . It has been the purpose in the present volume to trace the development of the theory of reflex action and to record the discoveries of the phenomena which the theory was designed to render intelligible.[36]

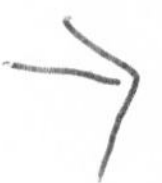

Taking his cue from Sherrington's 1906 synthesis, *The Integrative Action of the Nervous System*, he distinguished "the inhibition of reflex action" as a distinct thread in his story. The history of the reflex concept described knowledge of how organisms welded excitation and inhibition together into appropriate action. As Robert Boakes commented more recently, "Unlike a Cartesian reflex relying only upon excitatory action, one that includes inhibition might account in a mechanistic fashion for those integrated and apparently purposeful actions that had led others to believe in a spinal soul."[37] As Fearing and Boakes indicated, "excitation" and "inhibition" constituted a basic pair of terms for representing the organism's achievement of nervous integration. Sherrington also provided the framework for Fearing's own physiological research in the 1920s. In giving his book the subtitle, *A Study in the History of Physiological Psychology*, Fearing emphasized to his scientific contemporaries that the successful integration of neurophysiology and psychology would depend on an adequate theory of excitation-inhibition.

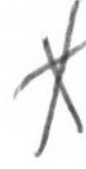

Fearing treated inhibition as a phenomenon observed by various early writers, demonstrated experimentally from 1845 and firmly established as a fundamental dimension of neurophysiology by 1870. Reflecting the focus of research in the 1920s, he organized his discussion around the great number of mechanisms proposed as explanations for inhibitory action, "none of which," he concluded, "offer an adequate interpretation of the observed phenomena."[38] However, he also set these mechanisms in a broader framework, reflecting a contemporary North American consciousness that inhibition had become a tangle of issues that, if unraveled, might unlock knowledge of how the brain subserved psychological processes. Similarly, his contemporary, the psychologist Raymond Dodge, provided a thoughtful overview designed to clarify the meaning of inhibition, to review its physiological basis, and thereby to contribute to a renewal of physiological psychology.[39]

Fearing's history was greatly dependent on others, notably on the still unsurpassed account by Conrad Eckhard, a physiologist at Giessen and a participant in the development of reflex theory in the third quarter of the nineteenth century.[40] These histories, like other histories of neurophysiology, suffered from not being able to bear the explanatory weight they placed on the notion of empirical discovery. I have suggested that some power to arrest action, equally with a power to excite action, has been implicit in the notion of control. Once such control was conceived in organic terms as a property of nervous structures, it was necessary to differentiate initiating and arresting powers. The very conception of what the nervous system meant for the life of the organism presupposed excitatory and inhibitory functions. Even before modern biological formulations, a general sense of a living being's self-regulation implied paired activation and cessation. Many writers pointed out that this was evident in ideas of equilibrium going back to Hippocrates. Nineteenth-century physiologists were fond of quoting a Hippocratic aphorism to illustrate this ancient lineage, and they quoted it to such an extent that it became hackneyed: "Duobus doloribus simula abortis nos in eodem loco vehementior obscurat alterum" (If a patient be subject to two pains arising in different parts of the body simultaneously, the stronger blunts the other).[41] In fact, nineteenth-century writers frequently described knowledge of inhibition as "inevitable." Mercier observed, "This hypothesis of a universal and ever-present inhibition . . . is of such indispensable necessity to a comprehension of the physiology of the nervous system, that we may say of it . . . 'If it did not exist it would be necessary to invent it.' "[42]

Such evidence creates great difficulties for a history of neurophysiology organized around the theme of empirical discovery. Existing accounts are unsatisfactory inasmuch as they have not clarified the relation between concept and experience in the construction of knowledge. They have failed to do this primarily because they have excluded the dimension of the social, that is, they have excluded reference to the means by which shared representations of reality compose a frame of possibility for even the most individual or most experimentally rigorous observation. Historical accounts, couched in terms of discovery, have all too often treated individual perception as unmediated by socially acquired categories.

There can be little doubt, however, that the dominant expressive idiom used by the nineteenth-century physiologists who published on inhibition was that of empirical discovery. Priority disputes, some involving the most intense feelings, litter the history of neurophysiology. Vagal inhibition, the spinal reflex, vasomotor nerves, reciprocal innervation of skeletal muscle have all been the subject of disputed claims. Discovery disputes were so common that they must be accepted as a significant social fact. Scientists exchanged intellectual property for status and career prospects, a situation fraught with emotion when competition for a restricted number of research opportunities was intense, as it was in the nineteenth century.[43] Making a discovery, and having one's peers agree that it was original, established the most clear-cut and prestigious form of intellectual property. At the same time, articulating scientific knowledge as the product of discovery expressed shared cultural values. Strongest of these was faith in scientific progress itself, a faith that expected those with the requisite training and personal qualities to uncover the facts of nature. The announcement of a discovery fulfilled the scientist's contract with society at the same time as it signaled expectation of reward. Discovery, as symbolic exchange, was thus central to the faith in science that so marked European society in the second half of the nineteenth century.

Since this ethos of discovery was such a strong social reality, it might be thought discordant to write the history of events as a process of conceptual shaping. The simple fact is, however, that discovery claims and priority disputes say very little about the way scientists form knowledge or why knowledge has a particular content, though they do say a great deal about scientific communities. I shall question the notion of discovery and, in doing so, restore to inhibition its richness of meaning in mediating between mind and brain, psychology and physiology, value and fact. These meanings, rather than the scientists' own representation of scientific progress as discovery, appear in the following chapters.

There has been intense scientific excitement about the potential of the neurosciences since the 1940s. Scientists became convinced that knowledge of the brain had become, or soon would become, sufficiently deep to answer psychological questions. A period of East-West scientific contact following the Cold War also made it appear that different traditions were coming together to create a common neuroscience. Computing and the associated "cognitive revolution" in psychology excited hopes that the means at last existed to create a unified science of mind and brain. This has influenced more recent histories.

In 1963, Solomon Diamond and his collaborators in the United States, supporting what they described as a "neurobehavioral approach," wrote the most comprehensive study of the history and contemporary usages of inhibition. As they commented, "Every penetrating observer of behavior has always been aware of the existence of simultaneous and incompatible tendencies in behavior, one of which can come to full expression only by suppressing the other."[44] Thus, they went on, inhibition is "a phenomenon comparable to excitation and every bit as important to the proper functioning of the nervous system."[45] This then led the authors to review what they considered to be references to inhibition across the centuries. They also stressed a comparison between the Russian physiologist Sechenov and the English physician Francis E. Anstie. Everyone would agree that, in some sense, Sechenov is central to the story of inhibition. Following the neurologist Jackson's citation of Anstie's study, *Stimulants and Narcotics* (1864), Diamond and his collaborators accorded Anstie similar recognition to Sechenov. They elevated to the status of a "new and insightful approach" and a "principle" Anstie's statement that "the apparent exaltation of certain faculties should be ascribed to the removal of controlling influences, than to positive stimulation of the faculties themselves" and therefore that the effects of hashish and alcohol "ought not to be called stimulant at all . . . they are, in fact, the results of a partial and highly peculiar kind of paralysis of the brain."[46] As they went on to explain, Anstie, and later Jackson, then deployed this "principle" of "loss of control" in a theory of nervous action presupposing a hierarchical system of control, with higher levels inhibiting lower ones and with inhibition being removed by drugs, alcohol, epilepsy, and so forth. This is indeed an important part of the history of inhibition. But Anstie's and Jackson's supposed "principle," as well as Sechenov's discovery of central inhibition, reformulated already widespread ways of thinking about human action. Anstie reexpressed a commonplace of Victorian moral understanding, and he was only one among many physicians to do so. Nevertheless, Diamond and his collaborators' book, *Inhibition and Choice*, remains the most wide-ranging and stimulating account of inhibition as science, discussing many of the sources that also appear in this study.

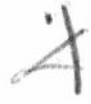

Inhibition has a more marginal and equally problematic position in other histories of neurophysiology. In a bold overview designed as an introduction to a major handbook of physiology, Mary A. B. Brazier ordered her material by picking out what she regarded as the major contributions to modern knowledge. Inhibition received significant notice under the headings of "spinal cord and reflex activity" and "physiology of the brain."[47] She has subsequently enlarged on one major theme, the history of discoveries concerning electrical activity in the brain and nervous system, writing an uneven account of the origins of modern knowledge.[48] The historians of medicine, Edwin Clarke and C. D. O'Malley, took such overviews further by compiling annotated extracts from sources selected for "inherent importance." Sources on inhibition played a part, again mainly under the theme of reflex action.[49] More recently, Clarke, in collaboration with L.S. Jacyna, has completed a detailed description of neurophysiology writings from about 1790 to about 1840, organized on the principle that empirical discovery in this period laid the foundations for the modern neurosciences.[50] Clarke and Jacyna did not discuss inhibition, since it featured in experimental neuroscience only after 1845. Other modern studies in the history of neurophysiology have a more selective character. The French brain scientist, Marc Jeannerod, for example, discussed the mechanism of action, distinguishing emphases on the promptings of the environment or on spontaneous events within the organism (hence serving as a basis for free will). He observed that scientists, in addressing such questions, have long assumed that the nervous system is a hierarchically organized structure. He referred to this assumption as a "principle which *constitutes* order, rather than being subject to it."[51] He identified Sechenov's discovery of inhibition in the central nervous system as a key step in understanding the way the organism achieved a dynamic order.[52]

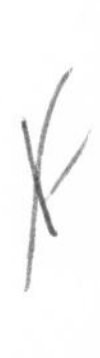

It is easy to accept that selectivity is necessary for clarity, though it brings its own problems. The history of neuroscience must consider the interrelations among anatomy, neurophysiology, psychology, neurology, psychiatry, and, not least, philosophy. Even using this language of the modern-specialist divisions is a problem. Further, since the brain is the substratum of the mind, a phrasing that it is historically appropriate to leave vague, it is a formidable problem to circumscribe any selected part of the area encompassing psychology or physiology. Histories relating studies of mind and brain have been as varied as opinions about the mid-brain relation itself. Brazier, Clarke, O'Malley, and Jacyna have in fact imposed selectivity by projecting back into the past the modern specialist disciplines, thus imposing a manageable order on the historical complexity. But how a field of research has been shaped as a communal activity and even how such a field became conceivable are themselves historical questions with special relevance to the study of mind and brain.[53] I do not think it is possible to write historically about neurophysiology independently of psychology, about brain science without reference to medicine, or on specialist knowledge isolated from lay understanding. History cannot but concern itself with how these relations existed in particular settings. Certainly, one important issue is the way neurophysiology became a separate research occupation and specialist body of knowledge, but we should not read this specialization back into the past. In an effort to take account of such matters, the present history of inhibition is a thematic study. In this limited sense, it follows such historical studies as Georges Canguilhem's on the reflex, Anne Harrington's on the bilateral brain, and Robert M. Young's on cerebral localization.[54]

Psychology has an especially difficult position as a branch of scientific knowledge. It has as its subject phenomena with which, as human beings, we all necessarily have an intimate familiarity. There is a labyrinthine quality about psychology, in which the subject claims to know itself and in which that subject is potentially every human being. This creates very real difficulties for the attempt to write the history of psychology. It is possible to refer to psychology as a discipline or specialist occupation only since the late nineteenth century. Before that, knowledge we might label "psychological" was part of a broader culture. Even in the twentieth century, it has not been possible for psychology as science to avoid being in complex dialogue with common understanding. It follows that the history of a topic like inhibition cannot be distinguished from debate about what might differentiate psychology as a science separate from common understanding. The point extends to the disciplines concerned with the physiology of the nervous system as well, since neurophysiology is about the material substratum of mind and conduct and hence has been intimately bound up with the history of psychology as science.

There is little agreement on the scope of the history of psychology.[55] Historians have most often focused on the establishment of experimental psychology as a distinct program of research. This occurred in Germany and subsequently in the United States in the last quarter of the nineteenth century. The classic account by E. G. Boring emphasized that psychology lay claim to having become a science through the extension of the experimental *method* to psychological topics. In his view, the scientific discipline of psychology came into existence by applying the techniques of physiological investigation to what had previously been philosophical questions about the mind.[56] Young and others have stressed that scientific psychology became a possibility after Charles Darwin's and Herbert Spencer's evolutionary theories created continuity between categories of nature and categories of mind and behavior.[57] Both approaches have argued that the development of experimental neurophysiology was historically crucial, institutionalizing an objective method of research that was then applied to psychological questions and supplying the vocabulary for a naturalized discourse about the human subject.

This picture is gradually becoming much more historically informed. In particular, the development of a sociohistorical approach to discipline formation in psychology has questioned the connections between late-nineteenth-century German and American psychology. It is clear that separate national and cultural settings fostered divergent patterns of discipline development. The differences of local context encouraged attachment to contrasting methods and enthusiasm for different bodies of knowledge.[58] Similarly, it is clear that the history of psychology in Russia has special characteristics.[59]

The German and American academics who argued for a distinct discipline of psychology in the late nineteenth century needed to show that the subject matter of psychology was distinct from the subject matter of neurophysiology. At the same time, they wanted to borrow techniques and prestige from the physiologists to construct objective methods for investigating psychological topics. The history of physiological psychology thus occupies a confusing but central position in the history of psychology. Historians have not written about the area in a systematic way.

Significant areas of nineteenth-century psychology developed without input from either physiological or evolutionary science. This was especially the case in areas influenced by idealist arguments in philosophy. Idealism, which conceived of reason as the means through which mind could know itself, could translate readily enough into psychological topics. In the German-speaking world, philosophical idealism affected the nature and direction of psychological argument even when the attempt was made to bring psychology into connection with the natural sciences.[60] Inhibition was also a feature of research in this setting. "Hemmung" was a familiar term, throughout the nineteenth century, for describing competitive interaction of mental elements or processes. This usage passed from analytic-philosophical to experimental-psychological studies. It was a usage that did not allude to either physiological or evolutionary hierarchies but rather to psychological dynamics (as in the work of J. F. Herbart).

The history of inhibition is thus largely a novel theme for the history of both psychology and physiology. In pursuing this theme, I hope to impose order on very complex historical developments, interpreting the shape and content of major fields of scientific knowledge. The theme continuously touches on psychology's contentious relation with physiology. It must also cover substantial psychological topics such as volition and attention and physiological topics such as the means of bodily control. All this one would expect given that inhibition denotes a controlling or regulatory relation. This meaning existed long before inhibition became a technical term in physiology, and it is therefore with early-nineteenth-century descriptions of human conduct that the story begins.

CHAPTER 2

Conduct, Loss of Control, and Mental Organization

The highest aim of Mental Hygiene should be to increase the power of mental inhibition amongst all men and women. Control is the basis of all law and the cement of every social system among men and women, without which it would go to pieces.

———T. S. Clouston, *The Hygiene of Mind*

THE MIND'S POWER OVER THE BODY AND THE BODILY ECONOMY

The word "Victorian" conjures up a British literature of order and disorder that stressed individual control and the individual's duty to society. Peter Gay has referred to "a vast and interminable outpouring of clerical and pedagogic polemics" in describing the literature of self-improvement.[1] This literature was sometimes theologically inspired and sometimes secular in intent; in the latter case, it used the language of mental regulation of the body rather than spiritual control of the flesh. The moral content, however, unified society across the religious divide. The early Victorian period in particular possessed a rich popular literature that brought a sense of the mind's controlling power—"self-help"—to a high degree of consciousness. "It is this persevering and remembered will, acting frequently in opposition to the animal nature, which it is my object to claim as the distinguishing characteristic of man."[2] As a mirror image of the will, this literature also projected a darker picture of the body and of the emergence of human baseness: "So man . . . becomes subject to evils greater than animals ever know, because his nature is of a higher order."[3]

Moral earnestness was linked to a sense of crisis in religious faith, to a fear of political disorder (given outward form, or so it appeared to the respectable, in the great Chartist agitations of the late 1830s and early 1840s), and to the middle-class critique of both aristocratic government and working-class indiscipline. The response focused these concerns on a struggle by the individual to achieve Christian goals in his or her life. As John Henry Newman wrote, "Unless you are struggling, unless you are fighting with yourselves, you are no followers of those who 'through many tribulations entered into the kingdom of God.'"[4] The physician and ethnologist, J. C. Prichard, therefore described certain kinds of suicide as not "the acts of a madman, but rather of a person possessed of reason, though under the influence of despair, of passions habitually ill-regulated, and uncontrolled by a sense of duty and religion."[5]

This struggle to attain perfect moral control was lifelong, though it had its greatest intensity in bringing up children. The parents had the duty of teaching the child habits of control, enabling him or her to lead the good life as an adult. The doyen of writers on "the Victorian mind," Walter Houghton, drew attention to the childhood of the clergyman Augustus Hare. As Hare's mother wrote in her journal, "The will is the thing that needs being brought into subjection."[6] Training the child therefore became a course of exercises in virtue's repression of desire. Hare remembered the consequences of his mother's views:

> Hitherto I had never been allowed anything but roast-mutton and rice-pudding for dinner. Now all was changed. The most delicious puddings were talked of—*dilated* on—until I became, not greedy, but exceedingly curious about them. At length *le grand moment* arrived. They were put on the table before me, and then, just as I was going to eat some of them, they were snatched away, and I was told to get up and carry them off to some poor person in the village.[7]

This struggle over the self prepared the adult for a state of virtue; equally, it prepared the adult to go out into the world and to struggle over others whose constitution, upbringing, gender, or race left them subject to desire and disorder. If learning control over oneself was the duty of the child, taking control over others was the duty of the man (and I mean "man"). The personal and the political were unified in language.

Questions of proper education were not restricted to children, as a lively historical debate about the cultural and political meaning of movements for adult education in the first half of the nineteenth century has shown. Organizations like the Mechanics' Institutes and the Society for the Diffusion of Useful Knowledge invested heavily in adult education, and there was an audience for popular works on phrenology, physiology, and health.[8] Steven Shapin and Barry Barnes have analyzed how, in this setting, the opposed categories of "head" and "hand" helped to articulate a hierarchical view of social relations.[9] Supposed differences in mental and manual competencies legitimated divergent education for different classes. Thus, the great Whig politician, Henry (Lord) Brougham, and the industrial apologist, Andrew Ure, assumed a difference in the psychological character of manual and mental workers, and they assumed that this justified the latter being in a position to regulate the former (like parents regulating children). This was reminiscent of the eighteenth-century jurist, Sir William Blackstone, who defended the property qualification for electors on the grounds that the poor would not be able to curb their desire for bribes: "The true reason of requiring any qualification, with regard to property, in voters, is to exclude such persons as are in so mean a situation that they are esteemed to have no will of their own. If these persons had votes, they would be tempted to dispose of them under some undue influence or other."[10] The marriage contract, also, implied a parallel relation between the active will of the husband and the passive position of the wife. The higher classes had a duty to control the involuntary, labile, and emotional activity of the lower classes since, as Ure wrote, the manufacturing classes are "the slaves of prejudice and vice; *they can see objects only on one side*, that which a sinister selfishness presents to their view; they are readily moved to outrage by crafty demagogues."[11] It was expected that working people would lead unregulated lives unless more refined and reflective minds exercised control from above. With suitable education, however, not least in basic physiology, it was hoped that working people would incorporate into themselves a power to control their nature.

Christian ideals had inculcated a view that human nature was polarized between higher and lower ends. By the early Victorian period, the imagery associated with this view had become intertwined with social and economic descriptions of the new industrial economy that portrayed control and regulation as features built into social relations by virtue of market forces. It was common to think of the economy as a self-regulating set of forces, with energy utilized at one point being balanced by the unavailability of energy at another. Self-regulating technology and physical theories of the conservation of energy added yet further dimensions. Thus, there were many resources available for thinking about control in terms of balance and reciprocal relations as well as in terms of hierarchical regulation. Indeed, reference to "the bodily economy" was to become a cliché of Victorian thought.

There were many ways in which bodily and societal terms and images constituted interrelated, or even identical, meanings. Williams drew attention to the fact that "consensual" initially had a physiological (as well as legal) meaning, referring to the way reflex actions coordinated automatic movements.[12] A healthy digestion was a rich source of metaphor for idealizations of social harmony, and so on. Popular physiology formed a distinctive genre of writing in the early Victorian period. As Roger Cooter has noted, the literature was not just utilitarian in content (like books of remedies or recipes) but presented a simplified summary of physiological knowledge as a guide to good living. It taught the laws of nature as a way to both health and success in life. The language of hierarchical control, praising regulation and balance, was perfectly illustrated in a contented digestion: "Nowhere else in human physiology can a regulated dynamic model be so readily illustrated and understood—the familiar upset stomach or constipation speaking volumes for believing in (and attending to) the naturalness of equilibrium and regularity."[13] Regulation was possible for a mind educated into a knowledge of bodily laws; left to itself, the undisciplined body was prone to excess. Order in the body and success in life were the inward and outward signs of virtue.

It is worth glancing ahead to note that it was precisely automatic bodily functions like digestion which encouraged physiologists in the 1850s systematically to introduce "inhibition" as a technical term. Both popular physiology and technical experimental physiology focused on the involuntary activities of the body. In developing conceptions of the body's balanced activity, physiologists of every level of sophistication contributed to thought in which "inhibition" was to become a key term.

The relation between popular physiology and the new experimental neurophysiology was evident in the textbooks of W. B. Carpenter, perhaps the most important writer in English on physiological topics for midcentury medical students. For example, though he used the technical language of reflex action in talking about the control of excretion, he described an aspect of everyday experience commonly understood to be central to a well-ordered life.

> The expulsors and the sphincters [i.e., the two sets of muscles] may be regarded as balancing one another, so far as their reflex action is concerned,—the latter having rather the predominance, so as to restrain the action of the former. But, when the quantity or quality of the contents of the cavity gives an excessive stimulus to the former, their action predominates, unless the will is put in force to strengthen the resistance of the sphincter; this we are

> frequently experiencing, sometimes to our great discomfort. On the other hand, if the stimulus is deficient, the will must aid the expulsors, in order to overcome that resistance which is due to the reflex action of the sphincters.[14]

Order, whether represented as the will's control over the body or as a learned balance of reflexes, was the key to the individual's comfort and efficient conduct in society. Such views were unremarkable and taken for granted. This character of embeddedness is just what we are looking for when we seek to explain the later interest in more precise concepts of control such as inhibition.

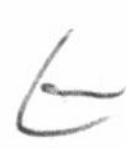

Belief in regulation also pervaded gender relations. An extensive and rich literature, developing feminist insights, has detailed the extraordinary extent to which the Victorians conflated the social and the natural in discussing women's place.[15] There was a concurrence of language and relations of value and power about mind and body, adult and child, master and servant, white and black, and man and woman. Just as there was a debate about the proper education of working men in the 1830s, so there was a debate about the educability of women in the 1860s.[16] Whereas, as it was argued, the working man's mind had to cope with an insensitive nature, the woman's mind had to cope with a pressing physiology of reproductive functions. The primary bodily identity of woman, defined in relation to reproduction and to the social institution of marriage, which many people conflated, created for man the rights and duties of a controlling power. Women's struggle to obtain education thus appeared to be a blow at the social order, since that order presupposed a harmonious division of labor under the regulating care of the male mind. This rational guidance, men argued, sustained a social world in which female impulsivity gave rise to virtue rather than vice. By a happy choice of words, we refer back to the "repression" of women. That women's nature did indeed require regulation and inhibition by a controlling mind was a point in Victorian belief where physiology and domestic politics met.

As many historians have noted, the question of control in personal life became especially concrete in the reaction to adolescent masturbation.[17] The Victorian concern to label this activity unnatural and to repress it as immoral is now a vivid symbol of oppressive inhibition. Masturbation was also a vivid symbol to the Victorians, but in the different sense that it betokened the assertion of the flesh over the spirit, the child over the adult, and the selfish act over service to the community. The literature on masturbation was also rich in capitalist metaphor.

Discussions of "the spermatic economy" entangled the moral and financial elements of indulgence and prudence. Exactly the same notions of the physiological economy were present in medical resistance to women's education: "When Nature spends in one direction, she must economise in another direction."[18] Male masturbation and female education both reduced reproductive capital. Only the saving of capital, the Victorians believed, permitted profitable work. Disciplining the child out of "bad habits" and "unnatural acts" thus justified severe measures. Further, a supporting medical literature portrayed prolonged masturbation as a cause not just of unmanly character but of insanity. In insanity, the individual finally surrendered all control and simultaneously became an economic burden. As asylum superintendents well knew, masturbation was a common and offensive reminder of just what the loss of control in insanity could mean.[19]

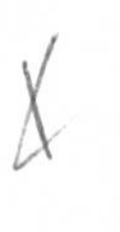

The morbid concern with masturbation, in its turn, was part of a wider response to sexuality. In discussing this matter, it is important to acknowledge possible distinctions between "repression" and "inhibition," though clearly the two words can mean the same thing. The Victorians at the same time criticized repression of the emotions and called for the repression of feelings in the pursuit of other ends, but they did not conceive of repression in a Freudian sense as a specific mental function. They did not use "inhibition" in its modern senses until the end of the century, when they borrowed the term from physiology. Both words were then associated with the control of sexuality, "repression" more systematically than "inhibition." It is by subsuming the words under the idea of control that we best convey their shared meaning.

Though the early Victorians excluded description of the "lower" instincts from public discussion, this exclusion accompanied a concentration of attention on sexuality. Studious public denial was the obverse of intense private contemplation.[20] What this reveals is not so much individual hypocrisy, though this was often real enough, but an elaborate culture of regulated sexuality. Medical and nonmedical writers on healthy living were more concerned with regulating the sexual economy than with simply repressing sex; their problem was the control of physical feelings, though, in the case of women, this could involve denial that such feelings existed. Repeated calls to duty, work, discipline, and self-denial were in substantial part a means of managing sexuality, just as they formed specific techniques for regulating individuals whose conduct threatened disorder—whether children, the working class, women, or criminals. It was this focus on regulation that created a popular social psychology in which the word "inhibition" was later to find its place. Social norms and collective values became the internalized controls in the body. At the same time, late-nineteenth-century physiology achieved an account of the body making control the very principle of life itself.

A concern with the bodily economy persisted in popular physiology throughout the century. The physiological legitimation of antagonism to masturbation or to women's education depended on an image of the body possessing finite reserves of energy. If resources were used in one direction, they could not be available in another. Thus, the husbanding and regulation of resources was a cliché of physiological moralism. Such notions fertilized ideas of inhibition later in the century, sustaining the integration of economic and physiological views. Spencer, most notably, covered the competition for resources in his systematic comparison of the social and physical bodies:

> The different parts of a social organism, like the different parts of an individual organism, compete for nutriment . . . great muscular exertion will determine such a quantity of blood to the limbs, as to arrest digestion or cerebral action, as the case may be. So, likewise, in a society, it frequently happens that great activity in some one direction, causes partial arrests of activity elsewhere, by abstracting capital, that is commodities: as instance the way in which the sudden development of our railway-system hampered commercial operations.[21]

This was a comparison of almost infinite flexibility, calling on a common experience of the everyday, both of bodily well-being and of earning a living. Just how flexible a resource this was is illustrated by medical concern that women's menstrual flow should *not* be arrested.[22] An extensive commentary attested to belief that this was a waste resource whose expenditure was a requirement, and an index, of healthy living.

Spencer reverted throughout his life to comparisons between political economy and the psychophysiological economy. Early on, it suggested to him the means with which to refute Malthus's strictures on progress. Spencer thought that the expansion of intelligence in civilized peoples would naturally limit their reproductive energies, reducing population growth.[23] This language comparing the balance of powers within individual character and within political economy placed Spencer in a dilemma. He systematically compared structures and functions in social and biological organizations, and he thus inevitably compared society's organs of control with the nervous system. The problem was that scientists considered the nervous system to be the central controlling power in the body, while Spencer's political commitments were exceedingly individualistic and opposed to centralized decision making. He therefore wished to minimize the significance of government as a controlling power in the body politic.[24] His dilemma brings out a confusing logical issue in the theory of the social organism and in other theories relating social to biological analysis. For some purposes, Spencer either drew or rejected analogies between social and organic structures and functions. For other purposes, he derived his descriptions of structure and function from general laws, and in this case, the biological and the social were related by an underlying identity. His "confusion" indicates the complex structure of a discourse in which terms articulated together according to meaning and not logic.

Nineteenth-century conceptions of control generally took for granted the individual's will as a real agency, even if it was agreed that it was difficult, perhaps impossible, to specify the nature of this agency further. The core concept was embodied in the common law, which presupposed the role of individual mental agency in preventing criminal or civil wrongs. The jurist Sir James Fitzjames Stephen conveyed this when he observed, "Every human creature attaches to the words 'to will,' or their equivalents, as vivid a meaning as every man with eyes attaches to the words 'to see.'"[25] If the will was such an essential faculty of human nature, it was clearly reasonable to think about human character and social relations in terms of dichotomies between controlling and controlled factors. Carpenter, for example, took such a dualism for granted: "We scarcely desire a better proof that our possession of this power [of volition] is a reality and not a self-delusion, than is afforded by the comparison of the *normal* condition of the Mind with those various *abnormal* conditions . . . in which the directing power of the Will is in abeyance."[26] As the following section will show, this frequently associated with, though it did not logically require, an imagery of the controlling power repressing otherwise innately active forces. As the Berlin medicolegal authority J. L. Casper observed, there were cases "of 'fury' without insanity in which the demoniacal nature of the evil principle breaks forth unshackled."[27] Writers on jurisprudence, legitimating social sanctions, conceived of the law as backing up or replacing the controlling power of the individual's will. By implication, undermining the rule of law—as radicals appeared to do by advocating atheism and materialism and thereby attacking free will—seemed to remove the very possibility of order.[28] Similarly, use of the insanity defense to acquit someone accused of a heinous crime appeared to critics as an encouragement for beastliness to break out elsewhere.[29] The individual will and the collective law were thus twin bastions against anarchy, bound together in a common purpose as the individual was bound into the social. The point need not be labored: we recognize an acute sensibility to the controlling will and to the regulated body throughout all walks of bourgeois Victorian life. To amplify the background to the social consciousness of inhibition, it is necessary to turn to the question of the mind's—or the will's—agency in the body.

Descriptions of human nature in the 1830s and 1840s showed an increasing interest in physiological matters. The early Victorians, more frequently than their predecessors, referred questions of conduct, of morals, of education, or of mental disorder to physiological conditions. By midcentury, it was common to state that progress in understanding the mind depended on revealing its relations with the body and, above all, the nervous system. Such beliefs fueled a debate about scientific materialism, though few of the more educated physiological writers admitted to espousing such a philosophy. The new physiological psychology had various weaknesses as a form of knowledge, but it did bring about a general consciousness of the intimate relation between mind and body, mediated by the brain.[30] This was to foster a profound change in representations of human nature. Writers on the relation of spirit to everyday life subsequently expressed themselves in terms of mind controlling, or being controlled by, the nervous system. Nervous physiology therefore became a prominent resource for reexpressing, and thereby reenforcing with apparent objective authority, the individual's responsibility to control himself or herself.

To be sure, physiology, particularly if we include ancient beliefs in the humors and in sympathy, had long been central in guides to well-being.[31] What was different about the new literature was its focus on the brain as the material condition of mind. It claimed a new, empirical authority for physiology in psychological questions.

Some of the new physiological authors were nonspecialists writing for a general audience. Others, while they did have a medical qualification, still wrote with an eye to a general audience or perhaps an audience of inexperienced medical students. There was no clear boundary between technical and popular works. Both popular and medical writers exemplified the portentous early Victorian search for the conditions of existence in natural law. The search was often deeply religious, many writers believing that natural law would reveal the benevolent authority of the Creator. For other writers, however, the Creator faded even as a remote presence, and natural law appeared to be self-sustaining and a source of authority in its own right. But whatever the religious differences, one value remained central: each person individually, and society generally, had a duty to acknowledge the dependence of life on natural law and to learn what this law was. Only in this way, it was argued, would mankind act in harmony with natural law and thus achieve individual and social well-being. Suffering, poverty, ill health, and social disorder revealed ignorance or indifference to that law. Physiology, particularly physiology of the brain, therefore acquired a crucial position in the creation of an improved future.

All these elements were exemplified in the extraordinarily widely read book by George Combe, *The Constitution of Man Considered in Relation to External Objects* (1828). Combe, like his Edinburgh friend, the publisher Robert Chambers, was a self-appointed educator. Perhaps more than any other single person, he raised consciousness that knowledge of the human "constitution"—by which he meant the physiological parameters of existence—was the foundation of progress. More particularly, Combe was the most influential exponent of phrenology in Britain, and phrenology emphatically focused both popular and medical attention on the brain. As Cooter has shown, the belief that the psychological faculties were localized in particular regions of the brain, and that the degree of those faculties' development affected the size of the relevant part of the brain and shape of the head, proved influential as a medium through which the natural laws of physiology became accepted as a guide for everyday life.[32] Nor was phrenology's influence limited to autodidacts or popular psychology: the way it conceptualized functional localization within the brain, when divorced from craniology, had consequences for mainstream psychological medicine and neurophysiology.[33]

The distinctive tenets of phrenology were discredited among most medicophysiological writers by the 1840s. By this time, however, the twin beliefs that existence was subject to natural law and that this existence was mediated by the brain had become an orthodoxy. After mid-century, a new generation of writers then reexpressed these beliefs in a more sophisticated fashion. Spencer was perhaps the most influential, and he was certainly the most systematic. His voluminous "Synthetic Philosophy" translated Combe's emphasis on natural law, the value of natural knowledge as the condition of harmonious progress, and knowledge of the nervous system as the underlying concomitant of mind into a systematic evolutionary philosophy.[34]

Combe's psychology of control or regulation, like phrenology generally, depended on the interaction between different faculties of the mind and corresponding regions of the brain. Phrenologists emphasized the individual's responsibility to exercise particular faculties and thereby to achieve a balanced life appropriate to circumstances. The stress was thus on education and balance as the means of control, rather than on anything specifically resembling inhibition, except in the weak sense that the development and exercise of one faculty necessarily lessened others. Phrenology nevertheless made a wide audience familiar with physiological laws as the ruling conditions of psychological function, and it also reinforced an understanding that the brain—as the seat of mind—was the "highest" organ of the body, lording it over the physiology of human nature. It was therefore a significant part of the background to theories of inhibition. In addition, many phrenological writers, including Combe (who was criticized for it by more radical colleagues), classified the mental faculties in a hierarchical way. Even while they emphasized the material nature of the human constitution, they preserved traditional values that placed reason and will higher than manual skill or emotion.[35] These writers thus reexpressed in partially physiological language a view of character that valued higher over lower faculties.

Phrenology was far from being the only expression of popular physiology. Moralizing about the material conditions of individual life existed alongside phrenology and continued long after the latter was discredited. This was exemplified in Victorian psychological medicine, discussed below. Medical men were especially prominent among physiological writers, most obviously because of their training and occupation but more profoundly because they also often sought a secular salvation in obedience to nature.

Turning meanwhile from medicine to physiology as a distinct occupation and division of knowledge, we must note that it had only a marginal position in Britain before the 1860s.[36] It existed not as a discipline but as a subsidiary of medical education. There was a relative absence in Britain of experimental physiological science of the kind well established in Germany from at least 1840 or skillfully practiced in Paris from at least 1820. Though it is therefore hardly possible to talk about institutionalized physiology in midcentury Britain, there were articulate individuals, associated with medicine, who argued the case for scientific physiology. They were impressed by Continental physiology and had faith in knowledge of natural law as a basis for social progress. Their main achievements tended to be writing textbooks, raising expectations about physiology within medicine, and loosely applying a physiological understanding to everyday questions of individual and social action and well-being. Two of the most prominent of these physiologists, Carpenter and Richard Todd, devoted considerable attention to neurophysiology.[37] In the process, they elaborated an account of the mind's hierarchical relation to the body and the higher brain's relation to the lower nervous system with every appearance that this was a framework of understanding that no one would question. Their writings exhibited a ready translation between a psychological language of control and a physiological language of nervous regulation. This was the area and the language that would underpin the reception of notions of inhibition in Britain.

Writers such as Carpenter and Todd assembled arguments from comparative anatomy and embryology to try to clarify functional organization within the nervous system. Developing ideas current in biological morphology, they described the neuraxis as a structure consisting of anatomical and functional units arranged in segments along its length. They supposed that the structure and function at each segmental level interacted with those at other levels and that the levels were arranged in a hierarchy from the top of the brain to the bottom of the spinal cord.[38] Neurophysiology therefore acquired the tasks of understanding functional units at each level and of specifying how the levels interrelated according to a serial order of dominance ascending to the brain. To provide the detail, ordering their questions as problems of empirical knowledge, physiologists drew on two areas of research. The first, made famous by the French physiologist P.-J. Flourens in the 1820s, discussed functional localization in the brain, differentiating levels but, specifically opposing phrenology, not localizing faculties within the cerebrum or higher brain. The second, associated especially with the claims of the English physician Marshall Hall in the 1830s, discussed reflex action and its structural foundations in the arrangements of the sensory-motor spinal nervous system. This portrayed the basic unit of nervous function in terms of linked but distinct incoming and outgoing nerves. Both areas familiarized researchers with a hierarchical conception of the nervous system (though the roots of this conception were much older). Hierarchical notions had a taken-for-granted quality in later discussions of inhibition. I will describe Flourens's work briefly here; reflex theory is discussed at greater length later.

There was a long history of attempts to discern different functions in different parts of the brain. Military surgeons correlated loss of function with brain injury, and there were studies of direct experimental damage to living animals.[39] Flourens introduced a new standard of experimental technique, giving his results a new precision and authority. He conducted what scientists know as a classic series of experiments with pigeons in which he progressively removed portions of the brain, taking out ("ablating") the cerebrum or cerebral hemispheres and then successive levels working down the brain, so that the last in the series of animals possessed only its spinal cord.[40] He also repeated experiments designed to excite nervous activity by pricking the different portions of the brain. He claimed that his results firmly showed that the cerebrum, unlike other parts of the brain, was both undifferentiated by function and unexcitable (i.e., direct stimulation did not produce movements). His conclusions entrenched a hierarchical view of nervous organization and mind-body relations in a list of "laws of nervous action" that included the following: "I. Nervous functions are subordinated one to another" and "III. The subordinate parts are the spinal cord and the nerves. The regulatory and primary parts are: the medulla, site of the principle determining respiratory movements; the cerebellum, site of the principle coordinating the movements of locomotion; and the cerebral hemispheres, site, the exclusive site, of intelligence."[41] He pronounced with all the force of his authority at the Académie des Sciences that this refuted phrenology and distanced true physiological knowledge from any imputation of materialism. Indeed, Flourens avowed both that the higher brain's equipotentiality confirmed its function as the correlate of the unitary mind and that its inexcitability left the mystery of mind's relation to body outside the scope of experimental investigation. He was explicit in stating that his research confirmed and gave empirical authority to a rigid Cartesian mind-body dualism, the unity of the self, and the freedom of the will.[42]

Flourens's work, and the respect it commanded in France, has to be set against the background of political reaction following the Restoration and the patronage system of the tightly regulated scientific community. Nevertheless, his experimental work was generally considered to be decisive. It appeared to most researchers throughout Europe over the next forty years to exclude the cerebrum, the seat of the mind, from analysis in the sensory-motor units evident at lower levels in the nervous system. His work therefore sustained a vivid image that the mind was related to the body at the highest level and via a unique structure. Neurophysiology thus incorporated a representation of the "highest" human attribute, the soul, into knowledge of the "highest" region of the regulatory nervous system, the cerebrum. There was much debate about function at the midbrain level, often adjusting Flourens's conclusions in detail, and there were even a few critical voices.[43] But all physiologists took for granted the hierarchical arrangement of the nervous system and the language of higher and lower as regards the brain. Comparative research on the neuraxis and experimental neurophysiology joined together on this issue.

In conclusion, we can observe that the language of higher and lower was simultaneously, and without contradiction, physiological and moral, or descriptive and evaluative. It thus formed a mediating language between the older psychological and Christian ideas of the soul's control over the body and the newer physiological ideas of the brain's control over the nervous system. The words "higher" and "lower" continued to have evaluative meaning in subsequent neurophysiological research.

Experimental physiology burgeoned. Concept and precept reinforced each other to confirm hierarchical regulation between mind and brain or, increasingly significantly, within the nervous system itself. For example, Flourens undertook other experiments to settle discussion about reports from J. C. C. Legallois that destruction with a needle of a particular area in the lower brain (brain stem or medulla oblongata) eliminated breathing. Legallois, and later Flourens, argued that this demonstrated the existence of a *noeud vital*, a brain center for regulating respiration, whose destruction ended life itself.[44] The technique used for demonstrating this center, and the model that belief in the center provided for thinking about the brain's differentiated control over basic bodily functions, proved highly influential.

In 1822, François Magendie reported his famous experiment on sectioning the spinal nerve roots, which gave empirical authority to the division of peripheral nerves into sensory and motor.[45] The late-nineteenth-century Viennese psychiatrist, Theodor Meynert, called this "the first fundamental thesis of neurophysiology."[46] Magendie's division, in its turn, again implicated the spinal cord and the brain as the intermediate structures, and hence seats of regulation, between incoming ("afferent") sensory and outgoing ("efferent") motor processes. Sensory processes, central organizing processes, motor processes—these were to be the terms that nineteenth-century neurophysiology used to map out the daunting complexities of nervous life. Yet, as Young has stressed, when Magendie himself considered the functions of the brain, "the experimental method which Magendie applies to the spinal cord is replaced by the introspective and analytic approach" of traditional nonphysiological psychology.[47] Thus, Magendie, like Flourens, contributed to the common attitude that separated the brain, portrayed as the "higher" organ of mind, from the analytic physiological constructs that he was simultaneously developing to comprehend the organization of life.

Sensory, motor, and other organizational terms became increasingly defined by the techniques and observational results of anatomy and experimental physiology. Their precise usage was hence increasingly restricted to the scientific community. Nevertheless, through physiology's continuing close links with medicine, through the extensive literature of medicine and physiology written for lay audiences, and—not least—through the fascination of scientists and nonscientists alike with the conditions of human nature, esoteric and vulgar knowledge remained connected.

DISORDER AND LOSS OF CONTROL

The simplest and most vivid evidence for the control of one part of a person's life over another was what occurred when such control was absent. Emotional outbursts, childish behavior, drunkenness, dreams—such common experiences threw into relief the ideal of a rational, conscious, and well-regulated life. Victorian descriptions of character and conduct contrasted order and disorder in everything between stereotypes of male reason and female sentiment and between the extremes of Isaac Newton's genius and hopeless idiocy. Disorder played a preponderant part in imagining order. As the eminent physician Sir Henry Holland commented,

> Dreaming—insanity in its many forms—intoxication from wine or narcotics—and the phenomena arising from cerebral disease, are the four great mines of mental discovery still open to us;—if indeed any thing of the nature of discovery remains, on a subject which has occupied and exhausted the labours of thinking men in all ages. . . . By the curtailment or suspension of certain functions, by the excess of others, and by the altered balance and connection of all, a sort of analysis is obtained of the nature of mind.[48]

There were numerous ways to conceive such alterations, but the point here is that disorder generally was a fertile breeding ground for ideas subsequently clarified by reference to inhibition. The Victorian language of "loss of control," which was both political and personal, conveyed the sense that the suspension of a higher power released the innate activity of a lower power. The existence of this commonplace meaning makes it difficult to refer to inhibition as an empirical discovery.

As has been indicated, medical and nonmedical writers created a literature on bodily health that merged insensibly into a literature on moral and spiritual well-being. Descriptions of the soul's power to discipline the flesh ran together with descriptions of the rational faculties regulating the instincts and emotions. It was easy, and irresistibly tempting, to moralize about these powers by holding up to the reader examples of what happened when control was lost, to lead the reader through a sequence of disorder, from the dreaming mind to uncontrolled emotion to drunkenness and finally to insanity. Midcentury writers increasingly used the language of neurophysiology to describe this loss of control. While this appeared to provide the literature with a new empirical authority, it did not alter or diminish its evaluative content.

Theories of sleep and dreaming were as varied as they were speculative. Nearly everyone, however, supposed that sleep suspended conscious reason and will, suspending what was often described as attention, leaving involuntary organic functions and undirected mental wandering. According to Carpenter's physiological summary, in sleep both the "hemispheric ganglia" (i.e., cerebral hemispheres) and the midbrain sensory ganglia became passive. This implied that dreaming was merely the arbitrary association of ideas in the partially reactivated but unregulated cerebrum. He argued that sleepwalking involved both the sensory ganglia and the cerebrum exhibiting some activity but that this activity was not dominated by conscious control.[49] The psychiatrist Henry Maudsley later wrote that the somnambulist was "a sensorimotor being, and very much in the position of one of those lower animals that are destitute of cerebral hemispheres."[50]

Mesmerism (or hypnotism) and trance—"which have served at all times to perplex the world by the strange breach they seem to make between the bodily and mental functions"—concentrated the attention of medical writers.[51] Mesmerists disturbed medical men with their mixture of public performance and therapy, a threat to individual responsibility coming together with a threat to medical interests. The British vogue for mesmerism, evident from the late 1830s, prompted physiologists to try to calm public excitement, particularly when it became associated with spiritualist activity.[52] Scientific writers argued that these phenomena, however dramatic they sometimes appeared, involved merely the removal of the regulatory power of the will, reducing a person to automatic functioning. The hypnotized subject, they claimed, was in a state of sleep akin to that of the somnambulist, and in this state a suggested idea could induce him or her to act without conscious control. James Braid, the Manchester surgeon who tried to make hypnotic therapy respectable among medical men, observed, "I have never witnessed any phenomena which were not reconcileable with the notion that they arose from the abnormal exaltation or depression of sensations and ideas, or to their being thrown into unusual and varied ratios."[53] The practice of hypnotism, or "nervous sleep," therefore involved suspending the subject's will but not the central connections between ideas and movements. Not surprisingly, many moralists and physicians viewed this practice with suspicion, especially as the subject of this loss of control was often female.[54]

A significant neurophysiological consequence of this interest was that it implicated the higher brain levels, including the cerebrum, in automatic activities, drawing the mind into closer relation with the existing categories for analyzing the functions of the nervous system. The phenomenon of mesmeric automatism caused Carpenter to extend his systematization of reflex functions to include a class he called "ideo-motor."[55] In ideo-motor action, he argued, an idea present in the mind automatically and involuntarily resulted in a corresponding movement. Examples occurred in hypnotized subjects but also as the result of acquired habits or in states of drunkenness or insanity. He integrated moral and physiological language in writing about these topics. Publicity for the reality of ideo-motor action was at the same time publicity for the training and discipline that would ensure that automatic actions would be moral actions. His moralistic conception of education focused on the power of attention: "It is solely by the Volitional *direction of the attention* that the Will exerts its domination; so that the acquirement of this power . . . should be the primary object of all Mental discipline."[56] Fixing the attention, he held, determined which automatic functions came into play. Lack or misdirection of attention fostered an involuntary life of bad habits or worse.

Thus, the absence of mental control in hypnotized subjects could be likened to the absence of will in people totally under the force of habit. These negative conditions served as a potent reminder that the will exercised an overarching controlling function in healthy and moral human beings. It is very interesting to note that when a later wave of enthusiasm for hypnotism passed across Continental Europe in the 1870s and 1880s, it also prompted physiological theorizing. On this latter occasion, physiologists specifically invoked the suspension of central inhibition to explain the phenomenon (as discussed in chap. 4).

However, it was the effect of alcohol that provided the firmest, the most concrete, and certainly the most familiar example of the loss of higher control over lower function. The loss of control evident in drunkenness was indeed so familiar that it provided something of a baseline against which writers compared other experiences.[57] The drunken person's loss of discrimination, delicacy, and reason, and the release of lower and unguarded sentiments and actions, stood for everyone to see as an allegory of the fallen human condition. To the moralist, drink and uncontrolled emotion had the same character: the reckless lover was drunk with love; the enraged man acted as if drunk; and the mob acted in a drunken fury. Excessive indulgence in drink or emotion (and writers extended the list to suit their purposes) revealed how easily health and reason could be overtaken by illness and disorder. Many Victorians feared that only a continuously active will and watchful attention stood between the mind and the animal powers of the body.

These views translated easily into physiological descriptions of the economy and hierarchical arrangement of the nervous system. Already at the end of the eighteenth century, the physician Erasmus Darwin had described a closed economy of increased sensorial and decreased volitional powers to explain drunken vertigo (or even a child's enjoyment of a swing).[58] The Victorian physiologist Carpenter was an ardent Unitarian and teetotaler who found in physiology a basis in natural law for his social views. He argued that alcohol progressively affected, first, the cerebrum to produce a loss of intellect and then the sensory ganglia to produce a loss of perception, and finally it produced stupor by suspending both higher and midbrain activity, leaving the lower brain and spinal cord functioning automatically.[59]

It was generally perceived that drink initially produced excitement, and this was of course the basis for its widespread medicinal use as a stimulant. This was explained either as a direct effect on the blood or an organ or as an indirect effect involving release of function, for example, in exaggerated language and movements. No writer, to my knowledge, described the latter effect as the release of inhibition before the 1860s, and the adjective "uninhibited" did not appear until the present century (least of all as a compliment!). Nevertheless, a dramatic sense of alcohol's power to release what was hidden within pervades Victorian language.

Alcohol was only the most common among many substances that

altered levels of function. Opium, for example, which was widely available in many different preparations, was used as a stimulant in small doses, as a pain killer, and in larger doses, it was known to produce a deathly stupor.[60] Anesthetics also provided an impressive confirmation of progressive loss of control in a hierarchy of physiological functions, correlating with the hierarchical arrangement of the nervous system. As Spencer observed (giving notions of hierarchy an evolutionary implication),

> It is admitted as holding generally of these various agents—alcohol, ether, chloroform, nitrous oxide, &c.—that when their anaesthetic effects begin, the highest nervous actions are the first to be arrested; and that the artificial paralysis implicates in descending order the lower, or simpler, or better-established nervous actions. Incipient intoxication shows itself in a failure to form involved and abstract relations of ideas, while it remains possible to form simpler relations.[61]

From the 1840s, when anesthetics were introduced, every surgeon became familiar with the progressive loss of mental activity, beginning with the powers of will, attention, and reason and producing a state where only organic functions continued. In the hands of Jackson (whose work is discussed in chap. 4), this serial loss of function became the key to unlocking the secrets of nervous system disorders in general. The concept of control that Jackson organized systematically in relation to the "dissolution" of the nervous system, with corresponding "release of function," and that he worked out in detail to the benefit of clinical neurology was embedded in earlier psychological medicine.

This leads to the Victorian view of insanity. The end point of madness, dementia, or loss of mind and—its obverse side—unregulated bodily function, provided a powerful imagery for nineteenth-century representations of psychological, physiological, and even social disorder. The Victorians tended to elide differences between dreaming, emotion, drunkenness, epilepsy, and insanity, since each of these states involved a loss of control. Each state provided ideas for thinking about the others. Equally, the prescriptive and moralistic language considered appropriate for discussing the regulation of emotion or drinking was carried over without remark into writing on insanity and nervous diseases. Sir Benjamin Brodie, a successful London physician, concluded a popular discussion of insanity with the admonition that "there are many dogs whose natural and original instinct leads them to run after and kill sheep; but a proper discipline teaches them that they are not to do so, and counteracts the instinct."[62]

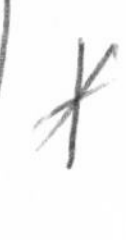

Medical men produced much of the literature on insanity, but their thought was not simply "medical." Insanity had been a public issue since at least the end of the eighteenth century, worrying philanthropists, local justices, the press, and the legislature. The English campaigns that made insanity so visible as a concern occurred alongside and in interaction with a novel account of insanity as moral disorder. The proponents of the "reformed" asylum, in both its private and public versions, intended that the new institutions should restore individuals to themselves, that is, restore their reason, morality, and power of control. The superintendents and staff of the new institutions were to impose the guidance that the disordered individual could no longer exert for himself or herself. This was the purpose of right habits, work, care, prayer, and discipline. The French figurehead of reform, Philippe Pinel, wrote, "We trace the happy effects of intimidation, without severity; of oppression, without violence; and of triumph, without outrage."[63] Restoration to health was marked by the inmate's internalization of such moral guidance. "Much of our own improved treatment of the insane, in the present day, turns upon the power of self-control which they can be induced to exhibit."[64] The degree to which such ideals were realized, or even realizable, is not the point here, though we can observe that they were distinctly ragged even before the major English asylum legislation of 1845. What is of significance is that "moral treatment" (or, as it became, "moral management") gave concrete expression, in terms of a social strategy, to a pervasive conception of how order was embodied in human nature.

A well-regulated life—this appeared to be the key to a Christian and a healthy existence. Emotional excess, drink, or insanity created disorder that made that experience impossible. It is no wonder, then, that a flood of publications, from religious tracts to medical textbooks, extolled the value of cultivating the right habits of control. If this were done when calm and in health, the individual would be able to face trials and tribulations without a loss of control. Without practice, the habits of right action would not be present: "It may be, that emotions and propensities which have acquired strength, by constant indulgence, become at length as irresistible, when the moment of temptation arrives, as those which are the result of mental disease."[65] A moral sensibility therefore held in tension the dignity ("manliness") of a firm will and the threat of base inclinations ("beastliness").

The Reverend John Barlow exemplified these views in the title of his lecture, *On Man's Power Over Himself to Prevent or Control Insanity*

(1843). His argument hinged on a dualism between "*Vital Force* by virtue of which [man] is an animal" and "*Intellectual Force* by virtue of which he is something more."[66] In his very characteristic view, degradation could result from either physical damage to the nervous system or wrong conduct—the "consequences of neglected education, of unregulated passions, of vice, of misery, and . . . of mismanagement also."[67] He then made the moral crystal clear to his listeners:

> Should my position, that the difference between sanity and insanity consists in the degree of self-control exercised, appear paradoxical to any one, let him note for a short time the thoughts that pass through his mind, and the feelings that agitate him: and he will find that, were they all expressed and indulged, they would be as wild, and perhaps as frightful in their consequences as those of any madman. But the man of strong mind represses them, and seeks fresh impressions from without if he finds that aid needful: the man of weak mind yields to them, and then he is insane.[68]

He stressed the continuity between psychological processes in healthy living and in insanity: at all times "wild" feelings were present, but in health there was a power to repress. The loss of this power constituted insanity.

Barlow gave his address not from a pulpit but from the lectern of a scientific body, the Royal Institution of London, when he was its secretary. His language and the social setting enabled him to convey without contradiction a physical meaning, citing disease, and a moral meaning, citing conduct. The Royal Institution had long been committed to education and social improvement through the study of the laws of nature.[69] Barlow was in this tradition in using naturalistic language to express truths about the human condition. Of course, for Barlow such truths were also part of an evangelical Christian outlook. As has been suggested earlier, many other contemporary lecturers in physiology and phrenology would have familiarized his audience with similar arguments.

The extreme disorder exhibited by a few insane people was a moving symbol for any kind of loss of control. As we have seen, medical men or clergy who were familiar with the insane were prone to hold up insanity as a general moral lesson. As the century wore on and the optimistic appeals for the moral reform of the insane were replaced by a leaden fear of insanity as an incurable disease, the moral struggle for prevention—aimed both at individuals and at society as a whole—became a major medical theme. This was to give rise to what was sometimes called the "mental hygiene" movement.[70] As the philosopher

F. H. Bradley commented, "Possibility of compulsion should make us see more clearly the need of so strengthening our will for good as to make that compulsion impossible for us, except in theory."[71]

The imagery of insanity as the breaking out of beastliness was evident in a fear that the insane could commit appalling violence. In extremis, violence welled up from below in an uncontainable act of savagery.

> Homicidal impulses may arise in the mind spontaneously, and prompt towards indiscriminate destruction and demolition or to solitary acts of murder. "The desire to energize" in a destructive manner arises as an intuition, and proceeds to the attainment of its end, excited by affinitive impressions from within or by vital changes in the nervous centres. The lower animals sometimes [also] exhibit impulses of this description.[72]

Medical writers also explained how less spectacular but more common forms of insanity involved loss of control in higher centers.[73] A poignant example was provided by cases of puerperal insanity, insanity consequent on childbirth, in which women and mothers gave vent to hideous sentiments, sometimes even killing their own children. A standard textbook description recorded how "explosions of anger occur, with vociferations and violent gesticulations; and, although the patient may have been remarkable previously for her correct, modest demeanor, and attention to her religious duties, most awful oaths and imprecations are now uttered, and language used which astonishes her friends."[74] The description revealed knowledge of a tension between public propriety and private foulness, a tension that much sharper when located in the constrained lives of polite women.

As physicians went on to explain, the physiological upheaval of childbirth made women an especially vulnerable class. Examples of the removal of women's respectability implied that women could not really be held innocent in nature.

> Every medical man has observed the extraordinary amount of obscenity, in thought and language, which breaks forth from the most modest and well-nurtured woman under the influence of puerperal mania; and although it may be courteous and politic to join in the wonder of those around, that such impurities could ever enter such a mind, and while he repudiates Pope's slander, that 'every woman is at heart a rake', he will nevertheless acknowledge, that religious and moral principles alone give strength to the female mind; and that, when these are weakened or removed by disease, the subterranean fires become active, and the crater gives forth smoke and flame.[75]

This almost medieval imagery of the pit existed alongside the most up-to-date reference to reflex action and cranial blood circulation. In the world of Victorian medicine, religious duty and healthy cerebral activity joined together to contain "the beast." Language itself carried both theological and physiological meaning. Men as well as women confronted the same circumstances, but it was assumed that men's greater strength of will and the absence of women's physiological upheavals created a different character and aroused different expectations.

While physicians observed obscenity in word and deed among the insane, a few specialists in nervous diseases were making a more precise record of the varieties of speech loss grouped under the term "aphasia." They found it very striking that the loss of voluntary, articulate speech did not necessarily eliminate the capacity to produce an apparently involuntary oath in response to a sudden pain or emotion.[76] The partial loss of language revealed the anarchy that threatened society from below. The language of polite society and the language of emotion thus existed as signs of the hierarchical relation between controlled and uncontrolled conduct. The further power of language to signal social strata hardly requires comment.

By midcentury, nearly all British medical writers on the healthy life and the prevention of insanity had self-consciously adopted a physiological idiom. We can observe writers translating moral and psychological terms into factual and physiological terms without any discernible discontinuity, carrying over the evaluative meaning of the former into the latter. Maudsley's skeptical account of the will provides an example:

> It is manifestly ordained that the will, as the highest mode of energy of nerve elements, should control the inferior modes of energy by operating downwards upon their subordinate centres: the anatomical disposition of the nervous system is in conformity with what psychological observation teaches. But the undoubted fact, that the will of a man can and does control inferior functions has led to a very extravagant and ill-founded notion as to its autocratic power.[77]

In fact, as regards inhibition, we will see that the language continued to describe both psychological and physiological regulatory processes. And this was not peculiar to English-language sources.

Experimental neurophysiologists working in the German language developed detailed accounts of inhibition. It is therefore necessary to say something about the background of the concept in medical psychology in this wider setting. Unfortunately, the extent and content of German-language writing for a general audience on bodily, mental, and spiritual health in the first half of the nineteenth century is largely unknown to me. I will therefore restrict myself to illustrating points with reference to a literature that already has an important place in our understanding of the history of psychiatry. The relation of this literature to a wider culture of "popular" physiology and psychology, comparable to what we find in Britain, must be left open. One small but significant example of the word "inhibition" in general use comes from Immanuel Kant's lectures on "anthropology" which he gave to nonspecialist audiences for many years in the late eighteenth century. These lectures were not systematic in a philosophical sense but commented on practical psychological and moral topics. In this setting, Kant discussed drunkenness, sleep, fainting, and asphyxia as "the inhibition, weakening, and total loss of the sense powers" and referred to "an inhibition of the regular and ordinary use of our power of reflection."[78]

Political circumstances in the German-speaking world were very different from those in Britain. There was an enormous diversity of states, from Hapsburg and Catholic Austria to the Grand Duchies of Weimar or Oldenburg to Protestant Prussia extending far to the East. These political structures had a long lineage, but by the late eighteenth century, imperial or aristocratic rulers depended on alliances with a university-educated administrative class to sustain economic and political order. This class fostered a consciousness of a larger German identity that depended on shared language and culture. In the wake of military humiliation by the French under Napoleon, this "idealistic" unity led to the academic world acquiring considerable significance in relation to political aspirations.[79] However, only after 1871 and on terms dictated by Prussian material and military success was this ideal unity to achieve political expression. Liberal attitudes, valuing the individual's autonomy as a basis for the general good, never achieved the political prominence they had in Britain. German-language writers stressed individual duty and responsibility, to God and to the state, as dictated by the position a person occupied in society. The educated elite, notably civil servants, a group that included university and gymnasium teachers as well as administrators, and professional men such as doctors, reflected at length on their own contribution to questions of social order. Kant's general lectures on anthropology were only one example of cultural activity that integrated thought about personal conduct with social ends. Nineteenth-century German physicians and physiologists inherited and sustained these practices. As the servants of civil society, they self-consciously accepted an elevated calling. As educators, they were committed to perpetuating German cultural values, even when their day-to-day research led into highly abstruse matters.

This sketch of the German-speaking world could of course be extended, with appropriate comparisons and qualifications, to the rest of Europe. As discussed later, Sechenov's research on central inhibition or Pavlov's research on learning had distinctive implications in the context of Tsarist Russia. In Russia, almost any non-Orthodox theory about human character or about bodily capacities could appear subversive of a political system legitimated by divine right. Following 1855, substantial sectors of the administration argued that Russia had to learn from the West to sustain its power. But Western systems of government, even those with the most minimal representation of the people, were steadfastly resisted until 1905. When some modernization was undertaken, as with the administrative reforms in the 1860s, maintaining the autocratic order remained paramount. This order greatly stressed individual responsibility, presupposing the ethical and spiritual duty of each person before God, before the tsar, and before the law. In this setting, even to suggest that human beings were in any way a proper subject for the natural-historical sciences provoked conservative opposition. Conversely, the "Westernizers" often looked to physiological and psychological science to provide new and authoritative ideas on human relations.

Though to support this argument would be the subject of another study, we can assume that German or Russian writers on the mind and body were as bound up with moral and political questions as their English-language colleagues. A few illustrations, taken from the history of psychiatry, may make the point. The discussion below of the philosopher and educator, Herbart, adds further support.

The Leipzig professor of psychological medicine during the 1820s, J. C. A. Heinroth, was derided in earlier histories of psychiatry because of his apparent avowal that insanity was sin. As both Otto Marx and Gerlof Verwey have argued, however, his views were rather more complex that this.[80] It is also historically uninformative to label his position "mentalist" in order to imply its backwardness vis-à-vis modern medicine. It is more positive to note that he contributed to debates on character, morality, and religious and civil duty which agitated the diverse German communities in the wake of the Napoleonic experience.

These discussions became particularly sharp in relation to medicolegal issues.[81] Just as contemporary German literature portrayed character as a question of balance among psychological faculties, Heinroth conceived of mental illness in terms of psychological disturbances. He divided systematic psychological medicine, first, into a characterization of the elements of the soul; second, into the "science of forms," a classification and description of disturbances to the soul; and third, into the "science of quality," an attempt to explain the types of disturbance.[82] When he described evil, he meant the working principle of disturbance, however generated in the mental life, whether through internal or external events (which, significantly, he did not clearly distinguish). Evil could not destroy what God had created in man's spirit, but it could and of course did disturb the spirit's search for perfection through reason (which he treated as a religious cognitive faculty).

In one passage, Heinroth described this disturbance of the good's striving as inhibition (*Hemmung*).

> Evil, despite all the inclination, is hardly able to *de*stroy something created by the Divine Spirit, though it is well able to *disturb* the development towards perfection, i.e., to arrest or inhibit it, and we encounter many such *inhibitions* in particular and general experience. . . . The Evil Principle, which is prevented by the power of Good from achieving its final objective, dissolution, annihilation, *de*struction, attains its objective at least to a halfway point, the point of disturbance, of inhibition. Thus it appears as an *inhibiting*, *retarding* principle, a principle pulling everything that strives upwards into the abyss in which itself abides.[83]

Inhibition here characterized the power of one principle to counteract but not eliminate another principle, with consequent retardation rather than development. Though the abstract sense of inhibition as a controlling relation is comparable with later usages, it is interesting to note that Heinroth's specific use referred to evil inhibiting good rather than vice versa. That Heinroth used the term in the context of describing the unfolding of an individual's spiritual development does not mean that he was not at the same time referring to processes of social or collective development. In his language, "development" or "retardation" of spirit represented both an individual and a collective interest. Thus, he believed that the mental physician worked to free "development" both for the individual and for the general good.

By 1840, most physicians were rejecting Heinroth's religious language as incompatible with the grounding of medicine in physiological reality. Nevertheless, considerable elements of traditional notions of balance and disturbance remained in the psychiatric literature, including the writings of the most famous of the midcentury German psychiatrists, Wilhelm Griesinger. His work shows how notions of individual character, particularly of disturbances to character, drew together a traditional concern with ordered relations and the new physiological science.

To describe Griesinger as "famous" is really to refer to his reputation with a later generation that considered him responsible for bringing the study of madness out of the asylum and into the academic setting. Belief in this achievement implied that he had also integrated psychological medicine with the new physiology of the nervous system.[84] Griesinger in fact had a somewhat limited experience of clinical and asylum psychiatry, and contemporary insanity specialists strongly rejected his claim to a position of leadership. Be this as it may, relatively early in his career, Griesinger published work that proved to be a powerful statement of the relations between neurophysiology and psychological medicine.

Though sometimes described as a "physicalist" in his approach to insanity (which draws a contrast with Heinroth's "mentalism"), Griesinger combined psychological and physiological approaches.[85] His psychology (following Herbart) referred to the interaction and combination of representations in the "Ego." His physiology approached actions as nervous processes, which he modeled following the idea of the reflex.[86] What held these apparently divergent tendencies together was a common vocabulary denoting the balance and conflict of forces as a system of organization. Griesinger utilized both an earlier Herbartian language of psychological forces and a new language of physiological organization to portray control and its breakdown.

Griesinger was one of a number of writers who were quick to see the potential of the reflex model, developed in the 1830s, for explaining many complex normal and abnormal movements. His aim was "to emphasize the parallels between the workings of the spinal cord (with the *medulla oblongata*) and those of the brain, in so far as it is an organ of psychic phenomena in the strict sense of the word, and to prove those parallels to exist by reference to normal and abnormal phenomena."[87] He went further than most, however, in his willingness to describe reflex functions subserving psychological—but unconscious—events even at the highest levels of the brain (which Flourens had ruled out). He also represented in physiological terms the psychological and teleological powers of the "I" to control or initiate movement. In this context, he developed a speculative *Hemmungstheorie*, or theory of inhibition, borrowing directly from the physiologist and physician J. L. Budge.[88] In Griesinger's view, volition, represented as a physiological event, involved higher brain regions intervening to lift or suspend the normal inhibited condition of lower brain and spinal reflexes, and these reflexes then proceeded to produce movements. How the higher levels acted on lower levels he could not say.

> The transition from the more or less conscious striving into muscular movement occurs in a way that appears to be much less a positive activity than the freeing from a resistance, from an inhibition. If, for example, we wish to walk or speak, this striving does not need yet another special act, a new positive impulse for the motor nerves, but the idea of walking or speaking passes into striving and striving into movement as soon as it is not hindered by anything.[89]

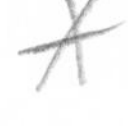

His conception of volition, as the freeing of inhibited reflexes, also reflected the common idea that drugs, such as alcohol, opium, or Nux vomica (strychnine), released movements organized at lower levels in the nervous system.

Such ideas provided Griesinger with the means to initiate a physiological psychology of insanity. As was the case with parallel work in Britain, familiarity with drunkenness was a potent source of ideas. In Griesinger's words, when one is drunk, "previously present inhibitions of ideas ['presentations' or *Vorstellungen*] dissolve, ideas long searched for readily appear, the pressure caused by adverse and sad thoughts gives way to high spirits."[90] This confirmed in his mind the value of a conventional classification of the forms of insanity into depressive and excited (the *Schwermuth* and *Tollheit* described by Albert Zeller, director of the well-known public asylum at Winnenthal).[91] He stated that depressive insanities were characterized by a state of exaggerated inhibition: "They arise . . . from the impression of an inhibition on the free flow of mental images, both in terms of their dispersion and their passing into striving. Whether these inhibitions are perceived or whether psychic pain grows from them is individually very different."[92] Moving between this psychological language of depression and a physiological language of interaction between higher brain regions and spinal reflexes, Griesinger also compared pathological mental conditions, such as the dominance of fixed ideas, with pathological nervous conditions, such as spasms or hemiplegia (partial paralysis). General conceptions of regulation, sometimes involving the specific language of inhibition, made possible a coherent way of thinking about a confusing mix of the psychological and the physiological in normal as well as in abnormal phenomena. As Griesinger commented,

> In man, the immediate transition of . . . sensations to movement is subject in a high degree to the influence of the understanding, and through it duty and morality intervene to control and govern the sensuous desires. But there are cases where these lose their power. In the insane, in whom the influence of the understanding over the instincts is enfeebled, and moreover the sensuous impulses perhaps strengthened, we often see, for example, the appetite for food or the sexual instinct showing itself with the utmost regardlessness.[93]

Normal moral controls thus involved the arresting action of higher powers over the automatic instincts. The new experimental physiology provided the terms to re-create this understanding as properties of the body.

Conceptions of health as a balance between excitation and depression were of course ancient and well represented in the Hippocratic tradition. It is therefore possible to draw a parallel between humoral medicine, with its nonspecific conception of illness and lack of sharp discrimination between bodily and mental processes, and more modern medicine, in which conceptions of illness as a disturbance of the excitation-inhibition relation also integrated physiological and psychological terms. The point may be illustrated with a few examples taken from general medicine in the nineteenth century.

Brunonian medicine had an extraordinary vogue, especially in the German world, in the early years of the century. John Brown was a Scottish physician whose writings reexpressed ancient conceptions of balance and health in terms of the strength, quality, and quantity of "stimulation." His *Elementa medicina* (1780) had divided disease into sthenic and asthenic, the former exhibiting an excess and the latter a deficit of stimulation. His claim that the very great majority of illnesses were in practice asthenic, and hence that excitation should dominate therapy, generated considerable controversy and enthusiasm at the time. It served as a lever against established orthodoxies whose therapeutic armory focused on depletion.[94] The details of such controversies about therapy are not important to the present story, but the terms in which they were conducted suggest great medical familiarity with a language of the interaction of forces and a common ability to envisage one force having a countering or inhibiting effect on others.

Such general notions, though obviously no longer in the Brunonian form, had a persistent value. Thus, for example, the English physician H. G. Salter, in his work *On Asthma* (1860), which is now regarded as the foundation of a modern approach, attempted to understand the disorder in terms of an excitation-inhibition model. Salter systematically treated asthma as a nervous disorder, rationalizing its symptoms of excitation and depression. Thus, he noted that the tendency of sleep to bring on asthmatic attacks was explicable in terms of the known effect of sleep in enhancing the intensity of spinal reflexes.

> It is just as sleep comes on, just as the will is laid to rest, or during sleep, that these different forms of involuntary muscular contraction most commonly occur. Any one, to convince himself of it, has only to fall asleep sitting on the edge of his chair, in such a position that it shall press on his sciatic nerves. As long as he is awake his legs will be motionless; but the moment he falls asleep they will start up with a plunge and suddenly wake him.[95]

Conversely, stimulants (such as coffee) or emotion (such as sexual excitement) acted as a countereffect to muscular spasms.[96]

As Salter's study of asthma suggests, the model of a balance of powers was particularly valuable in describing conditions where mind and body interacted. This was true for normal circumstances, such as those involving the passions and instincts, as well as for abnormal conditions. Much discussed hysterical phenomena provided particularly rich illustrations. As has already been mentioned, there was no lack of medical attention to the sexual powers, and a graphic picture of these powers at work in hysteria was provided by R. B. Carter in 1853. He portrayed hysterical fits as outbursts of emotional energy occurring when the conditions of a woman's existence—and the lack of a disciplined attention to controlling motives—released excitation, especially sexual excitation.

> The disease [is] . . . one of the misfortunes entailed upon the civilized female by the conditions of her existence, and the mobility of her nervous centres. . . .
>
> It is reasonable to expect that an emotion, which is strongly felt by great numbers of people, but whose natural manifestations are constantly repressed in compliance with the usages of society, will be the one whose morbid effects are most frequently witnessed. This anticipation is abundantly borne out by facts; the sexual passion in women being that which most accurately fulfils the prescribed conditions.[97]

Carter distinguished primary, secondary, and tertiary hysterias. In the first two forms, he believed, the emotion was so strong that its expression could not be prevented. In the most important group, the tertiary hysterias, however, he identified the cause of the fit as attention to a constant or fixed idea: "The occurrence of the fit, although not volitional, is yet a matter of surrender, and might be prevented under the pressure of an adequate motive."[98] He borrowed the term "ideo-motor" action from Carpenter to describe better what he meant.[99] An idea, for example, that the patient held about her body might become so fixed by attention that movements appropriate to this idea would occur automatically, almost as if such movements were involuntary and reflex in form. This was ideo-motor action. Hence, the male physician argued, it was the doctor's therapeutic duty to remove the hysterical woman from her home and to impose constructive moral training that would equip her with a motive adequate to repress emotional ideas. His idea of treatment was thus reminiscent of the ideals of the asylum moral therapists.

Carter's work shows clearly how notions of general physiology, psychological control, gender relations, and social order all ran together in a way that was mediated by a common language of hierarchical regulation. A literature about normality and abnormality, respectively viewed as successful control and as control released, endlessly reinforced its own presuppositions. The structural features of this language persisted into late Victorian medical literature and on into the twentieth century—in Pavlov, in Freud, and in many sources that provide the terms of our modern self-reflection.

REGULATION AND MENTAL CONTENT

The term "inhibition," or a conception of control that we would think appropriately described by that term, was not limited to the normative world of character and disorder. In the introduction, I drew attention to different notions of control, particularly distinguishing inhibition as the repression of a lower by a higher power from inhibition as the competitive arrest of one force by a qualitatively comparable force. The foregoing has illustrated the extent and richness of the former conception of hierarchical control in the relation between mind and body. Here, in partial contrast, I will describe the latter, dynamic type of interactive control as it was conceived to exist within the mind. This was also an important part of the background to modern ideas of inhibition. In many cases, however, the two types of controlling relations ran together.

What I call the interactive sense of inhibitory relations became a central feature of nineteenth-century writing on the organization of mental content. The ordered conscious world, achieved in the face of the theoretically limitless complexity of perceptual experience, implied that some discriminatory or organizational process must be active. The way this was understood depended on presuppositions about the nature of mind, its elementary constituents, and the manner in which they interrelated to create the mental content. Description of inhibition or the arrest of one constituent by another became a significant analytic tool. When psychology later began to be a separate academic discipline, drawing on experimental methods, it perpetuated this usage. These more modern discussions, however, were also deeply influenced by physiological research on inhibition. They will therefore be discussed later.

Accounts of inhibition in mental content were part of a technical topic that was, in our terms, both philosophical and psychological. The audience for this was restricted in a way that was certainly not the case in relation to discussions of inhibition and normal and abnormal conduct. Nevertheless, the basic premise behind the use of inhibition in understanding the organization of mental content was a commonsense one, resembling Aristotle's observation that a stronger activity of the soul arrests a weaker activity. This premise reappeared in a variety of forms in the work of the philosophers G. W. Leibniz, Christian Wolff, and Kant in the eighteenth century and in the experimental analyses of perception, memory, and elementary thought characteristic of early-twentieth-century psychology.[100] It was indeed a commonplace of both formal and informal psychological analysis.

The problem was to explain how it was possible for consciousness to exhibit an organization or focused order, given all the possible elements of mental content. There were two divergent traditions addressing this issue in the eighteenth century, though each was far from static or unified. The first, the sensationalist or Lockean tradition, tied the organizing property to the spatial and temporal relations of simple sensory elements. It was argued that such simple elements or ideas constituted the original material of mental content. David Hartley, Thomas Brown, and James Mill systematically treated organization as a function of the laws of "the association of ideas."[101] The second, the idealist or Leibnizian tradition, tied organization to the dynamic attributes possessed by mental content itself. Writers variously characterized the dynamic power in terms of the integrative unity of the soul, active mental faculties, or qualities appertaining to the stuff of mind. In this tradition, it was argued that mental activity constituted the organizing process. A search for properly explanatory psychological categories precipitated criticism of the idea of mental faculties and encouraged a conception of organization as a consequence of the dynamic life among more elementary mental powers. Herbart turned this approach into a systematic theory of the determination of consciousness that gave inhibition (*Hemmung*) a basic role. The way Herbart addressed the underlying question of mental organization then continued to be reflected in late-nineteenth-century psychology.

As professor of philosophy in what had been Kant's chair at Königsberg (now Kaliningrad) between 1809 and 1833, Herbart launched a system of metaphysics intended both to compete with Hegel in Berlin and to provide a rational basis for *Staatswissenschaft.* Such a science of government included pedagogy, the training of individuals into reason and into their rights and duties as political subjects, and state administration, the comprehension of the rights and duties of the state. Herbart was not successful in the tasks he set himself or in establishing a dominant school. His elaborate metaphysical undertakings were finally incoherent, while his pedagogy did not touch on the actual needs or possibilities of the Prussian school system. All the same, his discussion of the dynamics of mental processes proved highly suggestive for later educationists and psychologists.

Historians of psychology frequently cite Herbart, though with little reference to the historical context of his work. In his *Psychologie als Wissenschaft neu gegründet auf Erfahrung, Metaphysik und Mathematik* (1824–1825), Herbart rejected Kant's strictures on the scope of psychology as a "science" in Kant's rationally explicated sense of that term. He argued that he could deduce the nature of mental content from rational foundations, ultimately grounded in his a priori conception of the unity of the soul. Most famously, he contended that it was possible to develop a quantified science of mental dynamics, making psychology into a rational science like mechanics.[102] This led to the claim, in the retrospective view of the French psychologist Théodule Ribot, that "the first efforts toward a scientific psychology, in Germany, are due to Herbart. They constitute a transition from the pure speculation of Fichte and Hegel to the unmetaphysical psychology."[103]

Herbart understood the soul to be an indivisible entity that, nevertheless, in our comprehension, existed as a series of relations exhibiting perturbations (*Störungen*) and active self-preservations (*Selbsterhaltungen*). The perturbations and self-preserving relations took the mental form of "presentations" (the term commonly employed to translate "Vorstellungen," the German word widely used, especially in the later experimental psychology, as a description of the elements of mental content). Just as physical mechanics had constructed a science by abstracting quantifiable dimensions from "the real," so, Herbart argued, psychology could construct a science by abstracting the quantifiable dimensions of the dynamic mental presentations. Further, since the "simple beings" underlying the mental and the physical both existed in dynamic disturbing and resisting relations with each other, mechanics also provided a structural model for psychology.[104] Thus, the form of the mental that actually appeared in consciousness was a product of the dynamic interactions between the "simple beings" of the mentally real. A certain strength was necessary for a mental element to exist as a conscious, as opposed to an unconscious, presentation, since this strength gave it dominance over other elements. As Harold Dunkel noted, it was in this context that Herbart introduced the term "inhibition": "There is a psychological argument in favour of asserting that the presentations will tend to inhibit each other: if there were no such mutual resistance, all presentations would merge into one, and the content of consciousness would be a unity rather than that manifold of varied elements with which experience presents us."[105] Inhibition thus described the dynamic resistance that each presentation offered to every other. The activity of a presentation in overcoming such resistance generated its presence as conscious experience and constituted the organized character of that experience.

Equipped with this conception of mental dynamics, Herbart then attempted an a priori derivation of what other writers had referred to as the psychological faculties of reason, feeling, and will. One example was his description of our capacity to form abstract notions:

> It might occur to one that perhaps under certain circumstances the laws of arrest [inhibition] between concepts might effect a separation of the dissimilar from the common characteristics of concepts, such as logicians unhesitatingly ascribe to the faculty of abstraction . . . [but] partial concepts in a complex or blending carry every arrest in common, and hence remain constantly together.[106]

Herbart self-consciously used the mechanical terms *Druck* (pressure) and *Gegendruck* (counterpressure) to describe the force and resistance of presentations. When separated from its metaphysical underpinning by later German psychology, this became an attempt to specify the manner in which sensory elements relate, combine, and inhibit one another in forming conscious perceptions. This account thus fulfilled a role comparable to the laws of association in British empiricist psychology. Herbart translated the problem of the organizational unity of the "I" into a question concerning the dynamic interaction of presentations:

"This difficult metaphysical problem is, in a psychological sense, quite as simple as . . . how the apprehension of several characteristics together make up the concept of one object. . . . In the soul many representations merge into one act of representation when arrests do not prevent [it]."[107] This dynamic merging of mental elements, making possible unified experience, was to become the problem of "apperception" in later psychology.

It is necessary to stress that Herbart's apparently abstruse theory of mental dynamics directly underpinned his political or administrative and educational thinking. Though the metaphysical reasoning underlying Herbart's psychology was somewhat obscure, his description of the dynamics of ideas in conscious mental life was readily understandable. He intended that his empirical descriptions of the life of the "Ego," by which he referred to something individual and given to ordinary self-perception, should be readily applicable to practical ends.[108] He emphasized, for example, that each individual's consciousness was modified by separate presentations and therefore that there could be no practical psychology "in general": "There are no universal facts. Purely psychological facts lie in the region of transitory conditions of individuals, and are immeasurably far removed from the height of the general notion of man in general."[109] Practical psychology—that is, education, specifically, Prussian state pedagogy—must therefore take this into account.[110] Later educationists thus found in Herbart an individualized approach to the formation of the child's mental world.

The abstract way in which Herbart thought about relations made possible a common discourse among mechanics, psychology, and *Staatswissenschaft*. Each science articulated a dynamics concerning, respectively, mechanical forces, mental presentations, and the branches of the state. He thus introduced the second, analytic volume of his *Psychologie als Wissenschaft* with "fragments" of a statics and mechanics of the state, in which he utilized the concept of inhibition to describe the interaction between individuals in the constitution of political power. "The forces taking effect in society are undoubtedly psychological in origin. They come together inasmuch as they as manifested through speech and through actions in the shared sensory world. In the latter, they inhibit each other; that is the general spectacle of conflicting interests and organizational friction. Integration is also without doubt present."[111] It therefore followed that a rational science of politics depended on elaborating the relationship between individual and collective psychological forces. Nevertheless, just as Herbart had presupposed in his psychology that the soul had a metaphysical unity, so his account of politics presupposed that the state possessed a fundamental unity that in some sense logically preexisted the relationships among psychological forces. Only by comprehending these forces, however, could the state represent itself as a branch of knowledge.

Inhibition thus existed as a relational term in Herbart's systematic political psychology (as we may call it) as well as in the German literature of his time. It denoted the dominance of one element over another in the achievement of some organized end. Organized relations, whether in conscious perception, in individual character, or in state-administration, implied the repression of some actions through the activity of others. As one would expect, this language also covered the description of disorganized relations as the loss of a controlling balance of forces, allowing one power to express itself in exaggerated form. Thus, Herbart juxtaposed illusion, madness, dementia, and idiocy, suggesting that these states were the product of the abnormal exaggeration or inhibition of normal psychological processes. "From the innumerable cases which are narrated as very remarkable, the psychologist, as soon as he has recognized the psychical mechanism and its possible arrests, learns little or nothing new whatever."[112] Herbart may have felt that he was arguing rationally from philosophical and psychological premises in reaching such a conclusion. At the same time, he reexpressed in his own terms the conventional conception of health as balance and insanity as disorder.

Herbart's approach to psychology in terms of the dynamics of presentations was taken into mainstream psychiatric theory by Griesinger in the 1840s. As described above, Griesinger elaborated a psychology of the Ego in terms of contending ideas, and this provided a richly descriptive language for exploring emotional and volitional disorders. He referred freely to conscious and unconscious elements competing together. As a mid-nineteenth-century physician, he wrote about these elements being grounded in nervous processes; for example, by unconscious activity, he meant nervous processes unaccompanied by consciousness.[113] He thus transferred a psychological dynamics derived from Herbart to a theory of functional relations within the nervous system. "Griesinger was solely or primarily interested in Herbart's mechanistic psychology as a psychological theory which lent itself to being interpreted as an extrapolation of the physiological reflex model."[114] At the same time, he preserved the Herbartian psychological language that enabled him to write in terms relevant to the observation and experience of functional disorder in people. Griesinger took over Herbartian dynamics and used it to make a significant contribution to physiological psychology. This move was possible because the language describing the relations between forces, including inhibition, was amenable equally to physiological and psychological expression.

The main body of work continuing to address the issues that Herbart had raised was psychological rather than medical. Mid-nineteenth-century psychologists detached his mental dynamics from its original context and endeavored to make it more empirical. The mathematician, M. W. Drobisch, gave Herbartian psychology some credibility by arguing that it was possible to achieve the same kind of analysis on empirical rather than deductive grounds—an appealing move since Herbart's metaphysics appeared indefensible. However, this left unfounded Herbart's claim that psychology could be a systematically rational science, and it submerged a dimension of his work that had fundamentally influenced his conception of mental organization. Drobisch, along with F. E. Beneke, Theodor Waitz, and Wilhelm Volkmann, considered that psychology could be constructed as an empirical science through the introspective analysis of the organization of sensation and feeling in consciousness. This sustained one distinctive conception of psychology, largely independent of developments in physiology, into the last quarter of the nineteenth century. These writers did not form a socially coherent group, but together they established a significant precedent for the conception of psychology as a subject distinguishable from both philosophy and physiology. At the same time, they posed questions about perception and consciousness, as Herbart had done earlier, in terms that proved accessible to researchers coming to such questions after training in experimental natural science.

Beneke eschewed technical metaphysics and abstruse mental dynamics, aiming instead to write accessible, practical guides to psychological understanding and to conduct.[115] His work premised a commonplace recognition of the interaction of stronger and weaker mental elements in psychological life. He wrote for—and found—an audience looking for naturalistic psychological knowledge, knowledge relevant to the experience of the ordinary conditions of life rather than knowledge responding to the a priori requirements of theology or philosophy. Beneke specifically diverged from Herbart on the subject of the interaction of presentations in consciousness, arguing "that there is a continual redistribution of transferable elements within the total system of mental modifications," rather than arrest or inhibition between elements.[116] Drobisch, Waitz, and Volkmann, by contrast, argued that objective introspection required the postulation of the soul's unity and an approach to the formation of conscious mental content in terms of the combination and arrest (or inhibition) of the elementary presentations.[117] Drobisch, for example, "makes introspection his point of departure, obtains by induction the laws of combination and arrest, then finally infers from the existence of these laws the unity and simplicity of the soul."[118] He also made these ideas accessible, using inhibition, in the manner current in German literature, to discuss the relation between experience and feeling in the formation of character and individuality. Elsewhere, in a more technical book, he attempted to give new life to Herbart's mathematical analysis of psychological dynamics, but this too involved inhibition.[119]

Such approaches to the formation of mental content did not go unquestioned. One of the most prominent philosopher-psychologists over many years, Hermann Lotze, specifically criticized the image of consciousness "as *a space of limited extent*, within which the impressions struggle for their places." As he continued, "We thus smuggle in by the way, under shelter of a wholly unauthorized image, the idea of a mutual incompatibility of ideas, and of a pressure which they of necessity exert on one another."[120] For Lotze, conscious processes were to be understood in terms of the apprehensive activity of the soul, for which the language of force and resistance was wholly inappropriate. Not surprisingly, therefore, he made no reference to inhibition.

The problem of organized mental content, specifically, perception, which Herbart had hoped to resolve through a quantified psychological dynamics, reappeared as a major research area in German experimental psychology dating from about the 1870s. This new research was undertaken in an academic setting that did not require psychologists to contribute directly either to *Staatswissenschaft* or to a wider audience. The institutionalization of natural-scientific research, as a cultural value in its own right, permitted psychologists to focus on technical matters of direct relevance only to other academics. Further, by this time, the development of complex and high-status research on physiological excitation and inhibition had generated a tendency for discussion of the relations between psychological elements to take its cue from physiology. Yet, in this chapter, I have shown that concepts of control, including a concept of inhibition, were common intellectual resources *prior to* the development of physiological theories of inhibition. Most important, these resources continued to have life, particularly in psychological medicine, long after physiology had apparently given terms such as "inhibition" a precise, material, and empirical meaning. Nevertheless, physiology certainly did transform and vastly enrich discussion of inhibitory regulation, and it is to physiology that we must now turn.

CHAPTER 3

Inhibition in Neurophysiology

I flatten out the frog and look to see what is happening inside it; and as you and I are also frogs, only we walk on two legs, I shall know what happens inside us too.

———Turgenev, *Fathers and Sons*

REFLEX ORGANIZATION

Experimental natural science transformed academic culture and the status and authority of scientific knowledge in the nineteenth century. It was often natural science, rather than theology, philosophy, or the moral sciences, that provided intellectual leadership, attracted the brightest students, and commanded public attention. Rigorous scientific methods appeared to guarantee a cumulative body of knowledge and, in conjunction with technology, to be the very motor of progress. Physiological science, the study of the functions of living systems, shared in this high reputation. Indeed, some of the most eminent natural scientists, like Claude Bernard or Hermann Helmholtz, were themselves brilliant physiological experimenters. It was all a part of the pattern that experimental science, exemplifying objective methods and creating explanatory knowledge, should transform approaches toward mind-brain issues.[1] Moreover, the ability of natural scientists successfully to tackle such issues became something of a test case for the sufficiency of the scientific world view. Neurophysiology and physiological psychology expanded at a rapid pace, attracting substantial intellectual and institutional investment from the middle years of the century.[2]

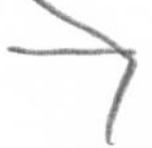

The concept of inhibition illustrates clearly the hope associated with experimental natural science: to transform thought about human nature and moral action into a natural-scientific mode. Scientists recast such topics in the terms of the new nervous physiology and psychology.

This inevitably generated problems in formulating relations between studies of mind and studies of brain. Choice of methods, decisions about explanatory concepts, division of labor between disciplines, and sustaining philosophical coherence became—and were to remain—problematic issues. Little was settled in the nineteenth century. Whether physiology and psychology were or were not the same subject and how these disciplines were to be related remained at issue.

For the scientists who hoped that physiology and psychology would become highly specialized, technical, and separate disciplines, and for their heirs in the twentieth century, such developments marked both the inevitable specialization of knowledge and the advancing "edge of objectivity."[3] Many believed that the new sciences would eliminate teleology (explanation by purposes) from the realm of animal or human action. It was anticipated that this would occur in the nineteenth century, just as seventeenth-century physical science had removed vital powers and final causes from the workings of the universe.

In reality, as many also accepted even in the nineteenth century, the outcome was less than straightforward since the scientific world view raised vastly complex issues, precipitating philosophical, religious, and moral questions. There were also stupendous difficulties facing the extension of scientific methods to encompass mind and brain. The introduction of physiological methods in relation to psychological questions did not involve simply the unproblematic application of an objective approach to describing nature. Indeed, in many ways, the new physiological discourse did not displace existing psychological meanings and teleological forms of explanation. That experimental science acquired unique authority as a source of knowledge did not necessarily mean that physiology's advance eliminated evaluative meanings from accounts of human nature. The intellectual investment in natural science did not in fact empty discourse about human nature of its rich content of values. This investment certainly generated a new, technical, and often esoteric understanding of detailed empirical questions. These questions became the substance of what researchers experienced as science, and they accordingly subscribed to the view that meaning was constituted by observation statements. As the history of inhibition shows, however, the conceptual framework of physiological science preserved a much richer content of evaluative meaning.

Inhibition became a major topic or cluster of issues in experimental and theoretical neurophysiology between 1840 and 1870. It was, of course, not coincidental that this occurred simultaneously with neurophysiology achieving authority as a specialist discipline. Neurophysiology, as research practice, and inhibition, as conceptual tool, were mutually constitutive. To understand the place of inhibition, it is first necessary to explore aspects of neurophysiology in the 1830s, insofar as it then existed as a specialty. For reasons that will become clear, it is reflex theory—by which I refer to the view that the reflex is the basic unit of function in the nervous system—that provides the starting point.

Modern notions of reflex action existed by the end of the 1830s. Physiologists argued that the reflex formed the simplest organized unit of anatomical structure and physiological function in the nervous system. It was understood that it consisted of a sensory nerve linked by the central spinal cord or lower brain regions to a motor nerve, the whole structure (subsequently known as a "reflex arc") acting together to produce a definite movement in response to a particular stimulus. The theory was to become fundamental to experimental practice and to theoretical argument in neurophysiology and physiological psychology.[4] It was taken up in varied and complex ways. It proved to be an extremely suggestive source of experimental questions and to be invaluable as a language with which to describe purposes or organized actions in mechanistic terms. Reflex theory was thus inseparable from the aspiration to find physiological answers in the search for objective psychological knowledge.

Marshall Hall forced the idea of his discovery of reflex action on his contemporaries. His belligerent and ultimately tedious claims tended, at least in Britain, to concentrate discussion on matters of priority, on the reality of what he claimed was a distinct "excito-motory system" of nerves, which he later called "the diastaltic system," and on speculative questions about the relation between sensation or other mental states and reflex events.[5] His views were distinctive, since he drew a rigid separation between the mechanistic reflex, "excito-motory" nervous system and the purposive, "sensori-volitional" nervous system. This placed him in conflict with the other major reference point for reflex theories in the 1830s, Johannes Müller's much cited *Handbuch der Physiologie* (which began publication in 1833). Müller, the famous Berlin teacher of physiology, took a much more integrated view of the nervous system than Hall. He treated the reflex as an analytically distinguishable unit rather than the mode of working of a distinct nervous structure. He considered its role in relation to the sympathetic nerve and hence to automatic bodily processes, some of which perhaps underlay the "sympathy" of one part for another. He believed that reflex actions might or might not be accompanied by mental states.[6] This enabled Hall to claim that Müller had no clear idea of, and had therefore not "discovered," the distinct reflex or "excito-motory system" that acted independently of mind.[7] However, it was Müller's integrated approach that was more suggestive to other researchers, and, though Hall's work was well known in Germany (partly through Müller but also through translation), it was rapidly overtaken by refined experimental and histological studies. By the end of the 1830s, the topic of reflex action was a substantial research area in its own right in the hands of experimentalists such as A. W. Volkmann first in Dorpat (now Tartu) during the period 1837–1843 and then in Hall and J. L. Budge, a *Privatdozent* in Bonn. It appeared that the study of reflex functions, linked to close anatomical study of sensory-motor structures, might provide the key to experimental analysis of the nervous system as a whole.

Hall and Müller described reflex action in different terms, but they both envisaged the mind's relation to its material organ, the brain, as the higher control of lower functions. This representation of hierarchical organization also expressed a hierarchy of values, as chapter 2 sought to make clear. By articulating reflex theory with reference to hierarchical organization, Hall and Müller made a significant contribution to translating a language ordering values into a language ordering structures and functions within the nervous system. This was a theme that returned in endless variations throughout the nineteenth century. That the mind, acting through the brain, regulated reflex actions—that "higher" regulated "lower"—became the core of inhibition theory.

Hall claimed to have discovered a distinct, material "excito-motory system" while simultaneously articulating an explicitly moral psychophysiological medicine. He believed that the reflex system explained automatic, instinctual, and some emotional actions; but, equally, he thought it threw into clear relief the distinctly mental, controlling "sensori-volitional" system. He described the latter system as "higher," both as a regulatory power and in the spatial arrangement of the nervous system.[8] While advancing physiology, Hall simultaneously preserved the ontological foundations of Christian morality in a causally active mental principle. By dividing the central nervous system into two halves, he literally embodied social values, elevating rational choice over automatic movements and providing a physiological vocabulary for prescribing conduct and character.

Using a physiological but still evaluative language, Hall reported clinical and experimental observations that indicated the normal controlling presence of the higher over the lower nervous system. For example, he explained an increased irritability to local stimulation in limbs that could not be moved voluntarily by reference to a disturbance in the economy of power between the brain and lower levels:

> I may affirm that in one kind of paralysis, that which removes the influence of the cerebrum, and which is therefore paralysis of the spontaneous or voluntary motion, there is augmented irritability. . . . We may conclude that, in cerebral paralysis, the irritability of the muscular fibre becomes augmented, from want of the application of the stimulus of volition.[9]

The lower levels accumulated a power to activity when the higher level was in abeyance. He confirmed such clinical conclusions by demonstrating comparable effects in frogs, reporting a series of experiments on decapitated frogs to show not only the independence but also the augmentation of reflex effects.[10] In turn, he argued, recognition of increased irritability provided a diagnostic criterion for "cerebral" paralysis (i.e., paralysis caused by a lesion in the brain), distinguishing it from paralysis caused by a lesion in the spinal cord (which would, in his view, diminish irritability).

Hall's theory of a dual, volitional and reflex, nervous system appeared to make clinical observations comprehensible. An English surgeon, W. F. Barlow, cited cases of abnormal spasmodic movements in patients in a hydrophobic coma, or in a hydrocephalous child, to illustrate how destruction of the power of the will increased the power of automatic movements. Pathology here revealed the normal harmony:

> Surely volition exercises a controlling power; and it is easy to conceive how muscles, under its influence, should be restrained by it from spasmodic action; the power of the will may act contrary to the nervous influence, which, were it not for its wholesome check, would throw the muscles into convulsive action on occasions when it does not take place.[11]

Thus, shortly before death, the spontaneous convulsions of the hydrocephalic child could be exaggerated by even a slight touch or by falling drops of water. Similar clinical reports acquired authority in the writings of the Berlin specialist on nervous disorders, Moritz Romberg. Discussing "spasms arising from increased reflex excitability," he concluded, "When the cerebral impulse is interrupted, and the conduction of the will arrested, the reflex phenomena not only become more evident, but they also break forth with greater force."[12] He also believed that there could be enhanced reflex excitability even where the cerebral connections were intact; indeed, he thought that this was a defining symptom of hysteria.[13] Pathology therefore joined with normality to confirm that the will was a power to hinder muscle movements.

Hall believed that the reflex "excito-motory" system was permanently in an excited condition, though normally overriden by the higher "sensori-volitional" system. This suggested to him, for example, an explanation for the body's normal muscular tone.[14] The reflex system was the mechanism responsible for the automatic life of the body. In his picturesque and evocative words, "By means of this system, the animal frame is constituted a casket, guarded at the upper part, and securely closed at the lower."[15] As the means of regulating the essential bodily functions, "the true spinal system *never sleeps*; respiration and deglutination, the action of the orifices and sphincters, are continued." In waking health, this system "is also constantly under a certain influence of the volition, as is manifest in the difference in the respiration, & c., during intense mental attention, sleep, and coma, and in ordinary circumstances."[16] In sleep, in drunken states, under intense emotion, during insanity, or in a host of other familiar circumstances, however, volitional control lessened or became absent. As the English physiologist E. A. Schäfer later summarized this commonplace: "It is a familiar fact that we are constantly in the habit of exercising voluntary control over, and arresting reflex movements; and that this function is exercised by the cortex [of the higher brain] is shown by its absence when from any cause the cortex is in abeyance, *e.g.* during sleep."[17] Hall's contribution was to suggest the terms in which this "familiar fact" became the subject of physiological experiment.

While Hall drew a sharp anatomical and physiological distinction between his two nervous systems, his description of the distinction used nontechnical and everyday language. Even more strikingly, he possessed no technical language at all with which to describe the relationship between the two systems. He stated merely that the brain system "influences" the spinal system and that removal of this influence explained automatic, emotional, instinctual, and pathological actions. Thus, he wrote with reference to dementia, "The patient lives a life of a mere excito-motory and nutritive kind. The cerebral functions are obliterated. The true spinal and ganglionic [i.e., autonomic] functions remain alone."[18] Similarly, the emotions dominated the lower system, but how they did this was "mysterious."[19] The higher psychical functions thus reflected the life of the soul, imposing on the body the purposes of the Creator. Hall's description portrayed a balanced economy between "higher" and "lower" in the body, but it did this without a technical, experimental language elaborating on the balance as a subject of knowledge in its own right. Rather, Hall restated nonspecific commonplace formulations of the relations between controlling and automatic capacities. This was evident in the following description of pathology:

> When the cerebrum is irritated, delirium ensues. When compressed, coma is induced. When lacerated, we have paralysis of *voluntary* motion. If the other phenomena are seen in diseases of the encephalon [higher brain], they arise from the extension of the influence of these to the true spinal and ganglionic systems, through *irritation*, or *pressure*, *counter-irritation*, or *counter-pressure*.[20]

What Hall could refer to only as the "influence" of the cerebrum was to become, in part, the technical question of inhibition. But inhibition was not a physiological term or a clearly formulated concept in Britain at this time.

Müller considered Hall's work carefully but believed that the latter's sharp distinction between the cerebral and spinal systems was untenable. Thus, for example, it appeared to Müller that Hall ignored the way the brain could act as a center of reflection in apparently automatic actions, as it appeared to do when the iris contracted in response to light.[21] Where Hall tried to define the "excito-motory" system *ab initio*, Müller tried to elaborate the reflex concept in the light of the known complexities of the sympathetic nerve, a structure that, at this time, did not have a clear anatomical or functional definition as part of "the sympathetic" or "autonomic" nervous system. It was well known that this nerve, which was associated with the essential or vegetative bodily functions, was independent of, but influenced by, the central nervous system. Müller considered whether reflex processes in the sympathetic nerve were important to these automatic levels of function and to their relations with the central controlling levels of the nervous system. In a broad sense, like Hall, he took for granted the existence of a hierarchical framework of functions.[22]

It was in this context, while discussing the relation between sympathetic and central nervous function, that Müller introduced the notion of inhibition. While acknowledging that considerable research was needed to clarify the point, Müller suggested that the sympathetic system might influence the organism in part through an inhibitory effect on voluntary motor impulses. Thus, he referred to a sympathetic "Hemmung des Willenseinflusses" (inhibition of the influences of the will).[23]

While Müller was unable to be precise about any of the interactions between the central and the sympathetic systems, he focused attention on such questions in neurophysiological and experimental terms, and it was significant that a concept of regulative inhibition had a part in this.

Müller's work combined an older tradition of physiological explanation in terms of nonmaterial categories with newer practices. Though his textbook and his teaching played an important part in creating a distinct discipline of experimental physiology in the German-speaking world, Müller himself did not separate psychological or even metaphysical questions about the mind's role in the body from physiological research. Hall thought that he had dealt with such questions by localizing the mind in the cerebral nervous system. Müller, by contrast, considered that the mind had a virtual presence throughout the organism, though he accepted that the mind's effects, in a material sense, were localized in the brain. "The vital principle and mind or mental principle of animals resemble each other . . . in this respect: they exist throughout the mass of the organism which they animate." However, it was the specific "property of the brain to have consciousness."[24] Further, in a famous—or we might say notorious—metaphor, he pictured the will acting downward on the central terminations of nerves in the lower brain regions. "The fibres of all the motor, cerebral and spinal nerves may be imagined as spread out in the medulla oblongata, and exposed to the influence of the will like the keys of a piano-forte. The will acts only on this part of the nervous fibres."[25] Using such imaginative pictures, Müller reinforced the conventional view that the sensory-motor organization of the cerebral nervous system extended as far as lower levels of the brain but not to higher levels.

These divisions between levels in the brain and between mental powers and nervous functions were part of a single, integrated language describing the hierarchical nature of psychophysiological life. Many other sources illustrate the same point. Carpenter wrote in one of his textbooks, "It seems well established . . . that the Spinal Cord, or small segments of it, may serve in Man as the centre of very energetic reflex actions, when the voluntary power exercised through the Brain over the muscular system is suspended or destroyed."[26]

Belief in a psychophysical hierarchy had long had a part in interpreting experiments on decapitated or brain-damaged animals, such as snakes, frogs, or kittens.[27] Experiments on headless animals revealed the existence of independent coordinated actions based on spinal cord function. Historians have therefore treated such experiments as crucial to the history of reflex action, referring particularly to the eighteenth-century dispute between Robert Whytt and Haller about the functions or faculties of the spinal cord.[28] As this debate illustrates, there was considerable interest in what such actions implied about mental principles. In addition, the debate inevitably raised questions about interaction and regulation between the brain and the spinal cord. As Sherrington later anachronistically observed, "This notion of the inhibition of the activity of one part of the central nervous system by the activity of another part had, from its psychological aspect, long been expressed."[29] Late-nineteenth-century physiologists such as Sherrington found in Whytt's work the first clear physiological report that destruction at higher levels augmented effects at lower levels.

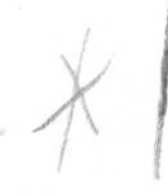

> When the hinder feet of a frog are pricked, or otherwise wounded immediately after cutting off its head, it makes scarce any motions with its legs, and shows almost no signs of feeling; but, if the toes be pricked or cut ten or fifteen minutes after decollation, the legs and thighs are not only violently moved, but sometimes also the trunk of the body.[30]

Whytt himself valued the observation for the support it gave for his argument, against Haller, regarding the independent sensibility of the spinal cord. Thus, he gave little attention to the organizational relations between higher and lower levels in the manner that later writers on inhibition, who cited Whytt, were to do. It was Whytt's point that he had shown the dependence of movements, in response to stimulation, on nervous connections through the spinal cord.

> When any of the muscles of the legs of a frog are irritated some time after cutting off its head, almost all the muscles belonging to the legs and thighs are brought into contraction, if the spinal marrow be entire; but, as soon as it is destroyed, although the fibres of such muscles as are themselves stimulated are affected with a weak tremulous motion, yet the neighbouring muscles remain at perfect rest.[31]

Whytt's manner of conceptualizing organization depended on positing vital powers and in mapping the distribution of these powers in different organs. By the time Hall reported similar results from similar experiments, however, it was possible to reinterpret Whytt's work as anticipating concepts of organization and regulation between parts of the nervous system. Whytt's "observation" of enhanced activity following damage at a higher level became common knowledge in physiology and clinical medicine, and Hall gave this concrete expression in his reflex theory.

Whytt had shown that a headless frog still moved in response to an irritation but—the *experimentum crucis* for reflex theory—that it did this only when the spinal cord was present. Later physiologists also found another of Whytt's observations to be highly significant. In the opinion of Eckhard, Whytt even initiated the observational understanding of inhibition: "The movements of the limbs of a decapitated frog elicited through stimulus of the skin begin not immediately after decapitation but only some minutes subsequently. One sees here [as reported by Whytt] the first observation that later became so significant a law of the inhibitory mechanism."[32] This requires some explanation. Eckhard was referring to what became known at the end of the nineteenth century as "spinal shock," the shock caused to the spinal cord by decapitation. This shock, it is argued in modern physiology, inhibits the normal reflex functions of the spinal cord for a certain length of time. Eckhard's elevation of Whytt's observation to the status of a discovery was anachronistic. Knowledge of shock, meaning knowledge of disturbed function caused by drastic damage to an animal, was of course common, not least because dying animals created endless problems in interpreting experiments. While Whytt appreciated the difficulties shock created for interpreting experiments on spinal cord function, it was really Eckhard's own generation of physiologists who characterized spinal shock as a specific inhibitory phenomenon.[33] Some twenty years after Eckhard wrote, in fact, Sherrington, who systematically studied the phenomenon, concluded that "whether such phenomena are best included under the head of inhibitions is very questionable."[34] Nevertheless, the general thrust of Eckhard's discussion, that decapitation experiments led to questions about the controlling relations between the brain and the spinal cord and that this was a major component in the background to theories of inhibition, can be accepted. It follows that it may be impossible to talk about inhibition being a "discovery," at any time, except in the most qualified sense.

As described, Flourens's experiments in the 1820s involving the decerebration of pigeons and other animals introduced a new level of precision into the research tradition. Physiologists in the second quarter of the nineteenth century therefore often addressed the hierarchy of structural and functional levels in the brain and spinal cord in the light of his theory. Flourens conflated the "highest" human attribute, the soul, and the "highest" brain structure, the cerebrum, and used his research to defend Cartesian dualism and a Christian idea of the human essence. Hall and Müller, though in different ways, perpetuated this

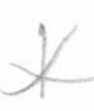

philosophy, even while they brought reflex action to the forefront of attention. Many observations and assumptions thus combined in the 1830s to establish the study of regulation, balance, and interaction between different parts of the hierarchically arranged nervous system as a major concern. Concurrently, the literature on moral character, popular physiology, mental pathology, and Christian ethics embedded the neurophysiological dimension in a wider culture.

The impact and significance of the famous experimental report by the brothers E. H. Weber and E. F. W. Weber on the vagal inhibition of the heartbeat in 1845 is described below. The object now is to make clear that their report had meaning directly in relation to a research tradition, and indirectly in relation to a moral culture, that had already begun to refer to inhibition as a regulatory property of the nervous system. Their report's catalyzing of a research program on inhibition, in the nervous system as well as in the heart, would probably not have occurred, and would certainly not have been so immediate, without this background.

Before turning to the reception of the idea of vagal inhibition, it is necessary to explore a little further the integration of reflex action theory and the theory of organizational levels in the central nervous system. Experimental research, exemplified by study of the reflex, gained a secure institutional footing and expanded rapidly, especially in German-speaking universities, around 1840. Research took on a collective rather than an individual character as each researcher started from and fitted into a network of related activity. A number of younger experimentalists or microscopists seized on Hall's and Müller's rather simple accounts of the reflex as opening opportunities for detailed work. A. W. Volkmann provided perhaps the most authoritative reviews, though he tends now to be remembered for having "observed" vagal inhibition in 1838 but then dismissing it as an unreliable artifact produced by his electrical stimulating apparatus.[35] More important, by refining experimental technique and by precisely formulating questions for such techniques to address, he made the reflex a detailed research topic.

Volkmann studied the effect of sectioning the cord at different levels, an experimental technique that was to remain important. He observed, for example, that stimulating a frog's sciatic nerve produced a reflex movement at the segmental levels of the body below where the nerve entered the cord. By contrast, in a brainless frog, the same excitation produced reflex responses at higher levels as well.[36] He concluded from this that the brain—and the volitional function that it served and that he specified in psychological terms—was a source of control over lower nervous levels. Decapitation removed this control, enabling reflex effects to spread upward in the cord. He did not refer specifically to *hemmen* in this context but used instead the verbs *hindern* or *verhindern* (to hinder or to prevent).

> The experience that in headless amphibia each stimulus causes reflex movements, which before decapitation did not occur, equally leads here to special considerations. It becomes clear from this that the brain contains the cause for the hindrance in the activation of the nervous principle . . . that deficient psychic influence [*Seeleneinfluss*] supports activation of the nervous principle, and, conversely, that the influence of the mind [*Seele*] possibly hinders this activation. The psychic forces, on which everything seems to depend here, are attention and will.[37]

Volkmann later explored this question of central control further in relation to reflex movements involving voluntary—but more especially involuntary—muscles. It was just this kind of research activity that suggested the sort of experiment in which the Webers observed vagal inhibition.

Volkmann's approach to nervous function was in the tradition of what we might call Müller's biological emphasis on the interaction of nervous conductions in producing purposive movements and on the integration of mental capacities with nervous physiological life. Their work exhibited a transitional psychophysiology, in which the conventions for describing mental control reappeared as the terms of research into integrated nervous action. The transition involved establishing social practices of empirical and experimental research in the relations between the brain and the spinal cord. It was assumed that the former influenced the reflex functions of the latter.

Volkmann articulated what proved to be a very profitable way of researching nervous functions when he turned the reflex notion around, asking why sensory excitation did not always produce a motor effect. The purposive nature of movements, rather than their continuous expression, appeared to require an organizing power. Volkmann tried to understand the causal nature of this power by suggesting that there were concentrated channels of conductibility in the nervous system. He thought that such channels might be created, for example, by the mental state of attention, which he envisaged (like a lightning conductor) as draining off incoming excitation and thus preventing it from automatically producing reflex movements.[38] Other researchers, a little later, developed the theory of inhibition to fulfill the same role.

One final illustration will confirm the manner in which conceptualizing the central nervous system in terms of control functions drew attention to the existence of inhibitory powers. Flourens's investigations of the brain had also concerned the functions of the cerebellum (a major lower brain structure). In what is now regarded as the classic study of this organ's functions, he reported how, following full ablation in pigeons, "volition, sensation, and perception persisted; the ability to carry out *general movements* also persisted; but the *coordination of these movements* in an orderly and determined manner was lost."[39] This was the starting point for later discussion of the cerebellum's role in organizing voluntary movements and posture. Discussing this topic in 1841, Budge straightforwardly argued that cerebellar coordination of movements required this organ to possess an inhibitory power (*Hemmungskraft*): "The cerebellum serves as the inhibition apparatus for the untrammeled power of movement."[40] He reported the results of some forty experiments designed to illuminate the controlling power of the cerebellum, and inhibition played a fundamental part in the interpretation of his results: "We have shown above how disturbed an animal's activity would be if these sensory and motor forces were uncontained; that these forces would be useless and disturbing if they acted individually. Such an inhibitory organ as the cerebellum was therefore absolutely necessary."[41] Beginning with this "necessary" assumption, he went on to discuss whether inhibition should be conceived as a general or localized property of cerebellar action, how it related to the organ's bilateral symmetry, what its place was in organizing bodily instincts, and so on. He did not seek to convey a sense of having discovered inhibition; rather, taking for granted accepted views on organization within the nervous system, he explored the properties of inhibition in relation to a specific organ.

Volkmann and Budge, of course, were only two among a large number of researchers, French as well as German, working in the 1840s on the organization of functions within the brain and spinal cord. Thus, for example, the young Brown-Séquard, who later played the major part in introducing the term "inhibition" into France, was then seeking to establish a reputation and a scientific career in Paris with a series of sectioning experiments on the spinal cord.[42] Such research rapidly became detailed and complex, and it involved experimental sophistication. Nevertheless, it inherited the conceptual framework of the earlier, less rigorous research that had explicitly interrelated physiological and psychological categories in describing control and purposive action within humans and animals and that had used a concept of inhibition in this context. This earlier research, in its turn, shared language with a moralistic discourse that integrated the individual body into collective order.

PERIPHERAL INHIBITION

Sensory-motor physiology, the reflex, and localization of function provided anatomical and experimental research on the brain and nerves with its technical language. In the 1840s, however, this language rarely excluded all reference to mind. Many writers envisaged, in the English phrase, a "mental physiology," or an account of the material conditions of mental life as a precondition for establishing scientific psychology.[43] This was not intended to be a reductionist explanation of mind by matter: advocates of a physiological approach saw themselves as enriching the explanatory potential of mind-body dualism, not abolishing it in the name of materialism. Müller, Hall, and Volkmann were in the mainstream in giving attention to the mind's controlling relation to its material organ. Their notions of this relation incorporated moral values, and this characteristic did not suddenly disappear when physiologists translated the mind's controlling relationship to the body into the terms of organization within the nervous system. This translation also left philosophical questions concerning the mind-body relation as confused as ever. What it did achieve was an academic specialization in which what had once appeared as imprecise psychological questions reappeared as precise physiological questions. To an increasing number of scientists after the middle of the century, the latter appeared to be the only interesting, objective, and scientifically rigorous issues. When universities created an environment in which neurophysiology could expand as a self-perpetuating and self-referential occupation, it became possible to ignore or forget the psychological and moral meanings that had originally informed physiological discourse.

Neurophysiology became a specialist research discipline, but this did not eliminate earlier intellectual issues or resolve once and for all physiologists' relations with medicine, philosophy, and lay culture. The individual researcher's own world tended, all the same, to have an increasingly narrow focus. How he, and occasionally she, thought about the mind-body problem or about where specialized knowledge was related to the wider culture, if such matters were considered at all, became secondary issues. Such topics were not central matters for scientific research in their own right. The historian interested in such matters must deal, for the most part, with arguments used in particular circumstances, often in idiosyncratic ways, rather than systematic theory. The reconstruction of the story of inhibition after 1850 illustrates this point.

By 1840, work on psychological and physiological organization had given the concept of inhibition prominence in a variety of ways, whether or not this term, or its cognates, was used. Yet the idea of control through hindering rather than exciting action, let alone the question of understanding the means by which this could be effected, remained ill-defined. It was not a research topic in its own right. This changed following the Webers' report of vagal inhibition in 1845. It was (and remains) a standard component in the education of physiologists to describe how they discovered inhibition in 1845. Their joint publication reported work that E. H. Weber later made clear had been his brother's, and we can therefore refer to it as E. F. W. Weber's experiment. He electrically stimulated a frog's vagus nerves (that part of the sympathetic nervous system consisting of a pair of complex nerves running from the hindbrain to the thoraxic and abdominal regions) and observed a decrease in the heartbeat.[44] This was the first persuasive report that a nerve might have a specific inhibitory as well as excitatory function. The experiment had great influence: it attracted immediate comment and led to a great deal of fruitful research both on inhibition within the nervous system and on the nature of the heartbeat. It also became a classic physiological experiment, a model of experimental insight taught to generations of students. As has been argued, however, its impact resulted from the existence of a broad context of psychophysiology, a context that existed long before and lasted long after Weber's particular experiment.

Weber, writing up the first extended discussion of vagal inhibition, assumed that his readers would be familiar with general inhibitory phenomena, with the evidence of altered reflex excitability in headless animals, and with knowledge of voluntary control over the reflexes. For example, he wrote,

> We have, it is true, examples of similar inhibitions [i.e., to vagal inhibition] of the involuntary activity of animal muscles, but these are produced by the fact that nerves are put not in but out of action, namely, by affecting the spinal cord, which supports their activity. Here there is, for example, the

> sphincters of the anus and the bladder, which by their activity hold closed their openings and when their activity is suspended allow the passage of the excreta. The experience that the will restricts convulsions, if they do not occur too strongly, and can inhibit the origin of many reflex movements, which occur more easily if the brain is deprived or stunned than with whole or uninjured animals, also demonstrates that the brain can have an inhibitory action on movements.[45]

Weber took it for granted that his readers were conversant with inhibition as a general feature of control within the body, or of the will's relation to the body. What was distinctive about the observation of vagal inhibition was that it demonstrated a localized inhibitory function in a specific nerve, though even this observation was open to various interpretations. It had not been clear in earlier references to inhibition whether there were supposed to be specific inhibitory capacities in the nervous system and, if there were, whether they were localized. It was just as probable that what was observed as inhibition was the effect of the interaction of different excitatory forces.

Weber used the continuous current of a "galvano-magnetic stimulator," or induction coil, to depress the heartbeat in a frog, initially by placing the electrodes in the nostril and on the spinal cord (sectioned at the level of the fourth or sixth vertebra). He then localized the effect by stimulating the medulla oblongata and vagus nerves in various ways, confirming the role of the vagus nerves by sectioning.

> *When the vagus nerves, or the parts of the brain from which they originate, are stimulated, the speed of the rhythmic impulses of the heart slows down and the heart can be completely arrested.* . . . [These observations] provide us with the first certain evidence that the heart beat can be influenced by the brain; second, that this influence is affected by a nerve not thought to be involved in heart function; and finally, [we note that] this kind of effect of a nerve upon muscular organs, whereby movements which occur independently are inhibited or even prevented completely rather than stimulated, is new and startling.[46]

The observations thus had two striking implications: that the nervous system was involved with the heartbeat and that the nervous system possessed a specific inhibitory capacity. Weber himself drew general attention to these implications in 1846, in the context of a comprehensive treatment of muscular movement.[47]

Weber claimed that the new observations supported an earlier neurogenic theory of the heartbeat, and accounts by the historians Hebbel E. Hoff and Gerald Geison have described the part played by this argument in focusing physiological research. The question of the heartbeat turned out to be much more difficult than had been thought in the late 1840s. It was only with the description and evaluation of nervous ganglionic centers in the heart and, later, in the aortic arch that the observations of vagal inhibition acquired a settled meaning. Geison has argued that the question of the heartbeat became the intellectual and technical organizing principle of Michael Foster's influential "Cambridge school of physiology" in the 1870s.[48] Understanding the regulation of heart action was to be the great achievement of Cambridge physiology in the 1880s.

Weber's description of vagal inhibition was hardly a simple case of discovery. First, alternative contemporary explanations for the effect did not involve reference to inhibition; indeed, the concept of an inhibitory function still had its critics thirty years later. There was thus no necessity to conclude that the experiment demonstrated the existence of inhibition. Second, as I have stressed, Weber's choice of terms to describe what he had observed drew on a conventional understanding of organization within the nervous system. Central to this, as Hoff has suggested, was the existing conception that the brain and spinal cord exerted a regulatory and even inhibitory power over reflex actions and voluntary and involuntary movements.

Volkmann, who had been a student of E. H. Weber's in Leipzig, made a notable contribution to such work while studying the control of phasic involuntary movements. Not surprisingly, he was one of the first to discuss the report of vagal inhibition, since he had himself tried to stimulate the vagus nerve directly. It is interesting to note that he interpreted the experiment in the light of his thinking about the regulatory activity of the nervous system as a whole. It was also clear by the mid-1840s that many difficulties in interpreting results from the direct electrical stimulation of nerves stemmed from the electrical apparatus used, which produced a stimulus only at "make" or "break" in the current ("galvanization"). The development of the induction coil permitted the experimenter to apply a continuous current ("faradization"), and Weber used this type of stimulus in his experiment.[49] He hoped that this would mimic the normal excitation of a nerve. Volkmann used this apparatus to explore the effects of excitation on nerves to involuntary muscle in the gut, and he reported that a normal nervous excitation produced a purposive movement rather than the continuous contraction of the muscle. This, he believed, indicated the role of central inhibition.

> Since with no other kind of stimulation does it happen that a constant stimulus produces movement (i.e., an alteration of contraction and relaxation), and since in all other circumstances a continuous stimulus produces continuous contraction, the central organ must contain the mechanism for the former circumstance. There is no doubt but the continuous stimuli would throw the muscle into uninterrupted contraction did not the central organ *inhibit* its influence at the right time and thus permit a purposeful movement.
>
> From the above, the continuous stimulation that affects these nerves would cause a constant contraction in the viscera of the thorax and abdomen, were the motor stimuli not interrupted by central organs that periodically *inhibit* and purposefully regulate them.[50]

Volkmann's sense of the purposeful and regulated nature of bodily functions thus led him to posit inhibition as a condition for the achievement of such ends, and in this 1845 discussion, he did use the verb "hemmen." In Hoff's view, this argument was also the immediate context for E. F. W. Weber's own interpretation of the vagal inhibitory action of the heart, the bodily organ that spectacularly exemplified regularity.[51]

Weber did not believe that vagal inhibition produced its effect by the direct stimulation of muscle; rather, he thought of the vagus acting (analogous to a central influence) on ganglia in the heart (analogous to spinal ganglia), thereby indirectly regulating the heartbeat.

> The fact that activity of an involuntary muscle can be inhibited by the influence of the nerves that supply it, is new, and would be entirely without parallel, if we considered the vagus nerves as the actual nerves going to the muscle fibres of the heart, and the inhibition as the direct result of their action on these. We have, to be sure, examples of similar inhibition of the involuntary action of animal muscles; but this takes place not because the nerves are activated, but because they cease to function because of influences on the spinal cord, which is at the basis of their activity.
>
> Just as the inhibitory activity in the skeletal muscles acts primarily on the spinal cord, so the inhibitory action of the vagi does not act directly on the muscle fibres, but primarily upon those [nervous] structures which are responsible for cardiac activity, but which here are found in the substance of the heart itself.[52]

Weber thus drew a parallel between central inhibition and vagal action on the heart. As Hoff rightly observed, "The theory of Weber, therefore, did not in reality offer an explanation of the mechanism of vagal inhibition, but, rather called attention to a phenomenon already recognized in the central nervous system, and applied it *in toto* to the heart."[53] Weber's discussion also anticipated the direction of research over the next three decades: to determine the cause of the heartbeat and to clarify the role of vagal inhibition, if such it was; and to determine whether there was central inhibition within the brain and, if there was, to understand how it related to psychological functions.

Before turning to questions of nervous organization, it is important to note the association between the study of inhibition and the study of *regulation* of the heartbeat. This is a very definite example of the way in which the regularly ordered workings of the body, that is, what were understood to be the conditions of its existence as an organic system, endorsed a language of control including the term "inhibition." Questions of bodily regulation continued to focus on balance, economy, and order, and physiologists thus continued to share a language replete with reference to the social world.

The study of regulatory systems—gut movements, swallowing, breathing, blood circulation, secretion, and so forth—was a major feature of experimental physiology. Such researches characteristically subsumed the subject of inhibition.[54] Once a nervous inhibitory effect, as many believed it to be, had been demonstrated for the vagus nerves, and confident in the reproducibility of results using faradic (induction coil) stimulation, physiologists began to search for other examples. Weber's experiment was a model for exploring the nerve supply to internal organs and involuntary musculature. The research, however, was by no means straightforward. The anatomical distribution of the relevant nerves, which were often extremely fine and difficult to trace, had first to be established. The sympathetic nervous system was complex, and the degree to which it was integrated with or independent of events in the central nervous system was obscure. It was always possible to point to lack of refinement in experimental technique.[55] But by addressing such issues, natural science acquired both intellectual and technical content and prestige as an expert occupation. The study of the regulation of bodily functions suggested topics that could be broken down into specific experimental questions. Answering these questions provided researchers with training, with the prospect of discovery, and with reasonable confidence in forwarding a professional reputation.

This program of understanding regulation by reference to inhibition acquired its most specific form following Eduard Pflüger's announcement in 1855 that he had succeeded in halting intestinal contractions by stimulating the splanchnic nerve. This was the topic of his second M.D. thesis, formally under Müller in Berlin. He immediately generalized this result, proposing the existence of a *Hemmungs-Nervensystem*, a special system of inhibitory nerves complementary to an excitatory system, for involuntary functions.[56] He thus attempted to draw together earlier observations inconclusively identifying inhibition acting on the gut, the lymph glands, and respiration as well as on the heart. Pflüger gave the following account of the relation between his general theory and Weber's work:

> While I later focused on the distinctive form of movement of the heart muscle, and its distinctive relation to the cerebro-spinal system, I asked myself the question whether such an arrest [of movement] might have deeper connection overall to a new principle. I searched and in this way found in the Nervi splanchnici the inhibitory nerves for the peristaltic movements in the gut. In the explanation, however, I followed Weber. Nevertheless, in recent times, there have been attacks against the interpretation concerning the inhibitory nerves.[57]

His systematization was not widely accepted. It was regarded as speculative, and it even led the Königsberg physiologist Friedrich L. Goltz to exclaim, "Let us resist this flood of inhibitory nerves."[58]

Pflüger's discussion was the immediate occasion for the introduction of "inhibition," as a physiological term, into the English language. Characteristically for the British setting, the occasion in 1858 was as much medical as physiological: an address by Joseph Lister to the Royal Society on the topic of inflammation.[59] Many years later, when discussing antisepsis as a form of inhibitory action, Lister claimed, "I happened, I believe, to be the first to use the word 'inhibitory' in English physiology, by the advice of my old friend, Dr. Sharpey."[60] Lister's interest had been in the process of inflammation and in following up work by Bernard and by Budge and A. V. Waller on the nervous control of peripheral blood vessels.[61] He had also been intrigued by a traditional problem of "sympathetic" action, namely, why inflammation should appear in an area of the body remote from the site of irritation. This led him to study visceral innervation and Pflüger's work and to question whether the experimental production of an inhibitory effect was, as Pflüger claimed, actually evidence for an inhibitory function under normal conditions. Lister believed that so-called inhibition was produced by excessive action of excitatory nerves: "The view which has been advocated by Pflüger . . . seemed to me from the first a very startling innovation in physiology . . . my suspicion [was] that the phenomena in question were merely the effect of excessive action in nerves possessed of the functions usually attributed to them."[62] It is not clear what impact Lister's dismissal of the existence of inhibitory nerves had on his British audience, or even whether that audience was sufficiently familiar with German research to perceive the potential significance of the topic of physiological inhibition. Certainly, there was no sustained experimental program to pursue the questions of regulation that Pflüger had tried to address.

Lister himself experimented with galvanic stimulation applied to the sympathetic or vagal nerves supplying the heart and gut in the rabbit. It appeared to him that Pflüger's belief in the existence of special inhibitory nerves was not only implausible but also contradicted by observation, since in his experience a mild stimulus caused *increased* action, which changed to decreased action only as the stimulus became stronger. Thus, the same nerve appeared to be both excitatory and inhibitory. This suggested to Lister that the experiment picked out particular effects from the normal setting of bodily functions. The viscera were normally subject to the overall activity of the nervous system.

> It appears that the intestines possess an intrinsic ganglionic apparatus which is in all cases essential to the peristaltic movements, and, while capable of independent action, is liable to be stimulated or checked by other parts of the nervous system; the inhibiting influence being apparently due to the energetic operation of the same nerve-fibres which, when working more mildly, produce increase of function.[63]

Lister concluded that "it appears very questionable whether the motions . . . [of the heart or intestines] are, under ordinary circumstances, ever checked by the spinal system, except for very brief periods."[64] He did think, however, that inhibition might help explain certain pathological symptoms, such as constipation accompanying some hernias.

The controlling relations between the nervous system and the viscera were researched extensively during the 1850s and 1860s. Experimental results diverged and made everyone conscious of the complexities produced by using different types and strengths of stimuli. They also directed attention to the differences between experimental systems and the normal workings of an integrated organism. It was the exiled German physiologist Moritz Schiff who criticized Pflüger's approach most systematically. Schiff was a professor in Bern in the 1850s, moving on in 1862 to Florence where he was a major influence on the development of Italian physiology and at the center of a row about vivisection.[65] His approach to organic regulation presupposed energetic rather than structure-function principles. He developed the earlier opinion—held, for example, by Volkmann—that the intensity and anatomical spread of a reflex effect was influenced by the overall channeling of forces within the nervous system and not just local anatomical connections. Schiff held that the relative strength, duration, and dispersion of reflex movements should be explained by the whole preexisting and concurrent environment of excitations.[66] He thus rejected approaches, such as Pflüger's, focusing on specific, local inhibitory properties. This critical stance established a clear point of reference for anyone wishing to debate the existence and nature of inhibitory effects. His challenge existed in relation to bodily functions in the 1850s or 1860s, and it continued in relation to the central nervous system after Sechenov's paper in 1863 (discussed below).

The argument between Pflüger and Schiff restated deep-seated alternatives regarding organic regulation: whether it should be understood in terms of localized specific functions or the general dynamic physiological state. In practice, the overt argument most often concerned the interpretation of experimental results, whose subtle complexities ensured a seemingly endless supply of controvertible empirical resources for reconstituting the more general claims. Thus, Schiff explained the observed increase in intensity of a decapitated frog's spinal reflexes in terms of reduced spread of excitation through the central nervous system, the excitation therefore resulting in a more concentrated reflex movement. He cited in support experiments in which he cut a lizard's spinal cord at successively lower levels, producing a progressive increase in the intensity of reflex responses. Thus, he concluded, the brain had to be considered a drain on reflex activity rather than a center for its positive inhibition. According to similar arguments, following simple dynamic principles, he expected that the preexisting tonic state (level of excitation) of the cord would also affect the intensity of a reflex.[67] These ideas were very different from those, such as Pflüger's, that attributed inhibition to the function of specific structures such as the splanchnic nerve.

What some researchers claimed was a positive localized function appeared to others as merely the negative consequence of another physiological process. Nevertheless, inhibition became a much discussed idea in these debates. This did not mean, however, that inhibition itself was necessarily a particular subject of attention. The significant studies in the 1850s on the nervous system and its regulation of flow in blood vessels and glands, for instance, developed largely without reference to the term.

Scientists and historians alike have attributed the major work to the most outstanding of all French physiologists, Claude Bernard. This has left something of a gap in the literature on related research or on the contemporary reception of Bernard's results, particularly in the German-speaking world. The difficulty of integrating Bernard's work into the wider picture is compounded by the way Bernard, particularly in his Paris lectures published as *Leçons sur la physiologie et la pathologie du système nerveux* (1858), arrogantly but brilliantly organized topics around his own research rather than around a conventional systematic framework. Bernard reported to his audience the results of his own activity, largely ignoring German research or questions formulated by other physiologists—except where his priority was at issue. Sechenov, who had discussions with Bernard in 1862, noted that the latter "did not know German and was only very little acquainted with German literature on physiology."[68] Thus, though Bernard was preoccupied by the subject of organic regulation, he never integrated his results with German accounts of inhibition, even if only to criticize the latter. Rather, in a series of experiments, which have become a model of experimental argumentation, Bernard elaborated his own theory of the double, antagonistic innervation to vessels to explain the anatomical and functional basis of regulated bodily activity. This experimental work underpinned his developing general conception of physiological control, *le milieu intérieur*, and his systematic physiology of organic self-regulation.[69]

It had long been known that cutting the branch of the sympathetic nerve to the eye was followed by the pupil's contraction. Bernard himself traced this observation to 1727. In the 1840s, various researchers suggested that the eye received a double innervation that made possible contraction and dilation of the pupil. Then, in 1851, the German physiologist Budge, working with the English physiologist A. V. Waller, suggested the existence of an associated spinal center, and this suggestion was the immediate occasion for Bernard's *systematic* investigation of reciprocal nervous action: "I have insisted on the point that in place of pursuing an exclusive explanation to account for the modification of the pupil, it is necessary to search for all the other phenomena that, coming and disappearing simultaneously, seem to originate under a common influence."[70] His investigation of regulation by reciprocal innervation led him to explore the observation that ablating the cervical (neck) ganglia of the sympathetic nervous system, or cutting the sympathetic nerve, increased blood flow and hence warmth in the head on the sectioned side. He then confirmed the observation by applying an interrupted electrical stimulus to the sectioned nerve to the ear in a rabbit, which reduced the ear's temperature. The stimulus contracted the blood vessels supplying the ear and opposed the effect of a rise in temperature produced by the initial sectioning of the nerve.[71] Bernard subsequently studied a parallel system in the innervation to the submaxillary (salivary) gland, concluding that stimulation of the chorda tympani nerve increased secretion while stimulation of the sympathetic nerve decreased it. "All this shows us the existence in the submaxillary gland of a kind of unstable physiological equilibrium, or a sort of continuous functional balance determined by the antagonism of the dilator nerve and the constrictor nerve of the blood capillary vessels."[72]

This work rapidly achieved status—which it has retained—as a model of scientific physiology. By demonstrating the vasoconstrictor and vasodilator functions of the different elements of nervous supply to blood and gland vessels, Bernard described the regulatory capacities of the nervous system in specific, concrete terms. Other researchers, such as Brown-Séquard, who had unsuccessfully competed for a career, for which there were very restricted opportunities in Paris in the 1840s, disputed matters of priority or argued over interpretive details.[73] The difficulty and subtlety of experimental technique provided plenty of scope for both kinds of dispute. What was not in dispute was a conception of physiological organization stressing the balance of opposed forces, mediated by reciprocal innervation and central controlling nervous ganglia. Bernard never referred to a counterbalance between excitatory and inhibitory functions as such in the nervous system. He referred instead to "une sorte d'interférence nerveuse," or reciprocal action, between paired nerves, affecting constriction or dilation of blood vessels, flow in glands, or the muscles of the iris.[74] Others approached such regulatory functions via notions of reciprocal inhibition and excitation.

Just as the evidence for vagal inhibition inspired a search for inhibitory nerves, evidence for paired nerves to blood vessels inspired a search for other examples of reciprocal innervation. In 1862, Eckhard reported studies on the sacral nerve and its role in regulating blood flow to the penis and hence on erection in the dog.[75] In the same year, J. Rosenthal assembled a considerable body of work on the control of breathing, hoping to clarify the function of the nerves in making possible rhythmic movement.[76] Breathing, of course, along with the heartbeat, was a fundamentally rhythmic vital function, and it is therefore no surprise that it offered particular scope to theories of reciprocal innervation and of balance between excitatory and inhibitory effects as such theories became current. It had been held that the central nervous system played a controlling part in respiration at least since the work of Legallois reported in 1812. Rosenthal integrated belief about the controlling center with the concept of regulation through paired excitation and resistance, describing a nervous circle between the medullary center and the thoraxic muscles. The existence of this circle, he argued, made possible perpetual rhythmic movement:

> The respiratory movements are excited by the stimulus of the blood on the respiratory center. The transfer of this excitation to the appropriate nerves and muscles encounters resistance, through which the continuous excitation is turned into rhythmic action. This resistance is diminished by the activity of the N. Vaegus and increased by the activity of the N. laryngeus superior.[77]

A detailed picture of the mechanism involved was gradually constructed. The Viennese physiologist Ewald Hering and his student Josef Breuer, later a prominent physician and early collaborator with Freud, contributed an important experimental technique for mimicking—and hence a means of studying—inspiration and expiration.[78] By means of this technique, they showed that distension of the lungs caused the inhibition of inspiration and the initiation of the process of expiration.

A particularly clear example of inhibition in the reflex control of rhythmic movements was provided by Hugo Kronecker and Samuel Meltzer in 1883, when they described a marked inhibitory effect at the onset of each deglutination (or swallow) in the esophagus.[79] They demonstrated the role in the process of a central inhibitory center in the lower brain, a center excited by afferent fibers from the glossopharyngeal nerve (from the throat). Meltzer subsequently claimed that "it deserves to be especially pointed out that in these observations it was proved for the first time that inhibition is an integral constituent in the normal activity of a function" as opposed to the product of an artificial stimulation.[80]

There was also an attempt to reconceptualize diseases of the nervous system in the light of knowledge of the inhibitory nerves and nervous functions. In 1866, two Viennese physicians, A. Eulenburg and L. Landois, proposed to supplement Romberg's authoritative division of nervous diseases into those exhibiting mobility and those exhibiting sensation with a new category, the *Hemmungsnervosen*.[81] They then divided the new category into disorders associated with the different inhibitory systems of the gut, heart, respiration, and reflex movements.

The considerable experimental claims made by the 1860s therefore confirmed that the nervous system played a fundamental part in the automatic or reflex control of organic functions. The existence of paired nerves, with a degree of antagonistic function, linked centrally by ganglia or spinal or lower brain centers, provided the anatomical basis for regulation. Sherrington later summarized half a century of detailed work on organic regulation when he wrote,

> A point of general interest in the physiology of the great "alimentary" nerve centre in the bulb [medulla] is the high degree to which it employs inhibition. Each subdivision of it is depressible by "inhibitory" fibres from some afferent nerve trunk or another; thus, the respiratory portion by fibres in the superior laryngeal nerve . . . and so on.[82]

As Bernard commented in reviewing reflex regulation, experimental work "certainly proved that the action of the nervous system is an antagonistic action [*une action de contention*]."[83] He believed that this was the key to unraveling the complexities of the sympathetic nervous system. Others concurred: Schiff's lectures in Florence elaborated a systematic theory of reciprocal nervous action in interpreting organic regulation.[84] Both Bernard and Schiff conceived of regulation as a function of the balance between antagonistic forces, and neither was inclined to describe such forces as inhibitory. Nevertheless, where Bernard referred to "contention," others believed that they had found evidence of positive inhibition.

Issues of automatic control were highly complex and generated an extensive technical literature. Yet they appeared amenable to experimental investigation with existing techniques and with current concepts. The result was a network of research papers on what was sometimes known as "peripheral" inhibition—the inhibitory effects of nerves supplying bodily tissues or organs. Physiological observations going back to Hall and beyond, and the general conception of the brain and spinal cord as regulatory structures, made it natural to ask whether there might also be "central" inhibition in the nervous system. This question appealed particularly to scientists of a more speculative bent, or to those keenest on reductionist physiological explanation, since it appeared to be a possible key to constructing a psychophysiology and a science of the mind's controlling relation to the body. This understood, it was obvious that devising experimental studies of function within the central nervous system, to yield incontrovertible results, would prove more difficult even than studying the functions of peripheral nerves. Nevertheless, during the second half of the century, a large number of researchers attempted to extend the scope of experimental technique in this way. In retrospect, it is tempting to see an inverse relationship between the broadness of the approach and the sustained authority of the conclusion. Only at the beginning of the twentieth century was a substantial body of refined experimental knowledge to come together under an overarching theoretical framework in Sherrington's description of the "integrated" nervous system.

The physiological scientific community increased substantially in size in the second half of the nineteenth century. Such communities came into existence for the first time in Britain, Italy, Russia, and the United States. Physiologists achieved considerable intellectual autonomy in the execution of research. This growth and autonomy fostered the splitting of earlier topics into ever more precisely defined questions, each of which appeared to researchers to have only empirical or methodological content. This was evident with respect to central and peripheral nervous regulation as with other physiological topics. A research physiologist's outlook was therefore increasingly formed through training and practice on narrow and esoteric questions. Similarly, the favored mode of expression became the formal research paper, which implicitly, sometimes explicitly, devalued wider theoretical or speculative discussion and gave much space to experimental protocols and lists of observations. In spite of these occupational developments, I have argued that scientists nevertheless carried meanings and values from their collective past and from a wider culture into their intracommunal practice. Many nineteenth-century physiologists were indeed conscious of, and significantly motivated by, wider questions, and this was nowhere more so than in writing on the physiological correlates of mind. However specialized particular experimental practices became, scientists still often devoted considerable energy to trying to state what the program of neurophysiological explanation implied for psychology. Sometimes, as with the British "mental physiologists," this was part of an effort to enhance recognition of scientific knowledge in the wider culture. Sometimes, as with experimental psychologists in Germany in the 1870s and 1880s, it was part of an endeavor to make psychology a science. We will return to these broader preoccupations in later chapters and show that language, exemplified by the word "inhibition," continued to serve as a mediation between technical and nontechnical cultures.

Here I have discussed the impressive specialization of research on nervous regulation, centering on the functions of the vagus and other sympathetic nerves. Weber's work introduced an experimental exemplar rather than the concept of inhibition. It was novel, however, to believe that a nerve might have a specific inhibitory as well as excitatory function, and this naturally encouraged a search for further examples, a search culminating in Pflüger's belief in an inhibitory nervous system. In the 1880s, there was a renewed flurry of interest in the possibility of distinct inhibitory nerves, following Pavlov's and Wilhelm Biedermann's demonstration of their existence in invertebrates. The subsequent significant failure to locate them in vertebrates then turned attention toward inhibition as a phenomenon associated with the central interaction of nerves.[85] In addition, many physiologists had begun by the 1880s to think about inhibition in terms of possible causal mechanisms. This turned out to be a difficult topic, generating questions well into the mid-twentieth century. The interest in mechanisms had the effect of integrating inhibition with a range of topics in both neurophysiology and general physiology; it would thus be wrong to describe research on inhibition as a unified subject. Some comments on physiology in general are therefore needed.

It is common to treat the 1840s as a turning point in the history of physiological explanation, since it was in this decade that the young scientists Emil Du Bois-Reymond, Helmholtz, Carl Ludwig, and Ernst Brücke, all of whom went on to hold chairs in major universities, laid down an apparently clear prescription for the exclusive rights of physicochemical explanation in the field.[86] The prescriptive ideal had great power in supporting specialized standards of argumentation, while the concurrent elaboration of conservation of energy principles lent it considerable authority. To understand what the ideal meant in practice, however, requires at least three qualifications. First, as P. F. Cranefield, the historian of physiology, pointed out, it proved impossible to provide physicochemical explanations for most phenomena, given the peculiar complexities and properties of organic materials and processes.[87] The commitment to physicochemical explanation was an attitude toward the pursuit of knowledge rather than a description of what could be achieved. Second, in the 1850s, reductionist explanation became associated with the materialism of radical-liberal popularizers of science, and most academic scientists took trouble to distance themselves from what they regarded as poor epistemology, inferior culture, and distasteful politics.[88] Finally, many other explanatory commitments persisted, in spite of the academic prestige of the physicalist physiologists, and this was very evident in what were often labrynthine discussions about the mind-body relation. Even within physiology, more narrowly understood, Bernard was only the most famous among several researchers to argue that the physiological level of explanation was distinct from the explanatory levels of physics and chemistry.[89]

Those physiologists in the 1850s who were interested in inhibition were therefore not concerned with physics and chemistry but with whether organic regulation should be conceived as a property of particular centers and nerves or as the effect of a dynamic balance within the nervous system. These alternatives could be compared to Hall's and Müller's positions, localizing reflex functions in an anatomically distinct "diastaltic" nervous system or attributing reflexes to the general relations of nervous processes. Canguilhem described Hall's and Müller's differences as an illustration of a general nineteenth-century debate between *les localisateurs et les totalisateurs* of nervous functions.[90] The same alternatives reappeared in the debates about the cerebral localization of function following G. Fritsch and E. Hitzig's success in producing movements by electrically stimulating the cortex in 1870. Thus, it was not a lack of clarity or insufficient evidence that led some physiologists to describe inhibition as a local, positive function of specific nerves and others to describe it as a general, negative function of interactive nervous processes. These alternatives were a structural feature of the search for cogency in neurophysiological explanation. And, to make the point once again, it was argument at this level, rather than at the level of physical or chemical mechanisms, that in practice formed the core of neurophysiological theory, at least until the end of the century. Such argument relied on a language permeated by meanings that transcended the confines of specialized physiology. Nowhere was this clearer than in the work that brought central inhibition into the limelight.

CENTRAL INHIBITION: I. M. SECHENOV

Research on sympathetic and spinal nerve regulation of bodily functions created knowledge about inhibition in the outlying parts of the nervous system. This research on peripheral inhibition was integral to the development of physiology in general, and it was not an autonomous subject. The research was also of interest to students of the brain and its pathology, however, and the very idea of peripheral inhibition was influenced by imagery of higher controls over lower processes. I have emphasized that, in Hoff's words, "in the neurophysiological literature at that time [1845] certain observations had already come to light which clearly indicated the existence of inhibitory processes in the central nervous system."[91] There is nevertheless no question that Sechenov greatly sharpened the focus on the subject of central inhibition in 1863. He stated that he had discovered a specific inhibitory center in the brain. The clarity of this empirical claim has encouraged historians and physiologists alike to regard the date as decisive. For Fearing, Sechenov's paper marked "an epoch in the development of theories of reflex inhibition"; for Brazier, "the experiments . . . were to mould his thinking and to suggest to him a concept of brain mechanisms later to flower in the hands of Pavlov into the theory that has dominated Russian neurophysiology ever since."[92] And the direction of experimental research and theoretical debate following Sechenov's paper supports Sherrington's view that "as a working physiological thesis [central inhibition] only became accepted doctrine after Sechenov in 1863."[93] For all this agreement about Sechenov's significance, however, there is still considerable scope for reassessing his historical position.

According to M. G. Vyrubov, who provided an introduction for a French edition of Sechenov's psychological work in 1884, "M. Sechenov was the first who had boldly addressed with purely physiological methods the study of the most complex psychological questions, the first who had ventured to reduce the highest faculties of intelligence to simple phenomena of innervation."[94] This claim was exaggerated. Further, Sechenov's hope that all aspects of mind could be treated in terms of reflex action proved untenable. Yet, as Vyrubov emphasized, simple ideas were necessary for launching a new approach to mind, and Sechenov's were certainly among the most interesting and intellectually challenging.

Sechenov's importance to the history of science in Russia and his status among Soviet writers as "the founding father" of both experimental physiology and psychology have created a secondary literature requiring careful interpretation. As is also the case with the even more famous Russian physiologist, Pavlov, there is no modern non-Soviet intellectual biography firmly grounded in the social context of his life and in the Russian-language sources. Fortunately, some studies by Sechenov's Soviet biographer, the historian of psychology M. G. Iaroshevskii, exist in English-language translation. In addition, North American scholars have begun to research the historical context, and David Joravsky has provided a major reinterpretation of the history of Russian psychology.[95] I will draw on these studies to relate Sechenov to the European debate about inhibition, a perspective that has not been developed elsewhere.

It was crucial to Sechenov's role that his early career coincided with the tentative liberalization and modernization of Russian cultural and academic life following the death of Tsar Nicholas I in 1855 and the shock of defeat in the Crimea. Sechenov qualified as a young doctor in 1856 at Moscow University. He later described himself as "an extreme idealist" when a student.[96] In the Russian context of the 1850s, this meant that he looked to Western psychology for a way of thinking about problems of practical, individual human concern. Like many other educated young Russians, he placed intense hopes in the humanistic content of Western thought. Specifically, he studied Beneke's pedagogical cum moralist psychology of character (not association psychology, as has sometimes been claimed).[97] A legacy freed him to study experimental science in Berlin, Leipzig, Vienna, and Heidelberg. He trained with some of the great institutional leaders of experimental physiology and chemistry—Du Bois-Reymond, F. Hoppe-Seyler, Ludwig, Helmholtz, and R. W. E. Bunsen—and returned in 1860 to an appointment at the Saint Petersburg Military Medical Academy. There he helped to introduce experimental physiology into the medical curriculum, a change that embodied "Westernizing" and enlightenment values. He brought with him from Germany an induction coil and a galvanometer, and he initiated students into the sort of work that could be done using such instruments. This created some elements of a "Russian school of physiology," though Sechenov's group had a quasi-identity only for a few years.[98]

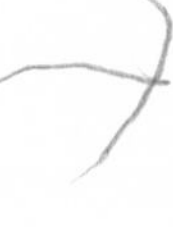

In the autumn of 1862, Sechenov traveled to Paris, where he worked for six weeks in the auditorium attached to Bernard's "laboratory," which was actually a small room equipped for vivisections. Here, where Bernard, who was recovering from serious illness, "regarded [his] work completely indifferently," Sechenov performed the experiments he claimed demonstrated a central inhibitory center.[99] Repeating his experiments before Ludwig, Brücke, and Du Bois-Reymond and then publishing the results in German, he attracted immediate attention.[100] Back in Saint Petersburg, Sechenov and his students elaborated and qualified the claim in a series of papers.

In the following summer, Sechenov wrote his brilliantly provocative essay, "Reflexes of the brain," which called for a *physiological* psychology. In Iaroshevskii's view in 1968, this was "the first plan in the history of world scientific thought for the construction of an objective psychology."[101] The essay appeared originally in two parts in Russian in the medical journal, *Meditsinskii Vestnik* (Medical Herald). For all its twentieth-century fame, therefore, this essay was to all intents and purposes unknown in Western Europe, at least until a French translation appeared in 1884. And even then an apologetic introduction explained that the essay's speculative character reflected the circumstances of the 1860s.[102] There is no evidence of the essay having any serious impact on scientists in the 1880s. "Reflexes of the brain" is now well known in the West through two English translations by Soviet workers from the revised edition in book form (1866). These translations were prepared to establish an official Russian pedigree for the major twentieth-century developments in Soviet physiology and psychology.[103] Sechenov's lectures to students, *Course of Physiology of the Central Nervous System*, were also published in 1866. The latter work has not been translated from the Russian; indeed, I have seen no systematic and reliable description of its contents.[104]

The tsarist censorship prevented the appearance of Sechenov's essay in the radical journal, *Sovremennik* (Contemporary), but not in a medical journal. This reflected a policy of treating differently specialist and lay readers.[105] In the version that did appear, only the title and concluding paragraph were altered:

> [I submitted] a small treatise to which I gave the title "An Attempt to Establish the Physiological Basis of Psychical Processes." The editor of the medical journal to whom I submitted the manuscript informed me that the censor's department insisted on a change of title (I rather think that the editor himself thought the title was not quite suitable for a purely medical journal). So I changed the title to "Reflexes of the Brain."[106]

The key change thus involved removing from the title the explicit reference to the physiological basis of mind. The government administration and the ecclesiastical authorities had a conflict of interest over censorship. The former, as opposed to the latter, was committed to modernizing medical services, and to this end, it had accepted the need for considerable "Westernizing" of medical research and training.[107] This commitment provided a significant opening in Russia for the introduction of science and of the world views and attitudes to social problems associated with it even when overt liberalization had gone into reverse after 1866.

In twentieth-century translation, Sechenov's essay comes across as an extremely bold and far-reaching scheme for representing mental life in terms of physical processes. It thus appears to be a radical attack on the philosophical idealism that legitimated the hegemony of tsarism and the Orthodox church. Sechenov's "physiological theory was created, not in the calm of the consulting room or laboratory, but in hard and unending ideological skirmishes with the opponents of materialism."[108] While his political views were undoubtedly very liberal, he was not in fact a radical materialist, even in the early 1860s, and he continued to publish and teach with only some slight restriction into the opening years of the twentieth century. However, as indicated, the government censor did change the title of his 1863 essay so it "less clearly indicated the final conclusions resulting from it."[109] The censor also cut the final paragraph that made explicit reference to morals, even though it was here that the author denied any attempt to undermine them. This last paragraph had begun, "In conclusion, I wish to reassure the moral feeling of my reader. The teaching which I have expounded does not destroy the value of human virtue and morals."[110] It was indeed this question of individual freedom and responsibility in morals and in law that touched a raw nerve, with liberals as well as reactionaries. Sechenov's critics associated his physiological determinism with moral nihilism, though this was an association that Sechenov emphatically denied. In the Soviet view:

> The publication of the "Reflexes of the Brain" made a tremendous impression on the progressive circles of Russian society. It became the handbook of the young people of the eighteen-sixties. People were deeply stirred by it, and it was the subject of lively discussion; and while it won many friends, it also made many enemies in the camp of the reactionary idealists.[111]

There were intense public debates in the "thick journals" about the relation between scientific understanding and questions of morality. Sechenov's work should therefore be seen as one component in the political and cultural ferment of the 1860s. It confirmed and reinforced the significance of scientific knowledge in Russian debates about human nature and social values.

In 1870, owing to dissatisfaction with conditions surrounding appointments at the Military Medical Academy, Sechenov left for a position in Odessa, which reduced his contribution to neurophysiological debates, though he continued his experimental studies of blood gases. He returned to active research in the area after he moved back to Saint Petersburg in 1876, this time to the university, but these later experimental studies were more narrowly focused. There was a general realization by the 1870s that experiments on stimulating central nervous processes produced very complex results. By this time, too, Russian and Western physiologists were directing research toward electrophysiology and the properties of nervous conduction as well as the gross effects of intervention in the central nervous system. Sechenov studied electrical fluctuations in the spinal cord under conditions of both inhibition and intensification of respiratory activity caused by direct excitation of the cord or by peripheral stimulation.[112]

Sechenov's thought, set in its Russian context, strongly supports the view that the concept of inhibition played a fundamental role in mediating between mental and physical explanation, thereby acting as a vocabulary through which the evaluative content of the former continued as part of the meaning of the latter. Sechenov's student enthusiasm for psychology had intense political connotations in the mid-1850s, and these fed into his interest in experimental neurophysiology. It is clear that he wasted no time in formulating a program, published as "Reflexes of the brain," that he hoped would enable psychological processes to be analyzed through the experimental study of physiological analogues. Sechenov was explicit that it was a broad interest in psychological questions, particularly a desire to bring volition within the scope of physiological science, that led him to attempt to prove the existence of central inhibition. Iaroshevskii, following Sechenov's autobiography, has argued that the work on inhibition emerged from the integration of his early idealistic psychology, which described the capacity of mental and moral forces to regulate the individual's life, and his medical thesis (accepted in Saint Petersburg in 1860) on alcoholism. Sechenov wrote,

> [Since] a candidate for a doctor's degree could not but know the tri-member [i.e., sensory, central, motor] composition of reflexes and the psychological significance of the middle member in acts concluding with a voluntary movement, it then follows that my thought about the transference of psychic phenomena, from the nature of their mechanism, to a physiological basis must have strayed through my mind during my first stay abroad, the more so since as a student I had studied psychology.[113]

In his thesis, Sechenov stated that "the most common characteristic of normal activity of the brain (as far as it is expressed in movement) is the discrepancy between the stimulation and the action and movement evoked by it."[114] He therefore turned to inhibition as a capacity that would substitute a physiological for a psychological cause in explaining this asymmetry in sensory input and motor output. Thus, when he went to Paris in 1862, he had a clear thesis to establish, namely, the presence of a physiological inhibitory capacity within the brain, a capacity that would subserve psychological control. Quite how Bernard figured in Sechenov's thinking is not clear, though perhaps the desire to work close to such a famous experimentalist requires little explanation, and Sechenov had already fallen in love with Paris. It may also be that Bernard's work on the depressor action of vasomotor nerves had suggested to Sechenov a line of approach to his own problem. Be this as it may, once in Paris, Sechenov, in Iaroshevskii's words, sought a physiological explanation for "the ability to resist external influences and put up barriers against unwanted impulses . . . [since] precisely this important feature could not be explained by the dominant ideas on the function of the brain."[115]

Sechenov's Paris experiments involved transecting the brain of a frog at different levels, observing first the consequences for the strength of spinal reflexes and then the consequences when he irritated the exposed end of the remaining neuraxis. He used a technique developed in Vienna by Ludwig Türck as a means of studying sensibility.[116] Türck had devised a way of lowering the hind limb of a suspended frog into a bath of dilute acid and accurately recording the time for the limb's withdrawal with a metronome. This permitted standardized observations of the intensity and speed of reflex actions. Sechenov's key result occurred when he observed a depression of reflexes following incision at the midbrain level. He then irritated the exposed end of the neuraxis with a salt crystal, at the level of the midbrain (especially at the thalamus). This irritation again depressed the reaction time of a reflex movement in response to a pain stimulus. He was not able to produce the effect with transection and irritation at higher or lower levels, and he devised experiments he thought showed that the depressing mechanism could not be in the spinal cord itself. He therefore concluded that he had produced a central inhibition and that there were central inhibitory centers at the midbrain level in frogs.

He summarized his conclusions in three points:

> 1). In the frog, the inhibitory mechanisms for reflex activity of the spinal cord have their seat in the thalamus, the quadrigeminal bodies, and in the medulla oblongata;
> 2). These mechanisms must be considered as nerve centres in the widest sense of the word;
> 3). The sensory nerve fibres form one, and probably the only one of the physiological routes for the excitation of these inhibitory mechanisms.[117]

These were striking conclusions. Whether there were such inhibitory centers and whether the excitation of reflex inhibition was central or peripheral in origin rapidly became disputed topics in research on the organization of nervous functions.

The eagerness with which Sechenov drew these rather dramatic and specific conclusions suggests that they fitted in with a preexisting plan for devising a physiological approach to human psychology. He also moved in his argument from frogs to humans and vice versa. Thus, he plunged his own hand into acid to see whether his sensibility to pain decreased (it did!) when he exerted a powerful inhibition over himself.[118]

Sechenov's paper, coming on top of the existing interest in inhibition, produced a flurry of related studies, many by Russians inspired directly by him. These studies soon began to qualify and refine his work.[119] His student, F. Matkevich, was the first to publish, and he accepted that Sechenov's experiments could not decide definitively how the inhibitory center, which Matkevich accepted as proved, was normally activated. It was not clear whether peripheral reflex or central brain mechanisms excited inhibition. He therefore attempted to study inhibition in animals that had not been operated on by experimenting on the effects of alcohol, strychnine, and opium, exploring the common but imprecise idea that such substances lessened higher levels of control.[120] Another of Sechenov's students, A. Danilevskii, distinguished pain and tactile reflexes and argued that it was only the former that were related to a midbrain inhibitory center in frogs.[121]

Matkevich's and Sechenov's work provoked emphatic opposition from Alexandre A. Herzen, the son of the famous Russian exile. Herzen was a student and close associate of Schiff, who (as described above) had already opposed theories of localized inhibitory function with his conception of dynamic and nonspecific nervous energization. In Iaroshevskii's words,

> The categorical profile of this school [of Schiff's] was formulated in the constants of mechanics and not those of anatomy, namely, stimulus strength, excitation strength, stimulus or excitation extensity, and so forth . . . the advocates of the "mechanical principle" viewed the organism as an open system that maintained only relative stability in the cycle of matter and energy.[122]

Schiff and Herzen rejected the idea of functional explanation in terms of nervous centers, referring instead to the balance and dispersion of nervous forces. Schiff had previously explained the heightening of reflex movements after decapitation by hypothesizing the transfer of the entire energy of the incoming stimulus to the motor nerves.[123] Herzen now published experiments designed to show that the effects Sechenov and Matkevich had attributed to *centres modérateurs* were produced by exhaustion or irritation of the forces of the gray matter of the frog's brain. His experiments, he believed, showed that "mechanical or chemical irritation of the posterior part of the spinal cord produces a considerable depression of reflex action in the anterior part of the body."[124] He was wholly opposed to the localization of function:

> I believe in the solidarity of the whole of the nervous system, for each irritation that impresses a point of the gray matter can be reflected from this point to all the other parts of the nervous system.
>
> The experiences I have described seem to me to prove in an irrefutable manner that a violent irritation of whichever sufficiently considerable part of the nervous system, central or peripheral, has the immediate consequençe of a large depression of reflex action in the whole organism.[125]

Thus, he concluded, the nervous system as a whole had a moderating function. Significantly, however, Herzen did argue that there was one part of the nervous system, the cerebrum, that had a special controlling role (*action régularisante*). As he observed, associating frogs poisoned by alcohol with everyday experience, "But we know alas! too well ourselves, how alcohol diminishes the influence of the will on our movements."[126] This loss of control occurred, he assumed, through the reduction of cerebral action.

Herzen implied that Sechenov had made no discovery at all. Sechenov and his associates responded with a series of papers that transformed Sechenov's original oversimple claims. Their research studied in ever-increasing detail the many variables affecting the nature and strength of reflex excitations following transection of the brain, the differing effects of different sources of experimental irritation, the problem of peripheral as opposed to central excitation as a source of inhibition, and the questionable comparability of frogs and mammals. For example, Herzen had argued that a salt crystal was too crude and strong an irritation to reveal anything about normal function and that a controlled electrical stimulus did not have the effect reported by Sechenov. B. Pashutin therefore repeated Sechenov's experiment, using an induction coil instead of a salt crystal as the stimulus source, to defend the inhibitory center theory. In a joint paper, Sechenov and Pashutin agreed that peripheral excitation produced inhibitory effects, though they argued that this occurred only when the midbrain region was intact.[127] It was also apparent that careful discrimination was necessary between pain and tactile reflexes and that a center for the inhibition of tactile reflexes had not been demonstrated.

Another of Sechenov's students, L. N. Simonov, extending the study of inhibitory centers from the frog to mammals, suggested that there might be inhibitory centers in the brain other than the ones posited by Sechenov and that this explained some variation in results. He specifically claimed to have elicited inhibition by electrically exciting the forebrain in a puppy, though later workers were unable to confirm this.[128] The researchers were soon forced to conclude that nothing was clear-cut: the conditions affecting the reaction time and the strength of reflex movements depended on interactions between segmental levels in the spinal cord and on preexisting or concurrent peripheral stimuli in the nervous system as well as on the excitation of a possible inhibitory center.

Sechenov thus qualified his own claims. In particular, he conceded Herzen's point that the strength of a reflex movement, such as the frog's hind limb scratch reflex, decreased when a peripheral stimulus was applied to affect the spinal cord at a level higher than that which was the center of the reflex process and at the same time as the exciting stimulus to the reflex. Tetanizing (applying a continuous excitation to) a sensory nerve markedly weakened an evoked reflex.[129] Sechenov therefore increasingly accepted that the source of the inhibition of reflexes might be peripheral rather than central in origin. He accepted also that there was evidence for inhibitory centers in the spinal cord. All the same, he continued to believe that the evidence for central inhibition remained. In 1867, for example, he worked for a period in Graz with Nadeshda P. Suslova, the first Russian woman to gain a medical qualification (by studying in Zürich), and she showed the delaying effect of central brain stimulation on the beat of the frog's lymph heart.[130]

Observing the beating of the frog's lymph hearts proved to be a relatively easy way of noting whether or not depression of activity occurred. Using this technique, Sechenov did a variety of experiments, causing inhibition by placing a grain of salt on the half-transected end of the spinal cord. This research opened up the question of inhibition pathways, a question that could not be answered simply by reference to a single, central inhibitory center.[131] Sechenov, however, remained firmly committed to the belief that there was a specific inhibitory center and a specific inhibitory mechanism and that this theory of central inhibition explained best the arresting power of volition.

Beginning in 1870, Sechenov's view of central inhibition was attacked in the city of its greatest influence, Saint Petersburg, by a physiologist who, two years later, occupied the same position at the Military Medical Academy. I. F. Tsion, like Sechenov, had spent some years training in Germany, publishing research especially on the regulation of the heartbeat. He judged that Sechenov's use of Türck's method rendered the conclusions invalid. Tsion argued instead that inhibition was a general "interference" effect within the whole pattern of nervous activity.[132] Not coincidentally, Tsion bitterly opposed the materialism he discerned in Sechenov and his students.

Sechenov's work on central inhibition, and the research papers that followed, focused on frogs and detailed experimental variables. At a more general level, this research contested the relative merits of different understandings of balance, economy, and regulation within the bodies of people as well as frogs, with those favoring the redistribution of energy opposing those favoring localized control mechanisms. At an even higher level of generality, the language that represented physiological order was also the language used to debate the material or moral conditions of social order. Discussing these layers in scientific papers is not the same as constructing a causal argument, perhaps an argument about social influence, but it does point out the interconnected nature of meaning within a common discourse.

These interconnections were strikingly apparent in the way Sechenov's programmatic writings brought a commonplace and value-laden psychology into relation with his technical neurophysiological research. My way of understanding the interconnections differs from that found in Soviet writers, but they too implied interconnections when they made Sechenov a crucial figure in what, in their terms, was the intellectual breakthrough to an objective science of human biology. The evidence supports Iaroshevskii's view that Sechenov transferred attention from the inhibition of internal organs to the inhibition of skeletal muscle because of his psychological interests.[133] Sechenov pursued the topic of central inhibition to establish a physiological correlate for psychological volition—the faculty that reactionary idealists held up as proving the impossibility of a physiological psychology. He had already become fascinated by empirical psychology as a liberalizing form of knowledge while still a student: he later alluded to reading psychology at the expense of his medical education. It is therefore not surprising that he criticized German physiologists for preferring research on sympathetic and spinal nerves to following up Weber's more provocative psychological comment on the tonic weak inhibitory influence of the brain on the spinal cord.[134] He hoped that his experiments in Paris would rectify the situation: "I set to work on experiments which had a direct relation to acts of consciousness and will."[135] He then immediately followed his 1863 experimental paper on inhibition by writing and publishing his theoretical program for the development of psychology, "Reflexes of the brain." This program relied heavily on the concept of inhibition, and it brought the day-to-day moral world of human action into a close relationship with neurophysiology.

Sechenov's translators have given us an English-language text impressed by the Soviet belief that it presaged a dialectical, biological, and unified psychophysiology, opposed to crudely materialist or idealist philosophies of human nature (both of which, in once current Soviet critical jargon, were "idealistic"). Sechenov was also interpreted as a forerunner of Pavlov. The biological approach was believed to be objectively correct, because it treated organisms, including humans, as centers of action in a continuous dialectical engagement with the environment, including society. It followed that research that distinguished processes as essentially physiological or essentially psychological engaged in abstraction, and to reify abstractions was a Western, "idealistic" practice. "Sechenov transformed both the concept of mental (feeling) and the concept of the reflex, supporting himself on the deterministic framework of the latter. Hence, he returned to the traditional idea . . . according to which the reflex was regarded as a psychophysiological category, and its basic terms were sensation and movement."[136] Sechenov's Soviet importance was that he redescribed the reflex as the basic analytic category for both brain and mind, so that it could serve to found a biological psychophysiology—later to be developed by Pavlov—in the most complex as well as in the simplest aspects of animal and human life.

It is extremely interesting to observe the significance that inhibition had for Sechenov's psychophysiology in the light of this Soviet interpretation. This is the clearest case in which the meaning of inhibition mediated the translation of mentalist moralism into physicalist science. To explore this, it is necessary to look in greater detail at "Reflexes of the brain."

Sechenov wrote, "I must confess that I have built up all these hypotheses without being well acquainted with psychological literature. . . . But my task was to show the psychologists that it is possible to apply physiological knowledge to the phenomena of psychical life."[137] Achieving his physiological program depended on understanding the three basic mechanisms that correlated with mental events: "viz. the mechanism of the pure reflex, and those of reflex inhibition and augmentation."[138] The potential contained in the concept of the reflex, to represent purposiveness in terms of the structural relations of the nervous system, was thus fully realized.

Sechenov's essay was written for a nonspecialist audience; hence he guided his reader from an account of the simplest reflex and involuntary movements to more complex voluntary movements and mental processes. To overcome traditional mentalist assumptions, he placed great weight on showing all movement ultimately originated with sensation, that is, with registering a change in the environment: "*The initial cause of all behaviour always lies, not in thought, but in external sensory stimulation, without which no thought is possible.*"[139] Similarly, Sechenov held it to be axiomatic that all external brain action—"the organ of the spirit"—manifested itself as movement. "All the endless diversity of the external manifestations of the activity of the brain can be finally regarded as one phenomenon,—that of muscular movement."[140]

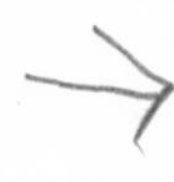

This statement, that action began and ended in observable physical changes represented in the body as sensation and movement, led to describing psychological processes as the middle terms linking sensation and motion in the brain. He argued that these processes were of two basic kinds: those that intensified movement and those that inhibited movement. If this were so, then the existing experimental research program on reflex action, particularly the study of conditions affecting the strength, reaction time, and dispersion of reflex responses in the frog, became the core practice for generating psychological understanding. Few of the technicalities of this program appeared in the essay, however, and Sechenov instead drew on everyday psychological illustrations familiar to general readers. This had obvious value for his exposition; in addition, it reflected the yawning gulf between the minute detail of neurophysiological statements and his sweeping psychological hypotheses. Be this as it may, Sechenov moved back and forth between physiological and psychological claims, arguing by loose analogy and by exploiting a mediating vocabulary.

A multilayered argument, combining references to headless frogs with everyday observations of people, enabled Sechenov to introduce inhibition. Everyone, he supposed, was familiar with involuntary movement following a sudden loud noise. Similarly, everyone was familiar with the attempt to brace oneself in anticipation of such a shock. "If the impressions come unexpectedly, the only nervous centre participating in the reflex is the nervous centre connecting the sensory and motor nerves. When the stimulation is expected, the activity of another mechanism interferes in the phenomenon, restricting and retarding the reflex movement."[141] A person who expected an external influence could exhibit resistance to it. This led Sechenov to ask "whether there is a physiological basis for accepting the existence in the human brain of mechanisms that inhibit reflex movements."[142] Referring first to the work of Weber, Pflüger, Bernard, and Rosenthal on automatic bodily functions, he then described his own experiments that he here claimed straightforwardly proved the existence of an inhibitory center in the frog's brain. No reader would have been in any doubt that he believed in the existence of a similar center in humans, since he moved freely between physiological explanation in the frog and psychological illustration in humans. "Knowing all these facts, contemporary physiologists could not but accept the existence of mechanisms which retard reflex movements in the human body (or, more accurately, in the brain, for our will acts only through this organ)."[143]

The same mixture of a priori argument, experimental detail, and everyday observation led Sechenov to argue for a balance between the mechanism of inhibition and a mechanism of intensification. "We therefore see that the cerebral mechanism which produces involuntary (reflex) movements of the body and the appendages, possesses two apparatuses in the brain, one of which inhibits movements and the other, on the contrary, augments them, changing the proportion between the strength of the stimulus and the size of the effect."[144] For example, involuntary movements became more pronounced in a frightened person or a hysterical woman who convulsed at an unexpected touch. Extreme fright, however, sometimes produced paralysis or complete inhibition. Sechenov believed that inhibited and intensified movements were excited by the same nervous pathways, and this supported his localization of the controlling mechanism at the center. He argued that intensification was probably always initiated by a peripheral stimulus, while he thought that inhibition might be either peripheral or central in origin. Thus, he attempted to spell out a theory of psychological control grounded in the physiological mechanisms of intensification and inhibition. "What other proof do we need that the mechanism of the involuntary movements . . . possesses two antagonistic regulators,—one suppressing movements and the other strengthening them?"[145] It was therefore up to future research to explore in detail the means by which intensified or inhibited reflexes regulated the life of the body.

Sechenov described the regulation of involuntary movements to provide a stepping-stone to a science of the higher aspects of human nature. He intended to confront idealism head on: "My task will be to explain the external activity of a man with an ideally strong will, who is acting on some high moral principle, and is clearly conscious of every step he takes."[146] Since the same nerves and muscles acted in voluntary and involuntary movements, it was reasonable, as well as in his interest, to inquire whether the same central regulatory mechanisms of inhibition and intensification were involved. His object was therefore to explore "whether there exist structures in the brain which participate in voluntary movements by retarding reflexes, and how they participate in them. We shall also look for structures which strengthen reflexes."[147]

This search proceeded by way of a lengthy demonstration that voluntary movements, in spite of subjective appearance and idealist tradition, originated in sensory stimulation. It was this argument that was to be central to his twentieth-century reputation, since it involved establishing the reflex as the basic unit of *all* psychological functions, tying a learning theory based on sensations and a pleasure-pain theory of action into the physiological program.[148] Having identified voluntary movements with reflexes, Sechenov could then claim that the mechanisms already known to regulate the reflexes were the physiological basis of psychological or voluntary control. In support, he simply conflated everyday knowledge of mental control with knowledge of physiological inhibition.

> Are there any phenomena in the conscious life of man which point to the inhibition of movements? These phenomena are so numerous and so characteristic that it is because of them that people call those movements which are performed with full consciousness, voluntary movements. Indeed, upon what is the common conception of such movements based? It is based on the fact, that under the influence of definite external and moral conditions, man can perform a certain series of movements, or can fail to do so, or finally, can perform movements of an entirely opposite character. People with a strong will may triumph over apparently irresistible involuntary movements; for example, one man will endure severe pain silently and without the slightest movement, while another one will scream and writhe.[149]

Such powers of voluntary control, Sechenov argued, were learned by limiting the scope of innate reflex actions and by grouping them into patterns. He believed that this required the action of an inhibitory center and could not be a consequence solely of inhibition by antagonistic movements. Acquired habits determined the scope of inhibition: "Our simple folk lead a life of toil and privations, and are known to endure terrible pain quietly and naturally. . . . the usual education of the children of the so-called intellectual class makes this coarseness of nerves unattainable for the adults of this class."[150]

Perhaps the most provocative implication of Sechenov's theory of inhibitory control was that it suggested that thought itself could be studied as a physiological process. He considered thought to be the subjective side of a reflex in which the last term, movement, was subject to a learned inhibition.

> Let us now show the reader the first and greatest advantage which man gains by learning to inhibit the last member of his reflexes. He thereby acquires *the capacity to think, deliberate, and judge.* For what is, indeed, the act of deliberation? It is a consecutive series of connected ideas and conceptions that exist in our consciousness at a given time, and that receive no expression in external acts. Now, a psychical act . . . cannot appear in consciousness without an external sensory stimulation. Consequently, our thoughts are also subject to this law; therefore, in a thought, we have both the beginning of a reflex, and its continuation; only the end of the reflex (i.e., the movement) is apparently absent.
>
> *A thought is the first two-thirds of a psychical reflex.*[151]

Inhibition, in Sechenov's hands, thus became the controlling mechanism that made possible those very functions, thought and deliberative action, that gave humanity dignity and independence from nature. The possibility of inhibition was the possibility that past associations rather than immediate sensations would sometimes initiate movements. It was the possibility that sensation might combine and recombine as intelligence and thought. Without inhibition, sensation merely exhausted itself in movement.

Inhibition was therefore the concept that mediated the ascription of the most valued capacities of mind to the natural world. We should recall the general task that Sechenov had set himself, faced by an official Russian attitude to psychological questions that presupposed that the individual mental will was a spiritual agency essential to social responsibility. He aimed to advance enlightened attitudes by applying physiology in the realm of human action. This had the ultimate goal of bringing about a predictive science of conduct, making possible a new social order. Toward the end of his life, indeed, he made a practical contribution to this project, albeit in a modest way, by studying the psychology of work and fatigue.[152]

Sechenov was well aware that his essay was speculative and unspecific in physiological terms. One can therefore sense the enormous intellectual investment that someone who was also a trained physiologist had in his detailed and technical studies of reflex inhibition. As he wrote in "Reflexes of the brain," "We have analysed only the external side of psychical reflexes,—only the paths which they follow. There has been no mention of the nature of the process."[153] Sechenov, along with some other physiologists of his generation, tended overoptimistically to believe that a precise understanding of reflex and inhibitory mechanisms was on its way and that this would provide a causal underpinning for psychology. In reality, physiologists became more and more preoccupied by the minutiae of each aspect of the causal mechanisms. The possibility of establishing physiological explanations for psychological phenomena became more remote since each generalization was called into question by new research revealing the complexities of central nervous function. Sechenov's program appeared enormously exciting to twentieth-century neuroscientists, especially in the Soviet Union. It is another matter, however, to understand the historical relations between this program and research in the last thirty years of the nineteenth century.

Sechenov's published experimental work after 1870 occupied a worthy but unexceptional place alongside related neurophysiological studies. While his approach has been cited in the twentieth century as opening up psychology as a science, his specific psychological views had few consequences within the scientific community in Russia or elsewhere in Europe.[154] The questions he had hoped to address through the direct study of inhibition fragmented into a range of detailed and refined issues. We must follow a cluster of not always related researches to trace the vicissitudes of inhibition in this period. Matters were also greatly complicated in the late nineteenth century by the beginning of an institutionally separate discipline of experimental psychology and an associated emptying of neurophysiology of reference to an explicitly psychological dimension. In addition, in medicine, both psychiatry and neurology attempted to be more circumspect about describing psychological phenomena. Even with all this specialization and refinement, however, it is still striking that the language of inhibition retained its power to advance discussion of the "grand" issues concerning mind and morality.

Sechenov himself was deeply disappointed by the failure of his theory of central inhibition to provide a royal road for the progress of physiological psychology. In the late 1860s, he contemplated but never wrote a work on medical psychology that would have exemplified the advantages of a physiological approach. At the same time, he admitted "that his work on inhibition had become shrouded in 'darkness.'"[155] When he subsequently returned to defend his psychology, he did so without reference to the details of experimental neurophysiology. Perhaps he was too well trained as a physiologist not to recognize that the fragmentation of the topic of inhibition left in a very vulnerable position his claim that it explained thought and volition.

In his 1873 essay, "Who must investigate the problems of psychology, and how," Sechenov restated his claim that "the analytical study of psychical phenomena is the business of physiology" and that it was the reflex concept that made this study possible.[156] In this entirely nontechnical review of the possibilities for psychological analysis provided by reflex theory, he restated his views on the central place of inhibition.

> But what about those cases when the stimulation of a sense organ produces the middle phase [of a reflex], but does not manifest itself by any external movement? Is not such an absence of the third [motor] phase a distortion of the very nature of reflex acts? Nothing of the sort! In these cases the sensation is followed by the stimulation, not of the motor organs of the body, but of inhibitors, so that the third phase does not lose its significance as a regulator of movement. . . . The actual existence of these inhibitors has been definitely proved by physiology; and it is these inhibitors that are responsible for the seeming absence of the third phase. The control of these inhibitors is commonly ascribed to volition.[157]

With these rather cryptic remarks, he struggled again to deploy the concept of inhibition as a physiological analogue for the mental faculty of the will. Nevertheless, since—as he readily conceded—knowledge in neurophysiology was still primitive, psychologists had to attend to the external manifestations of internal states, that is, to stimulation and movement, and not to the brain.

> Unfortunately, however, our knowledge of nervous processes,—even the simplest ones,—is almost nil. . . . The solution and detailed explanation of this side of nervous and psychical processes belongs to the distant future; and our research must be limited to the study of their external manifestations.
>
> Nevertheless, *we shall have to retain, as a principle, the conception of the psychical act as a process or motion, which has a definite beginning, course and end.*[158]

Having established the legitimacy of psychophysiology, Sechenov reverted to psychology. The reflex was the "ideal" basic analytic category, yet the "actual" account of reflex activity proceeded not in terms of nervous processes but in psychological terms, describing the three phases of stimulation, central regulation, and movement.

Sechenov then briefly discussed the child's psychological development, suggesting ways in which forms of reasoning, as well as the moral will, were acquired through learning and habit, all these being processes for which he presupposed a reflex foundation. He had, in the late 1860s, acquired at least a working knowledge of Alexander Bain's, Spencer's, and Wundt's psychologies, all of which had drawn psychology into relation with physiology. Sechenov hitched a developmental orientation to his approach, deriving complex psychological functions from elementary reflex units.[159] He continued to assume that inhibited reflexes were fundamental to the possibility of thought and will, but he had no more to say about the mechanism of inhibition than he had expressed in "Reflexes of the brain." It was evident that experimental neurophysiology and general psychology were already tending to go separate ways. It was not possible to use the research paper to address what ordinary people wanted to know about their mental life. But Sechenov's work showed how the meanings embedded in the wider world informed the direction and the content of both physiological research and the presentation of its value to a nonspecialist public.

CHAPTER 4

Inhibition and the Relations between Physiology and Psychology, 1870–1930

Moreover the entire drift of recent physiological and pathological speculation is towards enthroning inhibition as an ever-present and indispensable condition of orderly activity.

———William James, *The Principles of Psychology*

INHIBITION AND THE BRAIN

There is no straightforward story of the physiology or psychology of inhibition after 1870. Nor is it possible to fit an account of inhibition into an established picture: the relevant historical work has simply not been undertaken. The variety, complexity, and sheer quantity of research, especially in experimental neurophysiology, coupled with the way this research appears to twentieth-century scientists to underlie their own activity, has caused history to be in an underdeveloped state. Inhibition was not usually a research topic in its own right but existed as a significant element in a range of interests. It is not possible simply to catalog these interests, since they were of different kinds and represented increasingly specialized and distinct occupations. Neurophysiology, general physiology, neurology, psychiatry, experimental psychology, and philosophy tended to acquire separate identities, research traditions, and languages, and yet each had something to say about inhibition. The relations between these activities were themselves unclear and contested, particularly where they concerned the beginnings of psychology as a separate academic discipline, which was an important development in the late nineteenth century.

Even after acknowledging all this, however, there was still a great deal of thought in common across what, in terms of social arrangements, were diverging disciplines. The framework of understanding underlying the more general questions evident in the first half of the nineteenth century persisted into the second half and beyond. We can legitimately refer to a common discourse concerning regulation and control. Concepts of control continued to make possible the integration of detailed empirical claims into significant knowledge across the diverging specialties.

Inhibition sustained and enhanced its position as a key term in this discourse. It permeated the literature across all the relevant occupational areas. While, on the one hand, it had specific technical meanings for restricted, local audiences, on the other, it retained and indeed consolidated wider meanings. The concept of inhibition occupied a nodal position in the structure of the common discourse while also taking many different, specific forms in particular settings. It mediated between detailed experimental work and significant wider questions, and it held out the potential for communal understanding in the face of occupational and disciplinary fragmentation. In the first edition of his *A Text Book of Physiology* (1877), which marked physiology's coming of age as a separate discipline in England, Michael Foster thus introduced the physiology of inhibition with familiar medical examples:

> In ourselves the fainting from emotion or from severe pain is the result of a reflex inhibition of the heart, the afferent impulses . . . reaching the medulla [and hence the vagus supplying the heart] from the brain.
>
> Thus emotions are a very frequent cause of the progress of parturition being suddenly stopped; as is well known, the entrance into the bed-room of a stranger often causes for a time the sudden and absolute cessation of "labour" pains . . . [and this might indicate an inhibitory centre in the lumbar part of the spinal cord].[1]

Many other writers were to attempt to hold together physiology, medicine, and psychology through comparable examples and language. This was particularly characteristic of efforts to achieve a synthetic science of mind and body. As part of a language representing order, inhibition cut across disciplinary divides.

A growing majority of scientists, however, restricted legitimate knowledge to what was produced by the activity of experimental research. To these scientists, reference to a synthesis or to a wider frame of reference appeared remote and speculative or even "unscientific." Yet, however much experimental research acquired a hard-nosed ethos, scientists lived with the established conditions of theoretical discourse. This discourse resurfaced as an explicit concern in the theoretical syntheses of major scientists such as Sherrington and Pavlov. These syntheses restated the general ideas of organized control, including inhibition, while incorporating the experimentally constituted detail that was so characteristic a feature of the new specialties.

The first two sections of this chapter discuss the use of the term "inhibition" in experimental neurophysiology (though excluding work associated with Sherrington), first, in relation to the brain, and second, in relation to underlying causal mechanisms. The two subsequent sections then relate this research to the new experimental psychology and to the continuing medical-psychological interest in hierarchical control. The following chapter considers the major twentieth-century schools growing out of this work.

The main topics of physiological inhibition had been laid down by the 1860s: the regulation of automatic bodily functions involving the sympathetic or autonomic nervous system; the interaction and regulation of reflex actions; the question of central inhibition; and the mechanism of inhibition, associated with investigations of nerve conduction. These were to remain linked topics. By the 1860s, however, the high status and considerable institutional support accorded to experimental physiology ensured resources for exploring each aspect in detail and hence with a degree of isolation.

Goltz's papers, published as *Beiträge zur Lehre von den Functionen der Nervencentren des Frosches* (1869), were often cited as a judicious review of current knowledge on the organization of reflex actions. Goltz described clearly the contradictory experimental results that appeared to follow from the interaction of new and preexisting excitations at different levels in the spinal cord. Unraveling the factors that affected the spread, speed, and intensity of reflex actions created a relatively specific research program: many researchers could reasonably hope to contribute a detailed piece of the jigsaw puzzle. Goltz also reviewed Sechenov's and his associates' results concerning the relation between peripheral and central excitation as a source of inhibition. He suggested that the quantity of incoming stimuli affected the conductivity of the central links involved in a reflex. This implied that a process of "summation" occurred when a stimulus to a reflex followed on an existing excitation and that this process might be involved in the establishment of inhibition, possibly by activating Sechenov's midbrain region.[2] This led Goltz to the telling point that, if inhibition were treated seriously as a localized function, a great number and variety of centers of inhibition would be required to explain the interaction of reflex effects. Rather than refer to inhibitory centers, he therefore preferred to state that "a centre which mediates a definite reflex act loses excitability for this act if it is set in excitation at the same time by any other nerve tracts which are not concerned in that reflex act."[3] Goltz believed that his hypothesis could reconcile the idea of inhibition with the points made by Sechenov's critics, such as Herzen, in a way that Sechenov's inhibitory center theory could not. He believed it might explain the observation, made on intact frogs, that intense stimulation of sensory nerves caused inhibition of the back scratch reflex.[4] He also reviewed the control of bodily functions, reprinting his earlier report including the striking observation that a smart tap on a frog's belly caused the heart to stop. This suggested that sharp peripheral excitation produced an inhibitory effect through the sympathetic nerves.[5] Following Eckhard, he later added a comparative study of the excitatory and inhibitory regulation of the heart, the erection of the penis, and the evacuation of the bladder and anus.[6]

It is relevant to note that Goltz suggested that *psychological* knowledge of will power implied the existence of a central inhibition (which he preferred to locate in the forebrain), even while he regarded the physiological evidence as indecisive.[7] The overall direction of Goltz's physiological interpretation was toward describing inhibition as a general characteristic of nervous function rather than as a property of particular centers or nerve fibers, yet psychological considerations still inclined him to accept the possibility of the latter. For later physiologists, such as H. E. Hering, who treated inhibition as a general property of organic processes, however, "Goltz will probably have to be mentioned as the first of those who prepared the way for the right conception of the central inhibition processes."[8]

By 1870, no one seriously questioned the reality of peripheral inhibitory phenomena, in which stimulation depressed reflex excitability. This effect was often called reflex inhibition. As has been explained, experimental results still left considerable latitude in interpreting the extent to which inhibition might also be a central nervous phenomenon.[9] Opinion varied considerably about the reliability of Sechenov's claims. Some commentators concluded that there were two modes of inhibitory action, peripheral and central.[10] Another possibility was to accept that inhibition was a function of specific centers but to increase the number of such centers. Thus Goltz, followed by his student, A. Freusberg, extending the experimental study of reflexes from the frog to the dog, opposed the idea of one central center for inhibition, arguing instead that inhibitory stimuli could act at every level in the spinal cord.[11]

Everyone agreed that Sechenov had focused attention on crucial questions concerning regulation by excitation-inhibition in both the brain and the spinal cord. He had presented a challenging theory in concrete terms concerning the relationship between higher and lower nervous levels. Questions concerning the brain's relation to the spinal cord acquired new intensity in the 1870s following the papers by Fritsch and Hitzig (1870) and David Ferrier (1873) which opened up the experimental debate on cerebral localization of function.[12] The demonstration of the electrical excitability of the cortex, and the apparent correlation between different cortical areas and different sensory and motor functions, reconstructed the subject of regulatory control within the central nervous system. This new research subsumed large parts of Sechenov's more limited discussion of nervous control. At the same time, it inevitably raised the question whether the cortex had an inhibitory role, adding this possibility to debates about inhibitory centers at lower levels in the brain and spinal cord. As mentioned, however, Goltz had already raised the possibility of higher inhibition on psychological grounds, and psychological argument continued to have an influence on neurophysiological claims.

There were several attempts to draw together all these issues in the 1870s, balancing a commitment to the localization of function with a belief that the organism's activity as a whole required the integrated dispersion of functions. These opposing pressures in neurophysiological theory, toward localization and toward holism, were held in some kind of balance by the language of a hierarchy of levels and of excitation-inhibition, and this language continued to have psychological reference. There remained considerable disagreement, but such disagreement composed the field of practice for experimentalists and thus unified the field as an occupation.

Ferrier's book, *The Functions of the Brain* (1876), commented on many topics besides his own work on cerebral localization. While sympathetic to the general idea of inhibitory centers in the brain, he provided a careful summary of the ways in which the idea needed to be qualified to explain reflex regulation:

> Though as a rule the summation of stimuli increases the reflex action and makes it more general, this is only true of stimuli conveyed to the same part of the cord (Wundt). If, on the other hand, a sensory nerve in some other part of the body is simultaneously irritated, then the reflex action which would otherwise result from the first stimulus is altogether restrained or inhibited (Herzen, Schiff).
>
> This phenomenon seems to be of a similar nature to that which results from irritation of the optic lobes, or optic thalami in Sechenov's experiments; and it would appear that reflex action in general is inhibited when simultaneous impressions of different origins are made on the nerve centres.[13]

As was to be expected given Ferrier's preoccupation with the representation of sensory-motor functions in the cortex, he considered whether higher cortical levels might play a role in regulating reflex actions. His work on cerebral localization of function argued that the analytic categories applied to the lower levels—that is, the physiological analogues of sensation and motion—also applied to the highest brain levels that subserved mind. The excitation of precise movements by the direct faradic electrical stimulation of particular regions in the cortex apparently proved the point. He therefore believed that it was justified to extend ideas of regulation, based on the balance of excitation-inhibition, into the cortex. "This inhibitory influence of higher over lower nerve centres we shall see reason to extend into the region of the encephalic centres themselves."[14]

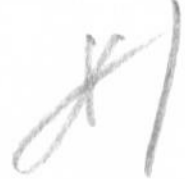

It appears that Sechenov's 1863 paper on inhibitory centers in the midbrain region was important for Ferrier's thinking. Ferrier combined this idea of inhibitory centers with an emphatic commitment to the hierarchical arrangement of levels in the nervous system which he acquired from Jackson. This then provided the basis for his physiological understanding of volition, a topic he did not hesitate to discuss in a physiological context. Ferrier and Sechenov started out from the same ideas of regulation and reflex action when they approached psychological questions, though Ferrier did not know of Sechenov's work on the reflexes of the brain. It was evident once again that physiological approaches to psychological activity drew heavily on the concept of inhibition.

> The primordial elements of the volitional acts of the infant, and also of the adult, are capable of being reduced in ultimate physiological analysis to reaction between the centres of sensation and those of motion.
>
> But besides the power to act in response to feelings or desires, there is also

> the power to inhibit or restrain action, notwithstanding the tendency of feelings or desires to manifest themselves in active motor outbursts.[15]

In an everyday illustration that Sechenov might have used, Ferrier invoked common sense, pointing to the reality of a voluntary inhibitory power: "Thus, by a strong effort of the will, some persons may succeed in restraining the movements of the legs which would otherwise result from tickling the soles of the feet."[16]

By referring to inhibition as a *psychological* "faculty" and at the same time treating inhibition as the *physiological* mechanism of mental attention, Ferrier made inhibition into "the organic basis of all the higher intellectual faculties."[17] He described inhibition at lower levels as either indirect (e.g., the effect of a second, stronger stimulus added to the stimulus exciting a reflex) or direct (e.g., vagal depression of the heartbeat). The former was "paralleled in volitional action by the inhibition or neutralization of one motive by another and stronger."[18] The latter was paralleled by inhibitory centers possessing a motor character, that is, by "volitional inhibition."

> As an illustration . . . we may take the power, accompanied with the feeling of effort, to rein in and inhibit the tendency of powerful feelings to exhibit themselves in action. The battle between inhibition and the tendency to active motor outburst, is indicated by the tension into which the muscles are thrown, and yet kept reined in, so that under a comparatively calm exterior there may be a raging fire, threatening to burst all bonds.[19]

It is hard to imagine a more direct integration of everyday psychology with the leading edge of physiological research. Indeed, in the second edition of his book a decade later, Ferrier was more circumspect about positing specific physiological analogues for specific psychological activities. Though he continued in a general way to correlate psychological processes with sensory-motor functions, he substantially removed the discussion of inhibition.[20] He perhaps thought it better to protect physiological science from the siren call of speculative psychology.

In the first flush of enthusiasm in the 1870s, however, Ferrier described the central inhibitory motor function as the physiological basis for the psychological power of attention, thereby associating the term "inhibition" with central questions in the mind-brain relation in British physiological psychology. British writers had often treated human action in reflex terms, envisaging that movements flowed automatically from the excitation of ideas. The mental control of movement and conduct, according to this view, depended on attention—a power to "modify and control the current of ideation."[21] Ferrier's speculations reconstructed this conventional emphasis on attention in British psychophysiology as a theory of inhibition. He argued, again in a manner reminiscent of Sechenov, that thought, physiologically considered, involved a sensory-motor act with the motor part in movement suppressed: "We think of form by initiating and then inhibiting the movements of the eyes or hands through which and by which ideas of form have been gained and persist. . . . We recall an object in idea by pronouncing the name in a suppressed manner."[22] The education of attention thus involved cultivating the power to inhibit movement: "The degree of consciousness is inversely proportional to the amount of external diffusion in action. . . . Hence, in deep thought, even automatic actions are inhibited, and a man who becomes deep in thought while he walks, may be observed to stand still."[23]

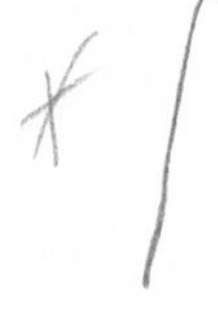

Ferrier did not doubt that "the nature of the inhibitory mechanism is exceedingly obscure," but he was prepared to list experimental and pathological data supporting the localization of inhibitory centers in the frontal lobes or forebrain.[24] He believed that the frontal lobes subserved attention and, although they did not directly initiate movement, that they were anatomically and functionally connected to lower levels that did.

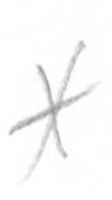

> Centres of direct inhibition and nerves of inhibition are . . . all centrifugal, or motor, in character, and it has also been shown that the frontal regions are directly connected with the centrifugal, or motor tracts of [lower levels]. . . .
>
> The removal of the frontal lobes causes no motor paralysis, or other evident physiological effects, but causes a form of mental degradation, which may be reduced in ultimate analysis to loss of the faculty of attention.[25]

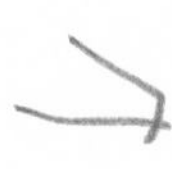

The concept of inhibition thus also appeared to be the key to extending the analytic categories of sensory-motor physiology into the functionally obscure—but in humans anatomically very prominent—region of the frontal lobes. It tied together the current emphasis on attention, which was held to be the basis of moral action, and the advancing edge of experimental neurophysiology.

Ferrier integrated his work with contemporary German research, notably, the physiological psychology of Wilhelm Wundt. Wundt is now renowned for the contribution he made to founding experimental psychology as a discipline. In the 1860s and early 1870s, however, he worked extensively on mainstream neurophysiological topics.[26] Subsequently, a focus on the relationship between nervous physiology and psychology remained characteristic of his psychological work, especially in the successive editions of the *Grundzüge der physiologischen Psychologie* (1874) which claimed to lay the groundwork for a new discipline of psychology.[27] This claim was central to German human science up until World War I. Wundt more particularly contributed to the debate on physiological inhibition. His views on this subject then became an important dimension of his psychology, and they can be used to illustrate some of its general features.

Wundt, like Ferrier, introduced his views on inhibition as part of an account of reflex action, referring reflex strength to the excitatory state of different levels of the whole system. He couched his discussion in terms of the debate between Sechenov and his supporters and Schiff and Herzen. While accepting the antilocalizers' evidence that the presence of a second peripheral stimulus increased the inhibition of a reflex action, Wundt wished to localize inhibition to the extent of pinning down the effects of inhibitory stimuli to the sensory spinal nerve ganglia or, in the brain, to Sechenov's midbrain region. Interestingly, he drew an analogy between the interactive effect of stimuli at lower levels, reducing the strength of reflex action, and the possible means by which one sensation displaced another in perception. At this point, he brought the physiological concept of inhibition into relation with the dynamic interaction of mental presentations.[28] Wundt was also prepared to suggest that the dynamic, and in part inhibitory, interaction between excitations at higher levels in the nervous system was the physiological basis for the action of will, and this is discussed further below.

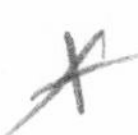

Wundt occupied a major position in German academic life, holding the chair of philosophy at Leipzig for forty years. The same elements underlay his program for a systematic science of psychology over all these years, even though he kept updating the details, as with inhibition. Rather than organizing his material around the topic of inhibition, Wundt subsumed inhibition under a more general principle in the nervous system, which he called "interference" (*Interferenz*), a term originally introduced to characterize the interaction of reflexes.[29] This principle was in effect a generalized statement describing the functional interdependence of all excitations, and it was thus comparable to Sherrington's later principle of "integration." Wundt described interference as dependent on (1) the relative phase of interacting excitations in nerve fibers (an effect elucidated in nerve conduction studies); (2) the intensity of the stimuli; (3) the spatial relations of the excited nerve fibers, notably, whether the excited fibers lay within the same nerve trunk or entered at the same level in the spinal cord; and (4) the state of higher brain levels, since any impairment, for example, by fatigue, strychnine, or cold, appeared to reduce their inhibitory effect on lower levels.[30] Each of these points had some significance in relation to understanding inhibition, but it was each point's detail, rather than descriptions of inhibition per se, that formed continuing research topics.

In 1873, Wundt noted that nobody had convincingly observed inhibition as a result of direct cerebral stimulation, though he thought this negative result was an artifact of the special difficulties associated with working on such a complex organ and not proof that the cerebrum was not involved in inhibition.[31] Researchers continued throughout the 1870s to question whether there were centers of inhibition in the brain, either at the midbrain level or at higher levels. Oscar Langendorff, for example, concluded that the cerebrum as well as the optic lobes formed such a center, suggesting that the cerebral inhibitory center was acquired as part of the process of learning control over the body.[32] As this example illustrates, it was in fact psychology rather than neurophysiology that prompted hypotheses about such centers. Thus, Wundt's account of interference, which addressed the inhibitory interaction of reflexes, went on to discuss the inhibitory action of the will through the higher nerve centers.[33] Wundt held that inhibition was a key physiological correlate of psychological apperception, which he localized in the forebrain. By locating physiological inhibition at the same site as psychological apperception, Wundt hoped to reconcile localization theory with the view that inhibition was a general feature of nervous function. The American psychologist Raymond Dodge later made this point:

> Since there is no mental phenomenon that may not operate to condition a decrement of some other, the inhibitory mechanism, whatever it is, must be as extensive as the neural conditions of consciousness. In the Wundtian schema the idea of a special inhibitory center is retained without encountering this difficulty by identifying it with an apperception center in the frontal lobes. According to Wundt's hypothesis, this center contains the "nodal points of conductions" whose abrogation produces disturbances that manifest themselves as impairment of intelligence.[34]

Wundt was thus struggling to reconcile physiological arguments for and against understanding control mechanisms in terms of localized centers while simultaneously taking into account features apparently required by psychological events. A term like "inhibition," with its ambiguous reference to physiology or psychology under a more general notion of control, proved invaluable. To see this, something further must be said about Wundt's general program for psychology.

Wundt's commitment to psychology was a commitment to what he believed to be a way of introducing objective methods into philosophy. He developed both an analysis of mind, which described mental processes in terms of voluntarist or psychical causal relations, and a physiological analysis of the nervous correlates of mental activity, which described physical causal processes. His training in physiology enabled him to develop experimental techniques as a means to report accurately on changes in the content of the conscious mind and to draw analogically on physiology in analyzing conscious processes. He exploited the concept of inhibition as part of the latter analogical activity. Both Wundt's question, how to understand the determination of the conscious world in terms of mental causality, and his approach to an answer were reminiscent of Herbart, with whose work Wundt was familiar. The problem of mental content for Herbart and Wundt became a search for law-like regularities in the inherent activity of mind. They argued that this activity gave rise to what appeared subjectively as the faculties of perception, attention, volition, and so forth.[35] The development of experimental technique and physiological knowledge after Herbart, however, obviously gave Wundt's work a different character.

Wundt relied directly on physiological analogy. He believed that the nervous system permanently exhibited a dynamic balance between excitatory and inhibitory forces.

> The state which we term the "state of rest" is really a state of oscillation—as a rule, of oscillations about a certain position of equilibrium—in which the excitatory and inhibitory forces counteract one another. It is a state in which, on the average, there is a slight preponderance of permanent excitation, though this may be transformed, under special conditions, and more particularly under the influence of antagonistic effects, into a preponderance of permanent inhibition.[36]

His psychological conclusion was that consciousness exhibited a parallel dynamic balance, that is, that mental processes were superinduced on a background or state of "tonic" perceptual awareness. Mental processes, he assumed, interacted in a way that was analogous to excitation and inhibition. Taking the analogy further, it followed that there was a hierarchy of mental processes, just as the balance of forces within the central nervous system depended on the relations between a hierarchy of levels. Wundt argued that it was the higher-level activity that integrated lower-level processes into consciousness. This higher mental activity was properly called voluntary. Active integration, in his terms, was "apperception." In William Woodward's words, "Wundt described the inhibitory and excitatory control of sensation and perception, cognition and volition, by successively higher centers for voluntary 'apperceptive' activity."[37]

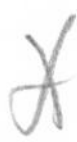

Wundt used the term "apperception" to refer to the active production of mental content, whereas he considered that the term "association," which was characteristically used in British empiricist psychology, denoted passive processes. In explaining this point, he again drew on the analogy suggested by excitatory and inhibitory physiological mechanisms. Woodward has described Wundt's argument in the following way:

> In his earlier physiological experiments he had defined excitation as movement following one stimulus, and inhibition as the difference in the movements following two stimuli sequentially presented. In the later psychological analogue, Wundt defined association as the principle underlying the reaction to one stimulus, and apperception as the principle underlying the reaction to two or more stimuli, simultaneously or successively presented.[38]

There are two relevant points here. First, Wundt was seeking to characterize mental processes in terms of experimental operations and hence to give an objective or scientific character to knowledge of those processes. Second, inhibition entered into the understanding of organization at both the physiological and psychological levels. It explained how differentiated movements, more complex than simple reflex movements, were possible, and it also explained the possibility of integrated perception, or "apperception," more complex than sensory association. Inhibition therefore described a principle intrinsic to the organization of consciousness and not just one mental process among others. Wundt did not refer particularly to inhibition in his systematic account of apperception. The dynamic organizing principle characterized by the term entered at a metalevel, and he explicated it through physiological analogy rather than through describing the role apperception itself played in psychological activity.

Reference to inhibition in Wundt's psychology also rested on much simpler, even commonsense, observations. Reporting on what informal introspection revealed about conscious dynamics, he repeated views common to much psychological writing, as when he described the competitive integration of sensory elements in conscious experience.

> A little introspection suffices to show that a sensation, in growing stronger or weaker, alters its *own* intrinsic character; while, if it grows clearer or more obscure, the change is primarily a change in its relation to *other* conscious contents. . . . These facts suggest that the substrate of the simple apperception process may be sought in *inhibitory processes* which, by the very fact that they arrest other concomitant excitations, secure an advantage for the particular excitations not inhibited. . . . The inhibitory effects are liberated . . . by certain excitations that are conducted to the centre; but their liberation is at the same time influenced by that incalculable manifold of conditions which, for the most part, we can merely group together under the indefinite name of the current disposition of consciousness, as determined by past experience and the circumstances of the time.[39]

He also constructed an elaborate and extremely speculative brain model that localized such activity in "*das Apperceptionscentrum*," but this really did little more than give spatial representation to the hypothesized dynamics of psychological processes.[40] As Ferrier recognized, Wundt treated attention as an extremely important phenomenon, considering it to be the active process of conscious or apperceptive awareness and relating it to motor activity in the brain.[41] In these related ways, Wundt attempted to achieve an analytic and experimental purchase on the traditional mental faculties such as perception, attention, and volition.

The further consequences of this kind of argument for psychology will be considered in due course. It is necessary now to stay with the development of brain research in the 1870s and 1880s to describe the claims that did most to refocus debate about localized inhibitory functions in higher brain regions. A "classic" paper by the professor of physiology at Breslau (now Wroclaw), Rudolph Heidenhain, and his Russian associate, N. Bubnov, published in 1881, provided detailed empirical evidence for such centers. The paper is now regarded as a classic because it anticipated the discovery in the 1940s by H. W. Magoun and R. Rhines of a limbic regulatory center, which has been a major plank of neurobiological research in the modern period.[42] Given this status, it is important historically to note that Heidenhain's and Bubnov's work, though much discussed, did not have the same unquestioned standing in the late nineteenth century.

Considered in historical context, the 1881 paper was part of Heidenhain's response to a widespread interest in hypnotism. The concept of inhibition once again proved its value as a means for drawing together psychological and neurophysiological topics, suggesting ways in which the former, which constituted the "real life" experience, might be explained by the latter, which constituted the "real science" explanation. Heidenhain was one of several well-established scientists who felt challenged both intellectually and socially by hypnotism. It was common for itinerant entertainers to exhibit spectacular hypnotic effects to large audiences. Heidenhain in Breslau, Wundt in Leipzig, Meynert in Vienna, and B. Danilevskii in Kharkov felt that these displays and the newspaper comment they aroused were a challenge to the dominance of natural science and rational understanding—and to professors as the official interpreters of this culture.[43] They therefore turned to physiological psychology to reassert a legitimate and sober view of the hypnotic phenomena that caused such public excitement. At about the same time, hypnotism became a dramatic feature of the medical approach to nervous disorders in France, with the highly public dispute between the Charcot school in Paris and the Nancy school led by H. Bernheim.[44]

Heidenhain adopted the standard view among physiologists that "so-called animal magnetism" was explainable in terms of the suspension in the hypnotized subject of normal conscious controls with the result that actions followed automatically from suggested ideas.

> For while, under normal circumstances, movements can be not only initiated by the cerebral cortex, but also inhibited, in the hypnotized subject both powers are absent.
>
> Normally, when the idea of a movement presents itself to our consciousness, we can carry that movement into effect or not. In the hypnotic condition, owing to the absence of the inhibitory power of the will, the unconscious perception of the movement irresistibly brings it about—a process in all respects analogous to reflex action.[45]

This explanation was comparable with physiological accounts of automatistic movement in the 1850s, but Heidenhain could take the approach further by drawing an analogy with the known role of inhibition in breathing or reflex movements. As G. J. Romanes observed in his introduction to the English translation of Heidenhain's book on the subject, "In hypnotism we are approaching a completely new field of physiological research, in the cultivation of which our previous knowledge of inhibition may properly be taken as the starting-point."[46] Heidenhain himself argued that the hypnotic effect was the product specifically of inhibition, that is, "*the inhibition of the activity of the ganglion-cells of the cerebral cortex*... the inhibition being brought about by gentle prolonged stimulation of the sensory nerves of the face, or of the auditory or optic nerve."[47]

The attempt to understand animal hypnotism already had something of a history in 1880. Johannes N. Czermak, a physiologist, and William T. Preyer, later famous for his writings on child development, had argued that the excitation of an inhibitory center, such as Sechenov had proposed to exist, would explain entertaining and spectacular effects like snake charming. Pressure to the animal's neck, they argued, activated an inhibitory center.[48] They referred back to the celebrated *experimentum mirabile de imaginatione gallinae* attributed to Athanasius Kircher, the display of laying an excited hen on its back in a state of apparent death simply by seizing it in a firm grasp, which had delighted audiences since the seventeenth century.[49] Heidenhain's research attempted to translate these interests into a precise description of functional relations between the cerebrum and lower brain levels. With Bubnov, he investigated possible motor functions of the cerebral cortex, using in tandem techniques for extirpating and for stimulating particular areas while observing the effect on the reaction time for muscular contraction. They concluded, "We have shown . . . that the reaction time as well as the duration of the muscular twitch is shortened when the cortex has been removed."[50] This implied, they believed, that the highest brain levels had an inhibitory function, and it could therefore be supposed that it was this function that was suspended in hypnotized subjects.

Bubnov and Heidenhain related their research to the discussion aroused by Sechenov's parallel "discovery" of a midbrain inhibitory center. Thus, they also explored the effect of previous or concurrent sensory and motor excitations on the cortical inhibitory function. They articulated important questions, such as "whether the voluntary interruption of muscular activity is due simply to the cessation of impulses from the motor centres or to positive antagonistic effects which inhibit the action of these motor centres."[51] Given the by then well-established evidence that peripheral stimulation could inhibit motor effects and given the research that had shown it was possible by direct stimulation to map sensory areas in the cortex, they suggested the experimental question "whether slight direct stimulation of the [cerebral] motor centres might not act in a way similar to slight peripheral stimuli and terminate an excitatory state."[52] They reported experiments that answered this question positively, laying the basis for the direct empirical exploration of the central inhibitory mechanism for regulating motor functions. In Schäfer's words, they showed that inhibition was "an active function of the cortex."[53]

Meynert was another scientist to be provoked by the phenomenon of hypnotism into speculating that higher levels of brain activity had an inhibitory function.[54] Of course, this claim also restated traditional views describing "higher" activity repressing "lower" activity. Meynert argued that the hypnotist first increased the blood flow in the subject's brain and then suggested mental images that, embodied as cortical representations, inhibited normal motor activity. He thought that the same process was common in mental illness. As an experimental underpinning for this argument, he had in mind the research by Goltz and others which had shown the inhibitory effect on one reflex produced by the simultaneous excitation of a second reflex.

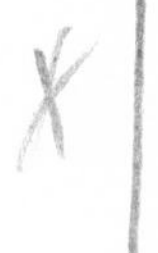

Bubnov and Heidenhain's paper received attention in the 1880s partly because their results opposed the prestigious neurological views of Carl Wernicke, Meynert, and Hermann Munk, who had argued that movements were induced by "motor images" in the cortex unless the movement was inhibited by some *extra*-cortical stimulus.[55] In undermining this specific point regarding the site of inhibitory action, Bubnov and Heidenhain in effect implied that the neurologists' general models of brain function were untenable. In response to Bubnov and Heidenhain's paper, Munk therefore queried whether they had demonstrated the presence of central inhibition rather than the action of antagonistic muscles. He distinguished "true inhibition" (e.g., vagal inhibition) from the inhibition involved in antagonistic muscle action, and he regarded the latter, not the former, as the basis of willed movements.[56] This controversy encouraged recognition of the dangers inherent in premature theorizing about brain function. As Bubnov and Heidenhain pointed out, their results indicated "an unexpected complexity of the process of central innervation."[57] This was a lesson that more and more researchers were taking to heart at the end of the century, and it encouraged the narrowing of research and skepticism about general models linking anatomy and function in the brain.

Bubnov and Heidenhain's paper also argued that the central nervous system was normally in an active or tonic state of excitation and inhibition. This was a view that had long been held, on both a priori and experimental grounds, however hazily expressed, when considering sphincter control, posture, and movement.[58] Bubnov and Heidenhain described a tonic condition of excitatory-inhibitory activity, a background against which particular contingent stimuli produced their effects. Sherrington later developed this understanding with greater precision. Thus, Bubnov and Heidenhain believed, the nervous system had to be envisaged as permanently organized in a functional as well as in a structural sense. Once this was understood, it became apparent that a phenomenon like hypnosis, or a drug like morphine, produced its effect by lowering an organism's ability to sustain tonic inhibitory processes. Experimental results, they argued, confirmed empirically what a theory of the nervous system as a system of control necessarily required.

> The assumption of inhibitions as part and parcel of the mechanisms of central innervation affecting by their relative value—i.e., by the ratio of their intensity to that of the excitations—the quantitative aspects of the process of excitation both in its intensity and its temporal sequence, enables us to understand many other things which heretofore were enigmatic. If we assume, as we are almost driven to do, that inhibitions delimit not only the temporal but also the spatial spread of excitation [then, many phenomena become clear].[59]

As they then portentously claimed, "the further development of a theory [of innervation in the brain] will largely depend on our progress in the understanding and evaluation of inhibitory processes."[60]

The basic claim that removal of the brain or decapitation enhanced reflex excitability had long implied the existence in the nervous system of tonic inhibitory activity. After about 1870, most physiologists, like Bubnov and Heidenhain, began to treat tonic excitation and inhibition as a background that had to be taken into account to interpret particular experimental results on reflex action. The disturbing variability and diversity of these results then began to fall into a general pattern: the relative excitability of a reflex action was a function of existing spatial and temporal relations among excitations and inhibitions in the nervous system. Wundt summarized this point. "The single transient reflex process is superinduced upon a reflex tonus, whose effects become apparent whenever there is interruption of the sensory paths in which the permanent innervation of reflex excitation is conducted."[61] This belief, that there was a tonic excitatory-inhibitory balance within the nervous system, in its turn, encouraged the view that excitatory and inhibitory forces were general properties of nervous activity. Whereas Pflüger had sought for specific inhibitory nerves and Sechenov had tried to locate inhibition in a specific center in the brain, by the late nineteenth century it was more common to conceive of inhibition as a problem of nervous function itself. At a more general level, however, the meaning of inhibition as the representation of control and balance remained, and through this language brain research remained part of a wider frame of reference.

MECHANISMS OF INHIBITION

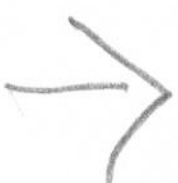

The view that inhibition was an intrinsic property of nervous function integrated brain research with questions concerning causal physiological processes. Considerable effort began to be expended in trying to unravel the mechanism of nervous inhibition. Success came in this area of activity, however, with understanding the mechanism of nervous conduction rather than inhibition. At the end of the century, many scientists believed that ideas about inhibitory mechanisms were still speculative, however much was apparently known about reflex inhibitory functions. There was a disturbing range of theories, and no one theory satisfactorily explained inhibition. This prompted several attempts to stand back and take an overview.[62] In its turn, the simple desire to review the possible causal mechanisms gave inhibition a rather misleading concreteness as a subject. On the one hand, inhibition became a technical problem in physiology connected with productive research on nerve conduction. On the other hand, however, the concept retained its creative ambiguity in the boundary area between physiology and psychology, an area that transcended technical concerns.

Here I present only a schematic guide to research on the mechanism of inhibition, since the area is secondary to my main theme. But this discussion does confirm that there was continuity of meaning, conveyed by reference to inhibition, across general psychological and specialist physiological contexts.

Views about the nature of inhibition were expressed in the earliest reports on vagal inhibition, and research on the heartbeat continued to stimulate ideas.[63] General theories of the organic economy were another significant source, with physical and economic metaphors often playing a leading role. This was therefore one significant way in which the study of inhibition continued to hold out the possibility that it would serve the grand questions facing a unified approach to mind and body even while becoming narrowly technical in character. Metaphorical language encompassed large questions concerning the balanced control of the organism, or the social human being, at the same time as it directed research on specific mechanisms. As will be seen, for example, physical metaphor was a potent resource for Freud's reconstruction of psychodynamics.

General physiological argument lay behind Schiff's outright rejection of Sechenov's inhibitory center. Schiff understood the body to be a balanced, energized system. In such a system, concentrating energy in certain channels inevitably directed it away from others, thus reducing some activities while intensifying others. In Schiff's view, as explained earlier, decapitation caused inflowing energy to be transferred in its entirety to motor channels, whereas normally some was diverted to the brain; this explained the appearance of released inhibition. Schiff similarly explained the apparent arrest of the heart by vagal stimulation in terms of exhaustion: he argued that weak stimulation accelerated the heartbeat, whereas strong stimulation had the opposite effect, analogous to the way excessive stimulation exhausted skeletal muscle.[64]

Though Schiff himself had finally to accept that his exhaustion theory could not explain vagal inhibition, approaches to physiological dynamics that adopted comparable explanations were common in late-nineteenth-century research.[65] The most distinctive was perhaps the attempt by Brown-Séquard to integrate psychology, physiology, and pathology in a general theory of the organization of nervous energy. His work had some influence in France but attracted little attention elsewhere, except perhaps in Italy. Late in Brown-Séquard's career, Bernard's death in 1878 opened up a position for him in the front rank of scientists at the Collège de France. He used his new position to expound *dynamogénie* as an organizing principle in nervous physiology.[66] In a long series of papers, rather than in a major text, he strung together a systematic alternative to both Bernard's physiology and German-language theories of localized nervous functions. These papers also introduced and popularized the word "inhibition" in French physiological circles and, from the late 1870s to the early 1890s, gave a distinct coloration to French discussions. "Inhibition" subsequently passed into psychological use in France.[67]

The belief that many parts of the central nervous system switched from excitatory to inhibitory action, depending on stimulus strength, was at the heart of Brown-Séquard's approach. Discussing the excitability of the occipitosphenoidal area of the cortex, he observed, "One knows that many parts of the nervous system are capable, under the influence of an excitation, of producing either a movement or an inhibition. M. Ch. Rouget has shown that the production of one or other of these two types of effects depends on the strength of excitation or on the degree of excitation of the part that gives rise to it."[68] This sense of the dynamic nature of nervous function went back to Brown-Séquard's clinical and experimental studies of spinal pathways and the sympathetic nervous system in the late 1840s and the 1850s. Like other physiologists at that time, he had attempted to develop reflex action theory to explain traditional medical notions of "sympathy" and the control of secretions or vasodilator and vasoconstrictor effects.[69] It was only with his lectures at the Collège de France in 1878–79, however, that he began explicitly to systematize his theory of nervous control around belief in the balance of excitation and inhibition.

Brown-Séquard tied all his work to clinical evidence, and he certainly intended his theory to create something of a revolution in neurology. His theory implied that pathological inhibitory effects should be attributed to the irritation (i.e., excitation) caused by a lesion, not to the lesion itself releasing some previously repressed motor effect. He provided evidence by reporting on a series of experimentally induced lesions and, in the process, elaborated a generalized theory of inhibitory function.

> Facts show that the excitability of a large part of a lateral half of the brain and the cervical spinal cord can disappear under the influence of an irritation caused by the transverse section of the lateral half of the dorso-lumbar swelling of the spinal cord or of the sciatic nerve, of the opposite side. The spinal cord can thus lose its excitability by an *arresting* influence (inhibitory influence) [une influence d'*arrêt* (influence inhibitoire)] coming from an irritation of the brain, just as the brain . . . can lose its motor excitability under the influence of an arresting influence coming from the spinal cord.[70]

Brown-Séquard therefore felt able to claim for himself the "discovery" of inhibition as a general property of the nervous system. While acknowledging that others had reported the existence of inhibition, he believed that only he had seen how to apply the concept to interpret the full range of normal and pathological effects in which it was implicated.

> There is an inhibition all the time which produces in a purely dynamic manner a disappearance immediately or nearly immediately, temporarily or persistently, of a function, of a property, or of an activity in nervous or contractile tissue, under the influence of the irritation of one part of the nervous system at a greater or lesser distance from the organ or tissue whence it arises.[71]

This suggested to him ways to understand such complex phenomena as tonic motor states, sympathetic action, the effects of drugs, and lesions. He did not attempt to describe *dynamogénie* itself in causal terms, and his theory thus discussed inhibition at an organizational rather than causal level. This may in part explain why his views were almost totally ignored by contemporary German- and English-language researchers who were physiologists rather than neurologists and who were increasingly interested in the causal basis of inhibition.

While physiologists did not adopt Brown-Séquard's theory of *dynamogénie*, they did elaborate several alternative conceptions of a dynamically organized nervous system. These attributed inhibition to the dispersion of energy released by a stimulus and the release of inhibition to the concentration of energy released by a stimulus resulting in an enhanced reflex.[72] Nevertheless, by the 1880s, the majority of physiologists were beginning to conceive of inhibition as a property of nerve action, though this action could itself be understood in dynamic physiological terms. The major exception was the "drainage" theory of inhibition advocated by the British physiologist and psychologist William McDougall. Significantly enough, McDougall discussed the physiological mechanism of inhibition with the requirements of psychological processes in mind, rather than developing an argument narrowly grounded in experimental neurophysiology. "Inhibition is essentially the result of a process of competition, and many psychologists have given expression to this conception in some such vague phrase as: The mind has only a limited quantity of energy, which will not suffice for the simultaneous maintenance of two mental processes."[73] As this passage suggests, drainage theory reexpressed in a more elaborate form the Victorian psychological commonplaces concerning the energy economy of the person. Popularizers, moralizers, and medical men had long drawn on a common repertoire of relational terms in political and physiological economy. This language, as illustrated earlier, was at its richest in Spencer's creative and influential portrayal of "the social organism."[74] Spencer had also urged that there was a finite quantity of "nervous force," meaning that when energy was consumed in one action it was not available for another. The implications for moral choice and psychological welfare were obvious enough. Toward the end of the century, references to the nervous economy still retained explanatory power for psychologists, since they invoked a level of explanation relevant for everyday circumstances associated with character and illness. The metaphor, however, tended to be too imprecise and insufficiently embodied in an experimental program to attract physiologists. Nevertheless, physiological concepts that they did use had the same roots.

McDougall defined inhibition as the necessary accompaniment of excitatory or active processes:

> It appears, in fact, that the inhibition of a mental process is always the result of the setting in of some other mental process, and, if we consider the under-

> lying physiological processes, we see that this means that the inhibition of the excitation of one neural system is always the result of the excitement of some other system, *that inhibition appears always as the negative or complementary result of a process of increased excitation in some other part.*[75]

He then exploited the analogy of the distribution of water from a reservoir to translate this general principle into physiological terms, since such "rough mechanical illustration . . . may aid us to conceive how the passage of the impulse through any one part of the system of higher level paths may inhibit by drainage the passage through any other."[76] McDougall continued to defend this analogy into the 1920s, but by then such looseness of expression contrasted unfavorably with the precise way Sherrington and his associates described both nervous integration and nervous conduction. Developments in the physiology of the nervous impulse, indeed, ensured that McDougall's thinking was largely ignored by physiologists.

In the period up until about 1900, however, it was common for psychological views of inhibition to interact in a creative way with speculation about its physiological mechanism. This was evident, as discussed, in a German-language writer like Wundt as well as in an English-language one like Ferrier, even though Germany had a more secure tradition of institutionally autonomous experimental physiology. Fearing retrospectively differentiated hypotheses about inhibition into what he called interference, metabolism, and refractory phase theories, though there was considerable overlap and interaction between the different positions.[77] As researchers attempted to investigate these theories in a rigorous way, they reinforced a growing separation between physiological and psychological practices and occupations. Argument for and against each theory increasingly depended on detailed results from experiments on the mechanism of nervous conduction, research expressed in abstruse experimental papers offering little of interest, even when it was comprehensible, to psychologists. Inhibition acquired its most technical meanings in this research. Finally, all of these theories were, in their turn, replaced after the late 1920s by the identification of inhibition with a chemical effect at the synaptic junction between neurons.

Goltz's review of the debate initiated by Sechenov in the 1860s made it clear that a spinal reflex center in the frog was inhibited when it received another afferent stimulus in addition to the one responsible for exciting the reflex. This led him to believe that inhibition was a modification of excitation rather than a distinct process. H. E. Hering later developed and summarized this view: "Inhibition is also excitation but an excitation that disturbs other excitations."[78] Hering therefore concluded that so-called central inhibition was really the result of a particular sum of excitations. He distinguished "*Erregungen H*" and "*Erregungen E*" (inhibitory and excitatory excitations) and referred to the central site of interaction between these excitations, the true locus of inhibition, as a "*Kollisionsort*" (point of conflict).

Goltz himself did not describe the process he had in mind as "interference." This was done by Tsion when he translated this functional theory into causal terms, hypothesizing that excitation and inhibition could be "interference" against a tonic background of nervous activity. Tsion was adamantly opposed to what he regarded as Sechenov's materialism, and, presumably not coincidentally, he also opposed the theory of centers of inhibition. Since nerve conduction had oscillatory properties, he argued, the coincidence of waves of conduction would intensify the stimulus, while the interference of waves would produce inhibition.[79] Many physiologists regarded this analogy as misplaced, or too speculative, or not even fruitful since it did not appear to translate into detailed experimental questions. Yet the analogies suggested by reference to "interference" retained a certain seductive quality.

A similar idea, developed independently, became well known in Britain through the work of the neurologist T. Lauder Brunton. His papers in 1874 and 1883 were also important in familiarizing English-speaking scientists with the actual term "inhibition." In 1874, Brunton, who, like Ferrier, was associated with research at the West Riding Lunatic Asylum at Wakefield, reported on his attempt to understand the inhibition of spinal reflexes and sympathetic action by reference to inhibitory centers. In a characteristically Victorian style, everyday psychology suggested inhibition as a topic, while experimental physiology suggested the means by which everyday subjects became science:

> Indeed it is this [inhibitory] rather than any other power which distinguishes the man from the boy, and its cultivation is one of the chief ends of education. . . . The first lesson that a child gets at school is one of inhibition; it is taught to sit still and restrain the movements which external impressions acting on its excitable nervous system prompt it to make. The whole education is, or ought to be a continuation and expansion of this lesson.[80]

Inhibition was a matter for daily education. But it was best understood through experiments on relatively isolated peripheral effects, such as the erection of the penis. Developing knowledge of these effects would then naturally return research to the hypothesis of central inhibitory centers in the brain, and this would, in turn, explain everyday psychological practices such as disciplining children.

Brunton had briefly attempted, using kittens and without success, to repeat Simonov's work in which he claimed to produce inhibition by electrically exciting a dog's brain. Brunton still concluded that, "although the experimental data regarding inhibitory centres in the brain is still defective, yet sufficient evidence has, I think, been adduced to warrant us to believe in their existence."[81] This "sufficient evidence" appears to have been Ferrier's claim that the frontal lobes did not possess a motor function, implying that their function perhaps involved the "higher" human capacity of inhibition.

In 1874, wanting to establish a common causal basis for all inhibitory effects, Brunton adapted loose ideas about the flow and transformation of nervous energy. As we have seen, McDougall carried these ideas into the 1920s. Brunton wrote,

> A violent emotion may only be restrained by opening a vent for it in some direction where it is not likely to do harm, but a feebler one may be suppressed altogether. I am inclined to think that this is effected through the agency of inhibitory centres in much the same way as reflex actions are arrested. . . . Certainly inhibition does involve great nervous waste. It is felt to be difficult, its continued exertion quickly fatigues, and it is one of the first powers to fail when the nervous system is depressed by exhaustion, disease, or the action of certain poisons.[82]

Psychological anecdote here became physiological metaphor, and the conclusion became embedded as a general organizational principle. Brunton portrayed mental action as being soothed by an outside excitation just as a reflex action was weakened by a second simultaneous excitation. "The soft touch of a woman's hand on her husband's brow seems not unfrequently to aid her words in clearing away painful impressions from his mind."[83] Woman, the civilizing influence, reappeared as the center of higher inhibitions.

In his later paper, Brunton described inhibitory organization as an interference effect rather than a property of particular centers: "inhibition and stimulation are merely relative conditions."[84] He suggested that there were direct and indirect pathways to motor centers in the spinal cord and that the route taken by an impulse was dependent on the strength of excitation. It was thus possible for a single stimulus to produce two (or more) impulses that interfered with each other in their effect on the motor centers. The interference of light waves provided a model. He thought that nerve conduction might indeed be likened to wave motion for a variety of reasons, among which were the results from Romanes's seminal work on elementary nervous propagation in the bell of the jellyfish. "We are justified, I think, by these experiments in considering that interference may occur in the nervous system, and that one part may exercise an interfering or inhibitory effect upon the other, which is constant under normal conditions, but will be modified when these conditions are altered."[85] As a medical researcher, Brunton was especially interested in the modification of interference conditions by drugs. He thus moved in his writing between clinical observation and what he supposed to be the mechanism of inhibition. This style contrasted with the detailed physiological and experimental reports characteristic of German-language researchers, who tended to be skeptical of the interference mechanism. Even Brunton himself did not consider interference to be the exclusive mechanism. He also referred to "diversion," a power to redirect excitations into different channels and hence to control movement, and he used an illustration that dramatically brought together the personal and the political.

> One of the most common of these [powers] is clenching the teeth, and it used to be a common practice in the army and navy for men to put a bullet between the teeth when they were being flogged, and at the end of the punishment this was usually completely flattened. . . . In children the motor channels into which diversion usually takes place are those connected with the respiratory system, and the sensory stimulus works itself off in loud yells.[86]

While Brunton argued that notions of interference and diversion could be tested physiologically by studying "the effect of alteration in the rapidity of nervous transmission upon inhibitory phenomena," it is clear that their appeal rested primarily on their explanatory potential for psychology.[87] He also believed that these notions could reconcile diverse observations on the excitability of reflexes and the effects of drugs. Physical analogy and psychological anecdote came together to generate thought about the processes involved.

Studying drug action was fast becoming a major research area in neurophysiology.[88] Substances such as strychnine or curare and anesthetics like chloroform had dramatic effects on nervous function, and these effects were often of considerable medical interest. The experimental investigation of the site and mechanism of chemical substances acting on animals became a major analytic tool, relating to the question of inhibition as well as to the study of nervous processes generally.

It was argued, for example, that quinine's effect in lowering reflex excitability provided the best evidence in support of Sechenov's inhibitory center.[89]

The metabolism theory of inhibition was both more general in its implications for physiology and more widely discussed than the interference theory. The theory or, more accurately, the group of related theories, subsumed excitation and inhibition as states within a metabolic cycle involving the building up and utilization of energy in the nervous system. This approach was initiated independently in the 1880s by Ewald Hering, generalizing his chemical assimilation-dissimilation theory of color perception, and by Walter Gaskell, arguing from knowledge of conditions of fatigue affecting the heartbeat.[90]

Gaskell, working at Cambridge in the 1880s in the laboratory established by Foster, investigated the mechanism of the heartbeat at great length and ultimately with great success. This research problem set the terms in which he commented on more general physiological questions, including inhibition. In his view, referring to the nerves of the heart, it was "in their case only [that we have] sufficient data on which to build a theory."[91] He proposed that the visceral nerves existed as pairs, the members of each pair having opposite assimilatory ("anabolic") and dissimilatory ("katabolic") effects. This implied that there must exist a distinct set of inhibitory nerves.

> The inhibitory nerves are of as fundamental importance in the economy of the body as the motor nerves. No evidence exists that the same nerve fibre is sometimes capable of acting as a motor nerve, sometimes as a nerve of inhibition, but on the contrary the latter nerves form a separate and complete nervous system subject to as definite anatomical and histological laws as the former.[92]

Gaskell further expected that this system of organization by double innervation would extend to skeletal muscle, though such innervation had not been discovered in vertebrates. This was the context of assumptions with which Sherrington, working in Gaskell's laboratory, began to study nervous organization. His argument that Gaskell's hypothesis could not apply to skeletal muscle led him to reformulate the question of inhibition as a function of central integration.[93]

The Viennese researcher Sigmund Exner also laid the theoretical basis for a treatment of the *Grundphänomene*, or ground phenomena, of psychological activity as a balance between excitatory and inhibitory physiological forces. He introduced the term *Bahnung* (later translated as "facilitation") to describe a nervous process that was the opposite of inhibition, whereby excitation increased the conductibility of a pathway.[94] He then used these ideas rather speculatively in constructing a model of nervous activity that might, at least in principle, explain psychological activity such as attention. Exner's erstwhile colleague, Freud, made a similar attempt at model construction, and for parallel reasons, in his "Project for a scientific psychology."[95]

In the hands of Max Verworn, a professor at Göttingen from 1900 to 1910 and in Bonn thereafter and sometimes regarded as the founder of general cellular physiology, this approach to inhibition was integrated into a comprehensive theory of the properties of living substance. Verworn initially believed that inhibition could be regarded as a particular aspect of general depressive metabolic processes. From the late 1890s, however, he was persuaded that experiments had failed to support E. Hering's view that inhibition correlated with assimilation processes in nerves, and he argued instead "that all the conditions necessary for the genesis of inhibition are realized in the refractory period" of nervous conduction.[96] He still held that inhibition was the consequence of general physiological processes, but he now believed that it was due to the period needed by a nerve for recovery after conduction rather than an assimilatory process. The German physiologist S. J. Meltzer, who emigrated to the United States, developed another version of the assimilation theory, based on the supposition that the increased use of one energy-consuming process (excitation) was necessarily in balance with the decreased use of another (inhibition). As he concluded, "All the actual phenomena of life . . . are the resultants of the two antagonistic forces; there is no absolute rest in a living part, and there is no action without any admixture of inhibition."[97]

These theories about living systems related somewhat uncomfortably to the exacting experimental practices that were the norm in neurophysiology during the last quarter of the nineteenth century. It was this experimental work that gave rise to the major alternative to assimilation theories, the refractory phase theories. These theories related more to what became a program of research on the nervous impulse than to the specific topic of inhibition.[98] Until the second decade of the twentieth century, questions about the nervous impulse and questions about inhibition were, at many points, interrelated, though continuing confusion about the mechanism of inhibition contrasted with progress in understanding the nervous impulse.

Refractory phase theories overlapped with interference and metabolism theories at many points, as, for example, Verworn's changing views made clear. They all shared something with Schiff's antilocalizing, dynamic view of nervous capacities, and they all sought to explain gross functional effects as the properties of nervous tissue. Schiff himself had reported that the rapid, repeated stimulation of a motor nerve weakened and finally led to the disappearance of the contraction of a muscle. Researchers on the heartbeat in the 1870s observed that the heart, after contraction, went through a period during which it was inexcitable (the "refractory period").[99] Beginning in 1885, the Russian physiologist N. E. Vvedenskii, who had been a student of Sechenov's in the late 1870s but who abjured his teacher's speculative bent, researched the effect that Schiff attributed to nervous fatigue.[100] Applying successive electrical stimuli to an isolated nerve-muscle preparation, Vvedenskii showed that it was either strong or rapidly recurring stimuli, rather than exhaustion, that caused a failure to transmit. The effect could be demonstrated most easily in partially narcotized nerve. He and others concluded that this phenomenon might be the physical basis of inhibition, and the phenomenon became known as "Wedensky inhibition." "If the nerve of a nerve-muscle preparation is excited by an interrupted induced current, an apparent inhibition takes place when the rapidity of interruption is increased beyond a critical point."[101] Vvedenskii went on to relate such phenomena to a general physiological theory of "parabiosis," which attributed excitation and inhibition to different phases of neuron activity. He concluded that inhibition could be compared to the narcosis of nerve and that this was induced by arriving impulses.[102] This approach continued to be important in the Soviet Union into the 1940s, in part characterizing what was sometimes known as the Vvedenskii-Ukhtomskii school.[103]

It was also possible to interpret Vvedenskii's results as due to something like the interference of overlapping stimuli or to the metabolic assimilation process in nerves following the dissimilation conduction process. Proponents of the latter approach to living systems, notably Verworn, elaborated these ideas into a fully fledged explanation for inhibition in general.[104] While this theory continued to have adherents into the 1920s, Verworn's publications were contemporary with Anglo-American researches that reinterpreted "Wedensky inhibition" in the light of the "all or none" principle of nervous conduction. Work by Keith Lucas, developed by E. D. Adrian, redescribed the refractory period in nerves as an effect of the conduction of impulses as discrete, uniform packets and of the time required to restore nerve to a conductible condition after each impulse. As Lucas and Adrian pointed out, there might be different forms of inhibition, "one depending on the extinction of impulses [Wedensky inhibition] and another on a general depression of function in the inhibited tissue, as in the action of the vagus on the heart."[105] It was the latter kind, physiologists began to conclude, that really deserved to be called inhibition.

The Lucas-Adrian approach to nervous conduction thus split from a physiological phenomenon associated with inhibition, the refractory phase of nerve, while leaving the question of functional inhibition where it was. The research tradition they exemplified, in addition, directed attention to the microprocesses of nerve action for a solution to the latter problem. This meant that the problem of inhibition became a problem in the chemical and electrical properties of nerves. By the mid-1920s, this was sharpening the focus on the synaptic junction between nerve cells (neurons) as the site of inhibition. Otto Loewi, working at the University of Graz, discovered that the vagal effect on the heart could be mimicked by a chemical, acetylcholine, and this and many other studies gradually persuaded scientists of the role chemical transmission played in carrying nervous impulses across the synapse.[106] It subsequently became possible to study chemical transmission in facilitating and inhibiting the reception of impulses by the postsynaptic neuron. Sherrington and his associates had already identified the motor neuron as "a collision-field for joint algebraically summed effect" of convergent excitatory and inhibitory systems.[107] Synaptic transmission thus became the locus for understanding nervous integration in physicochemical terms. The development of the electron microscope made it possible to picture the structure involved.

In this context, discussion about inhibition appeared to be restricted to a clearly circumscribed group of highly trained scientists. The scientists themselves certainly saw the matter this way. Their activity consisted of mastering and advancing detail in a language only they could comprehend. Their discourse, as they saw it, was constituted solely in and through experimental practice.

If we look at the wider context of their research activity, however, it is apparent that their discourse retained its broad nineteenth-century frame of reference even in the 1920s. It was this broader frame of reference that ultimately made it intellectually significant to investigate inhibition. Further, physiological psychologists like Fearing in the United States or Pavlov in the Soviet Union continued to use inhibition, understood as a physiological mechanism, to create theories that answered questions about the organization and psychological life of the organism as a whole. Reference to inhibition continued to make the fundamental point that a language of limitation as well as of excitation was intrinsic to understanding organization. This reference was often conveyed in a highly technical language, as in theories of synaptic transmission. But it was also a reference deeply embedded in moral representations of character, the economy, and society. To see the extent to which this was the case, it is necessary to return to the late nineteenth century, to experimental and medical psychology, and to the wider culture that looked to science for an understanding of order in human affairs.

PHYSIOLOGICAL AND EXPERIMENTAL PSYCHOLOGY

Experimental neurophysiology became an active and well-supported research specialty. It exemplified what in the English-speaking world later became known as "pure science," the intention to pursue knowledge for its own sake. Yet, as I have argued, the research—however specialized—never completely detached itself from open-ended psychological matters. Sechenov or Heidenhain addressed questions to the internal workings of the central nervous system which were weighted with psychological implications. Even causal theories of inhibitory processes, such as "parabiosis" (Vvedenskii) or synaptic transmission (Sherrington), drew on concepts of organization that were as indebted to psychology as they were to physiology. While there was increasing institutional separation of research specialties in the late nineteenth century, many reflective writers still sensed that physiological and psychological research was interrelated.

The division between what was properly a physiological and what was properly a psychological subject was contested. There was no consensus. It appeared that dividing up topics in one way implied materialism, while dividing it up in another way implied idealism. Any attempt to settle the issue seemed to lead into a philosophical, and often an emotional, quagmire. In these circumstances, many scientists adopted a pragmatic modus vivendi, accepting the conventions of a particular research tradition and taking the philosophical legitimacy of that tradition for granted. They then variously conceded or denied the legitimacy of other traditions, when they did not actually ignore them. Many scientists also worked as if all significant questions were empirical in form, thus making the question of the relations between physiology and psychology a matter of the relations between two bodies of empirical knowledge. The question could therefore safely be left to the future progress of empirical science, and it did not make problematic their current practices. Whether such assumptions were philosophically justified is, of course, another issue.

Psychology has been a substantial and distinct academic natural science discipline in Europe only since the 1940s. It had some disciplinary standing earlier, on a large scale in the United States and, in diverse ways, on a much smaller scale elsewhere.[108] It has been common to portray psychology as first achieving disciplinary status through a double separation, detaching experimental psychological methods from philosophical inquiry in one direction and differentiating psychological from physiological questions in another. This occurred in Germany between about 1860 and about 1880. Young English-speaking scientists, having acquired postgraduate training in Germany, then transferred the new discipline to North America. There is now a rich historical literature about these events; two points are especially relevant. First, though it was German-speaking academics who contributed most to constructing experimental psychological methods, they did not thereby construct an institutionally separate discipline. Most German researchers engaged in experimental psychology continued to hold appointments in philosophy well into the twentieth century. The academic discipline of psychology, therefore, first had a separate social existence, in the 1890s, in North America. Second, the North American discipline reflected distinctive, local intellectual and social characteristics. The new North American experimental psychologists greatly altered what they had acquired from Germany: their psychology was much more positivist in character, and, in response to its patrons' expectations, it sought to become a practical mode of thinking about the individual's relation to society, especially in the realm of education.[109] What did transfer from the German to the American setting was an experimental ethos, modeled on the natural sciences and hailed as the realization of objective methods in studying psychological phenomena. In Germany, the experimentalists had to compete with other groups, each claiming the means to achieve rational understanding in psychology, and they had to struggle to obtain a lasting position. In North America, they achieved dominance.

German and American researchers who advocated experimental methods also argued for a distinctive subject. But there was considerable disagreement about what it was that psychologists should study and what made psychology distinctive. Psychologists were in an especially awkward position in relation to the established experimental discipline of physiology, which had inspired many of the experimental techniques of the new psychology. Experimental psychologists generally rejected the reductionist aims of some earlier proponents of a physiological psychology, claiming instead that psychology had its own distinctive subject matter: mental content, language, behavior, or whatever. It was obvious, however, that something had to be said about this subject matter's relation to the body. Further, the historical dependence of technique on physiology, a shared training and research ethos, and the quest for social credibility and authority as a new natural science ensured that the question of psychology's relation to physiology remained absolutely central. Many reflective observers also accepted that an answer to this question was needed if there was to be any coherent solution to philosophical disputes about the nature of psychological knowledge.

The complex and unsettled relations between physiology and the new psychology are especially evident in the history of a term like "inhibition" which had both physiological and psychological meaning. "Inhibition" was a common term in the new psychology, and this requires some discussion. It was noted that this usage was confused and vague. The term sometimes referred to a specific effect comparable to physiological inhibition, and it sometimes referred generally to opposition. "In fact, inhibition seems to be a general term for the psychologist. He has used it to signify all kinds of opposition."[110] The writer of this complaint in 1899, the American psychologist B. B. Breese, analyzed critically five types of psychological usage: "inhibition as an expression of the power which ideas, as such, exert upon each other"; "as obstructive association"; "as logical contradiction"; "as a mode of the will's activity"; and "as a psychophysical phenomenon."[111] He persuasively rejected the first for hypostasizing ideas, the second as an unnecessary and unwarranted extension of the powers of association, the third as simply a misuse of language, and the fourth as actually referring to motor adjustment. Thus, he concluded, "I am satisfied that its use in psychology should be confined to psychophysical phenomena. . . . Almost universally the instances of inhibition cited . . . involve definite bodily activities, either within the field of sense perception or bodily movements."[112]

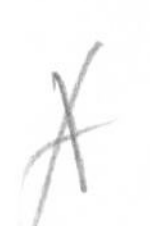

Breese's strictures were not taken to heart. Reference to inhibition in psychology, throughout the nineteenth century and into the twentieth century, involved argument by analogy from physiological or physical processes to psychological ones, just as belief in the arresting power of the will over the body encouraged argument in the opposite direction. Medical psychology, in particular, perpetuated the richly evaluative connotations of the term, in interaction with both physiology and experimental psychology. To understand the adoption of inhibition as a term in scientific psychology as it developed in Germany and North America, it is illuminating first to consider the situation in Britain and, to a lesser extent, in France. This will allow me to bring out the full range of discussions concerning psychological control. To tell the story of inhibition is to weave together many different strands and not to unwind a chronological thread.

Experimental psychology hardly existed in Britain in the nineteenth century, though there were attempts to imitate the Germans right at the end of the century.[113] Association psychology, which was a deductive rather than an empirical way of thought, occupied the place of a scientific psychology in intellectual debate. Its two great Victorian exponents, Spencer and Bain, greatly enriched its content, the former by restating it in evolutionary terms and the latter by bringing it into constructive relation with knowledge of the nervous system and by equipping it with a new theory of action. Their work later made a significant theoretical contribution to the new "functionalist" psychology in North America.[114]

Bain, who is sometimes said to have written the first specifically *psychological* volumes in English, restated the associationist principle that the order in mental content reflected the order (contiguity and similarity) of sensations in experience.[115] He simply did not refer to possible dynamic relations between conscious contents in the manner of Herbart or Wundt, who explained order by reference to one idea's presence excluding another's. Bain did not use the word "inhibition" in either a physiological or a psychological context. Nevertheless, there was an important sense in which Bain did deploy a concept comparable to inhibition. He rejected the view that the activity known as "the will" was the product of a mental faculty, arguing instead that it was the indirect consequence of motives, that is, feelings of pleasure or pain, associated with sensations, thoughts, movements, or other feelings. Bain supposed that such indirect action often followed from attention, a phenomenon he sometimes described as if it were a faculty, though he intended the description to refer to a product of association between feelings and thoughts. The relevant point is that Bain referred to attention causing particular thoughts or feelings as a power to "suppress" or "overpower" other thoughts or feelings.[116] This reflected a conventional Victorian view of attention, and Bain was also conventional in building attention into a moralistic psychology of individual development and conduct. It was argued that attending to one complex of associations rather than another was a basic "volitional" means by which the individual took control over his or her life, forming sound habits and exchanging an instant pleasure for the satisfaction of the long-term good.[117]

Bain treated attention as both a positive and a negative process—positive in making possible certain abilities (e.g., remembering) and negative in controlling other activities (e.g., suppressing instincts). His treatment was evaluative in a moral sense as well as descriptive in a psychological sense, and Bain did not distinguish these modes of expression. He took for granted a moral and psychological economy, supposing that the energy available to a person could be directed one way rather than another, and that moral habits formed through different outlets competing for this energy. For example, Bain referred to the way children slowly acquire steady work habits in the face of incoming sensations:

> We have to be put under training to resist those various solicitations [of sensation], and to keep the mind as steadily fixed upon the work in hand as if they did not happen. The process here consists in becoming indifferent to what at the outset caused pleasure or pain. We can never be free from impressions of touch, but we contract the habit of inattention to them. The occupation of the mind upon things foreign draws off the currents of power from the tactile susceptibility.[118]

He therefore advocated the constant exercise of the thinking mind to build up habits that reduce the energy of our emotional nature. "The originally powerful intellect, by asserting its own exercise, more and more deepens the penury of the emotional nature."[119]

The moralistic setting fostered representations of the power and desirability of one kind of mental process existing at the expense of another. British psychology was a study preparatory to ethics, and it therefore emphasized cultivating good habits, the conflict of motives, and the control of appetites and instincts. The word "inhibition" later described such control. Beyond this, Bain's language—like the language of inhibition—encoded a hierarchical psychological dynamics that clearly derived from social values. Bain provided a charming example:

> Take the practice of regular early rising. Here we have, on the one hand, the volitional solicitations of a massive indulgence, and on the other, the stimulus of prudential volition as regards the collective interests of life. . . . What

> the individual has had to act so many times in one way, brings on a current of nervous power, confirming the victorious, and sapping the vanquished, impulse.[120]

He described habits of mind and body as the individualized and internalized conventions of social order. In developing habits, one chain of associations became "checked" or "overborne" or "curtailed" by another.

Though Bain argued that psychology had to be brought into relation with physiology if it were to sustain its claim to be a science, he contributed nothing to working out this relation at the level of empirical detail. He provided no physiological analogues for the conflict of motives and the formation of moral habits. It was Carpenter who attempted this in Britain. Carpenter, who was not an associationist, since he believed that the will was a real agency in mental processes, elevated attention to the high position where it mediated mental purpose in human existence. As discussed earlier, Carpenter also described a hierarchy of nervous levels, characterizing reflexes at each level as the basis for organized functions. Attention, in his writings, referred to mental activity causing one idea or feeling rather than another to control bodily life by energizing one reflex system rather than another. This moral psychology was comparable to Bain's in many ways, and Carpenter too emphasized that moral character depended on the cultivation of right habits. Building habits involved embedding particular patterns of reflex processes (or, in his words, "ideo-motor" actions) into the nervous substrata of mind. Carpenter did not use the term "inhibition" either, but he did contribute to the discourse that was to provide a ready home for this term.[121] Victorian conceptions of mental and moral order presupposed a selective quality in human character, a quality produced by one action reciprocally suppressing another. German experimental psychology, as it developed, attempted to represent such assumptions as the precisely observable interrelations of the elements in mental contents.

Bain, and Spencer, also noted the way that the presence of one kind of mental element sometimes lessened the strength of another and thus affected associative links. Spencer referred, for example, to what he called "the antagonism" of current and remembered feeling. It indicated the important role that physical models had in his account of psychological processes that he attributed this phenomenon to the capacity of nerves to sustain only one discharge at a time.[122] Bain referred to the power of positive association being reduced both by feelings and by what he called "obstructive associations": in the former, "in minds very susceptible to emotion, the more purely intellectual bonds of association are perpetually combined and modified by connections with feeling";[123] in the latter, the mechanical interaction of competing mental elements produced "the distracting influence of too many ideas."

> The principle of compound association necessarily involves this efficacy to obstruct. If two ideas, by both pointing to a third, constitute a prevailing bond of restoration [of a memory], it must likewise happen that if these two present ideas point in opposite directions, they will be liable to neutralize one another's efficacy. The power of assisting implies the power of resisting.[124]

Building on an argument developed by the Scottish philosopher, William Hamilton, that there was a necessary antagonism between sensation and perception, Spencer turned the relational contrast generated by successive sensations into a precondition for consciousness at all. "Consciousness of the changes [i.e., perception] is an antagonism with consciousness of the states [i.e., sensation] between which they occur. So that perception and sensation are, as it were, ever tending to exclude each other, but, never succeeding. Indeed, consciousness continues only in virtue of this conflict."[125] Spencer argued that consciousness necessarily had a relational composition and that the source of this composition lay in the contrast between one sensation and the next. Change between sensations correlated with physical change. He then attempted to derive from this a priori argument all the complex phenomena of mental life. This derivation presupposed the "antagonism" of mental elements. One element's resistance to another established the contrast of sensation that was the foundation of thought and the contrast of feeling that was the foundation of emotion. Similarly, sensory contrast was also the ultimate origin of the subjective experience known as volition:

> When, after the reception of one of the more complex impressions, the appropriate motor changes become nascent, but are prevented from passing into immediate action by the antagonism of certain other nascent motor changes appropriate to some nearly allied impression; [then] there is constituted a state of consciousness which, when it finally issues in action, displays what we term volition.[126]

Spencer's analysis did not refer to anything that might properly be called inhibition. Nevertheless, when he described the antagonistic or competing presence of different mental elements as the stuff from which mental life was generated, he was recognizably addressing the same issues as German psychologists when they sought—drawing on the concept of *Hemmung*—to determine the pattern of conscious contents.

Bain and Spencer were certainly not interested only in esoteric psychological questions, as sometimes appeared to be the case with the German experimentalists. Like their mentor John Stuart Mill, they both discussed psychology as a foundation for ethics, and ethics and psychology intertwined in practical theories of human character and individuality.[127] Spencer's account of the antagonism between mental elements in complex psychological processes therefore, for example, also provided him with a ready means for classifying human types. His classification incorporated conventional discriminatory values into what he thought were empirical descriptions. According to Spencer, associative structures in the mind and brain in lower human types, such as savages or women, were relatively simple. Sensation or feeling was likely to result in action without much antagonism in such people. In higher types, by contrast, complex associative patterns made antagonism to the direct production of action more likely. Delay in action characterized the rational man.

> The brain of the uncultivated man as compared to that of the cultivated man, must be one in which the routes taken by nervous discharges are less numerous, less involved, less varied in the resistance they offer—one, therefore, in which the number of ideas that can follow a given antecedent is smaller, and the degrees of strength with which they can present themselves are fewer—one, therefore, in which the possibilities of thought are more limited, and the balancing between alternative conclusions less easy.[128]

The hallmarks of the cultivated man were antagonism between associative links, the contrast of thought and feeling, and reflective rather than spontaneous action. Spencer's politics was a sustained assault on the unreflective hope that government could solve problems. He embedded in the concept of "antagonism" between mental elements the defining characteristics of what he admired in Victorian sensibility, the psychology of individual control and the politics of self-help, and this in turn provided a classification for different types of human beings. "Antagonism" was virtually the foundation for the moral life.

British empiricist psychology became well known in French progressive circles through the writings of Hippolyte Taine and Ribot.[129] Ribot, especially, borrowed extensively to publicize a nonidealist, non-Catholic analysis of mind and character. Though neither original nor deep, Ribot's many publications in the last quarter of the century brought together the findings of experimental neurophysiology, empiricist psychology, and clinical neurology, making naturalistic psychology into a challenging and viable program with implications for education, the care of the insane, criminals, and other social questions. He relied significantly on inhibition, especially when outlining his scientific approach to the key psychological topics of attention and volition. While conceding that the mechanism of attention was obscure, Ribot was in no doubt that "the whole problem consists in this very power of inhibition, of retention," and that an understanding of attention would therefore come from physiology.[130] He thought of inhibition as a general nervous property, propagated by nerves at the same time as excitation, a view that experiments on nerve conduction appeared to confirm. "On this hypothesis, then, every excitation would determine in the nervous substance two modifications, the one positive and the other negative: a tendency to activity on the one side, and a tendency to the inhibition of this activity on the other side."[131] These physiological properties, in Ribot's view, were the vehicle for psychological volition. Conscious volition or effort was the mental awareness that accompanied the resolution of conflict between alternative associative links and their corresponding conclusion in action. The will was "a power of arrestation, or, in the language of physiology, an *inhibitive* power." Effort "always occurs when two groups of antagonistic tendencies are struggling each to supplant the other."[132]

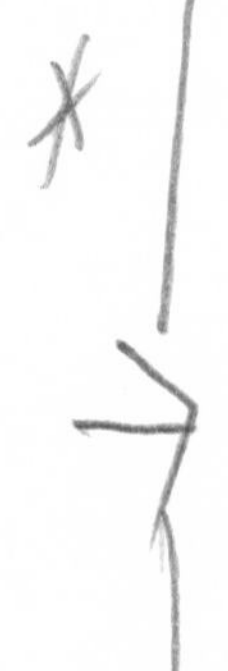

Ribot's view of the will was developmental, not static: inculcating the power of attention, making it possible for one train of ideas to dominate another, was therefore the crucial step in socializing the child. Children were thoughtlessly active without this power. "Attention is the momentary inhibition, to the exclusive benefit of a single state, of this perpetual progression [of ideas]."[133] Teachers should therefore understand the physiological processes of inhibition if they were to hold the key to education. Ribot here followed Preyer, the influential German writer on child development (and investigator of animal hypnotism), who had voiced similar views. Voluntary inhibition and character required training, beginning with "the very humble form of inhibition of natural evacuations."[134] When training failed to establish inhibition, then the child was simply not educable.

In Britain, the long-standing but always controversial clinical category of "moral insanity"—a state in which the mental incapacity was believed to lie wholly in the emotional or volitional faculties—was also discussed as a failure of inhibition. The Edinburgh psychiatrist Thomas S. Clouston taught medical students that insanities demonstrating incapacity of will could be classified as "states of defective inhibition." He included such forms as erotomania and homicidal impulse, as well as moral insanity, under this heading.

> I knew one such case (F.K.), who was continually breaking every commandment of the decalogue. He went through a form of marriage with four women, to each of the three last having told that he was unmarried, and I just saved the fifth by a few hours from going through a form of marriage with him! Several members of his family had been insane, and others subject to various neuroses. He took his heredity out in immorality.[135]

This was a lack of inhibition with a vengeance. By the end of the century, prison medical officers were describing repeat offenders in similar terms. There appeared to be a class of mentally inadequate prisoners who were not educable by punishment.[136] Similarly in France, recidivism became a prominent political issue in the 1880s and 1890s, and Ribot and others linked the phenomenon to the psychological incapacity of individuals to respond to punishment. "If, in spite of repeated menaces, the inhibition be not produced, the individual is little or not at all educable in this respect."[137] It was even suggested that a scientific understanding of inhibition might provide the courts with an objective definition of criminal responsibility, since a measurable loss of inhibition implied a measurable loss of responsibility.[138]

Ribot edited the *Revue philosophique*, an influential organ advocating a naturalistic approach to philosophical and social questions in the Third Republic. Ribot also advised Alfred Binet early in his career, and Binet went on to play an important part in establishing experimental psychology in France and in founding *L'année psychologique* in 1895. Binet, like Ribot, initially accepted a strict associationism, but his work on hypnotism gradually led him to argue for the role of a synthetic, coordinating mental power that could not have an origin in associations.[139] Binet believed that experiments on perception showed that suggestion affected hypnotized subjects partly by causing them not to see. He referred to this as an example of induced inhibition: "Provisionally one could surmise that . . . the experimenter induces in the subject a mental impression that has an inhibitory effect on one of his sensory or motor functions."[140] Such an effect, he argued, could not be the product of association. Experiments illustrated the general phenomenon of antagonism between images (such as those that might be suggested by a hypnotist) and sensations, or between different images, or between two simultaneous perceptions.[141] Though he acknowledged that antagonism of this character was not strictly analogous to the interaction referred to by physiological inhibition, Binet suggested nevertheless that it was properly called psychological inhibition.

F. Paulhan was another French writer on psychology who, like Ribot, elevated inhibition to a fundamental position. He wrote for a general audience, and his work may have helped create familiarity with inhibition as a psychological term in both France and Italy. Acknowledging that Brown-Séquard had named physiological inhibition, Paulhan described analogous psychological phenomena in perception, judgment, emotion, and so forth, outlining what he called "the laws of systematic inhibition." He defined inhibition as "a mental fact which tends to prevent the occurrence . . . of the elements which are not susceptible of being united for a common end."[142] Inhibition was thus the systematic opposite of association.

Bain's, Spencer's, and Ribot's neuropsychologies were derivative and soon dated. Similar associationist principles of analysis were also used, however, by researchers who did claim originality in the brain sciences. Meynert, for example, was a prominent creator of neurophysiological analogues for associative psychological processes. The result was a speculative and stylistically obtuse discussion of brain functions, in which one can observe him relating psychological commonplaces, such as the inverse relation between thought and sensory awareness, as physiological truths. He cited this relation to justify a belief in the cortical inhibition of lower centers:

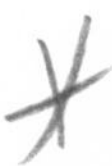

> The greater the cortical excitation following upon the independent revival of cortical memories and of associations, and upon the exercise of thought, the more the influence of the subcortical centres will be diminished. *This is cortical inhibition.* I wish at this juncture to call particular attention to the incommensurability of cortical reminiscences with sensory perceptions.[143]

It would be hard to find a more concise illustration of the power of esoteric language to reexpress the ordinary and thereby to clothe values in the authority of science. Meynert literally embodied values.

Tightly focused research in experimental psychology became a novel feature of academic life in the late nineteenth century. With some exceptions, notably in the United States, however, there was little institutional support for such work in non–German-speaking countries until the new century. Many writers referred to "psychology" as a subject, but when they did so, they covered a nebulous group of interests and investigative methods. Their subject continued to be accessible to an educated but nonspecialist audience. This body of work, exemplified by Paulhan, referred frequently to inhibition and, in doing so, perpetuated long-standing views about the economy and hierarchy of psychological processes and about the nature of instincts, attention, emotion, and thought in determining the differences between humans and animals and between different human types.[144] Reference to inhibition enriched the representation of both control and difference, as the following examples illustrate.

Popular writers on science and medicine found in the physiology of inhibition a new way to describe the old truth that health depended on harmony and balance. A writer on hypnotism in the English *Fortnightly Review* commented that "all the higher manifestations of mind are correlatives of the harmonious co-operation of numerous brain elements."[145] Inhibition between the parts of the brain was essential to this harmony: it is "at the root of the higher exercise of our faculties. . . . Thus, when we say that anger or fear paralyses, we allude in very accurate language to the inhibitory influence which powerful emotion exercises upon the other cerebral functions."[146] The physiological view, common in the 1830s and 1840s, that the higher human accomplishments depended on suppressing those movements that tended to follow sensation or emotion, reappeared at the end of the century. Thus, Max Nordau, in his obsessive study, *Degeneration*, explained that artistic expression was a subtle form of psychological imitation and that imitation was the nervous system's natural tendency to discharge excitation in movement. Consequently, "if every representation be not embodied in perceptible movement, the cause is to be traced to the action of the inhibitive mechanism of the brain, which does not permit every representation at once to set the muscles into activity." It followed that "healthy men" were "possessed of well-working inhibitory mechanism."[147] When inhibition was inadequate, art held out a means of self-deliverance from emotion.

Such views on mental economy persisted well into the twentieth century. McDougall's extensively republished books, especially *An Introduction to Social Psychology* (1908), which attempted to lay the foundations for social analysis with an account of human instincts and character, continued to use a model of dynamic energies to analyze psychological processes. He wrote that the effective integration of a person's character hinged on inhibition, that is, on the sublimation of diverse energies to a common purpose. Inhibition, he stated, always involved the positive expenditure of energy. "We inhibit our output of energy in one direction, along one line of action, by adopting another line of action . . . and by concentrating our energies along that line, as when, under sudden pain, we grind our teeth and clench our fists in order to inhibit the impulse to cry out."[148] Such beliefs may well have played a significant part in the 1920s in "popularizing" psychology and, more specifically, Freudian "sublimation." If so, then the question of popularization becomes in part a challenge to understand the complex metaphorical and evaluative interplay between dynamic economic beliefs in psychological and political spheres.

As was discussed in the context of causal accounts of inhibition, McDougall's more specialist papers combined popular psychology and physiological reference in exactly the same way. He consistently regarded inhibition as a process involving nervous energy draining away from an excitable part. Thus, he attributed psychological attention to "reciprocal inhibition," a process in which excitation in one reflex arc in the brain decreased energy in other areas. He therefore argued that sensory attention was not functionally restricted to the motor side of nervous activity, as some experimental psychologists were arguing.[149]

Natural history and evolutionary theory came together in the second half of the nineteenth century to create a relatively systematic approach to animal and human instincts. This then became an important part of North American experimental psychology, contributing to its characteristic functionalist and behaviorist orientation. Animal instinct, learning, and attention proved to be a rich vein for exploitation by new experimental techniques. Such research elaborated ways of talking about psychological processes that referred frequently to inhibition as the competitive action of different elements. This psychological language proved persistent.

It may well have been the philosophical writer and vice-chancellor of Bristol University, C. Lloyd Morgan, who introduced the term "inhibition" into the study of animal learning. His study of trial and error learning in chicks described movements that successfully obtained food as "reinforced" and those that were unsuccessful as "inhibited." This was congruent with what was known about human learning.

> What we term the control over our activities is gained in and through the conscious reinforcement of those modes of response which are successful, and the inhibition of those modes of response which are unsuccessful. The successful response is repeated because of the satisfaction it gives; the unsuccessful response fails to give satisfaction, and is not repeated.[150]

This was the pleasure-pain principle of utilitarian theory restated in terms of experimentally observable variables. The subsequent attempt completely to eliminate the subjective, mental element of "satisfaction" in the principle was to create behaviorism. Morgan himself, however, attempted to understand how mechanical trial and error learning had evolved into the "higher" human abilities. Having made it clear that "the physiological faculty on which [suppression of action] is based is inhibition," he suggested that this might relate to intelligence.[151] He defined intelligence: "the ability to perform acts in special adaptation to special circumstances, the power of exercising individual choice between contradictory promptings, and the individuality or originality manifested in dealing with the complex conditions of an ever-changing environment."[152] Intelligence, on this definition, became possible in animals when inhibition interrupted the automatic flow from stimulus to perception to emotion and to fulfillment in action. Suspending action permitted other processes, those we call thought, to inform the achievement of an action. "Through inhibition, through the suppression or postponement of action, there has been rendered possible that reverberation among the nervous processes of the brain which is the physiological concomitant of aesthetic and conceptual thought."[153] Morgan thus turned to physiological inhibition as the key mechanism in the evolution of the higher psychological abilities and ultimately of volition itself. "I believe that volition is intimately bound up and associated with inhibition. I go so far as to say that, without inhibition, volition properly so called has no existence."[154]

A committed evolutionist like Morgan thus drew on the meanings of inhibition to mediate between the world of automatic animal behavior and volitional human conduct. The same meanings tempted others into a comparable search for reconciliation between the new physiological psychology and idealist belief in human freedom. The American philosopher James H. Hyslop accepted that "modern psychology considers such [reflex] action as the original type of all our later modes of activity."[155] Action based on conscious deliberation therefore depended on the existence of some physiological mechanism for holding up the reflexes. Inhibition was such a mechanism. "Inhibition is thus an antagonistic force against the direct agency of stimuli and sensations to produce muscular activity, and thus establishes more or less of the equipoise necessary for deliberation and the formation of ideational motives."[156] Hyslop followed the common Victorian view that it was the person who had cultivated habits of calm reflection, rather than the impulsive person, who was subject to immediate impressions, who acted freely, that is, deliberately. "Freedom is proportioned to the extent to which the higher forms of consciousness inhibit the causal agency of the lower forms."[157]

These strands, along with many others, were woven together by William James in his tapestry, *The Principles of Psychology* (1890). James attempted to create a seamless whole out of German experimental psychology, neurophysiology, the natural history of animal and human action, and a philosophical and evolutionary approach to mind. The strands unraveled even in his own work, and few other psychologists contemplated anything so grand. North American scientists increasingly became specialists in neurophysiology, animal behavior studies, pedagogical techniques, or whatever. James, for his part, touched on inhibition in several different connections.

Referring back, like Morgan, to studies of instinct by Douglas Spalding and Romanes, James emphasized that the instincts were not as immutable as they had sometimes been taken to be. Indeed, he thought that some flexibility in instinctive actions was a necessary consequence of their evolutionary origin. He believed that instinctive behavior could be modified by habit and, in this context, referred to "the law of inhibition of instincts by habit." "A habit, once grafted on the instinctive tendency, restricts the range of the tendency itself."[158] He illustrated what he meant with a coy comment on the sexual instinct in Boston life: "The possession of homes and wives of our own makes us strangely insensible to the charms of those of other people."[159] James also constructed a theory of learning to account for "the education of the will," a process in which habit formation mediated between instinctive and consciously chosen actions. He argued, significantly on a priori grounds, that this education involved training in inhibiting, as much as exciting, movements: ordered life was possible only if movements were ended as well as started. "We should all be cataleptics and never stop a muscular contraction once begun, were it not that other processes simultaneously going on inhibit the contraction. Inhibition is therefore not an occasional accident; it is an essential and unremitting element of our cerebral life."[160]

James described this requirement for the achievement of control in neurophysiological as well as psychological terms. If the organism was "a machine for converting stimuli into actions," then stimuli must inhibit as well as excite if the resultant actions were to have a shape.

> The *effect* of the wave [of impressions] through the centres may, however, often be to interfere with processes, and to diminish tensions already existing there; and the outward consequences of such inhibitions may be the arrest of discharges from the inhibited regions and the checking of bodily activities already in occurrence. When this happens it probably is like the draining or siphoning of certain channels by currents flowing through others.[161]

Once again, inhibition was constituted through the metaphor of a closed system of energies, activity in one place reducing activity elsewhere, and interaction making for organization. The metaphor fostered psychological and physiological speculation alike. Thus, James linked inhibition to feelings of displeasure: "The displeasure seems to dampen the activities. The psychic side of the phenomenon thus seems, somewhat like the applause or hissing at a spectacle, to be an encouraging or adverse *comment* on what the machinery brings forth."[162]

Fellow psychologists did not always approve of playing fast and loose with the concept of inhibition in this way. There were attempts to give the term precise content, either through studying perception and attention experimentally or by tying psychological knowledge to the physiological mechanisms of inhibition. Thus, Breese argued that "it is within this field of psycho-physiology that the conception of inhibition has meaning from the psychological point of view."[163] This implied that the displacement of one mental element by another should be treated as the consequence of the *physical* necessities he thought it really was. Breese felt that the imagery should not be allowed to become detached from its roots. To study inhibition, he therefore began extended research into binocular rivalry in visual perception. Nevertheless, even Breese was tempted into discussing wider implications when he stressed the relationship between motor activity and consciousness. Developing a point of educational significance, he argued that suppressing motor activity suppressed conscious processes: for example, inhibiting word articulation inhibited learning words. Claims like this returned the meanings of inhibition to the sociopsychological setting where they had originated. Whatever its ideals concerning rigor, the new psychology in America remained closely tied to the educational purposes that justified its institutional support.

North American psychology at the end of the century was already an institutionalized discipline. It had taken and adapted experimental techniques and scientific training from Germany and an empiricist and evolutionary outlook from Britain. By contrast, in Germany, the subject did not have equivalent disciplinary standing, and in Britain, it simply did not exist. The German case was complex since there were competing claims about what scientific psychology should be, as well as a pressing need to define and defend the new experimentalism against its philosophical critics. Wundt's work stood out as a relatively comprehensive, and certainly forcefully presented, discussion of the new psychology, but it was not alone or uncontested. As described earlier, his program involved drawing complex comparisons between physiological inhibition and "apperceptive" psychological activity. The historical work has not been done which would enable us to describe in detail the reception of his theories or the subsequent utilization of inhibition in experimental psychology. One example may be cited. G. E. Müller, a professor at Göttingen, was a second major influence on the institutionalization of experimental technique in psychological research. Unlike Wundt, however, he did not attempt to create a comprehensive new philosophy incorporating objective psychological methods. Following Hermann Ebbinghaus's pioneering and still famous study of memory in the 1880s, Müller and his student A. Pilzecker studied some related processes that Ebbinghaus had ignored which concerned forgetting or difficulties in memorization brought about by interaction between memorization and other learning activities. To explain their results, Müller and Pilzecker introduced a parameter in memorization that they called "interference."[164] They then classified the different modes of interference as different types of psychological inhibitory processes.

Inhibition was generally available as a relational term for researchers exploring the organization of mental content. Sechenov casually observed that the pain of placing one's hand in acid was diminished by being simultaneously tickled.[165] Exner devised optical experiments to illustrate sensory inhibition or the suppression of one sensation by another. He then systematically analyzed attention in terms of inhibitory and facilitatory physiological analogues.[166] The new experimentalists took for granted the reality of inhibition in the achievement of organized states. The Austrian physician Heinrich Obersteiner commented, "It appears . . . that in every mental act, whether it be in the domain of sensation, volition, or intellect, there is seen an inhibitory power, essentially the same in all cases. This inhibitory power on which depends all consecutive mental action, is Attention."[167] As he indicated, the question of mental order was intimately bound up with interest in attention, and this linked German experimentalists and the British, French, and North American empiricists. Further, the very idea of attention seemed to presuppose an inhibitory relationship between one mental activity and another.

Descriptions of competitive interaction between mental elements in forming mental content ran through the literature from Herbart to Wundt, Spencer, and the later North American experimentalists. This history became bound up with the topic of attention and with the assumption that the higher mental processes, in some way, involved a physiological process suspending the translation of excitations into movement. Wundt and the other students of sensory psychophysiology pioneered the attempt to reconstruct these questions in experimental terms. Their programs were continued into the twentieth century. G. Heymans, who was an important influence on the development of academic psychology in the Netherlands, conducted an extended experimental investigation into sensory attention. He concluded that there was a general law correlating the power of a stimulus to inhibit another stimulus and its intensity.[168] Other researchers used the study of reaction time, the variation in speed of response under different conditions, as another would-be objective route into these issues.[169] Psychologists in the United States quickly found applications in education and in psychotherapy for the results of studies on perception and attention. "Progressive relaxation" technique, for example, attempted to utilize the power of one sensory mode to inhibit another as a means to cope with stress.[170]

Inhibition, in studies concerned with perception, attention, child development, and animal behavior, thus became a common feature in experimental psychology in the period before World War I. It proved invaluable in many different settings since in each it referred to the constructive organization of wholes through the competitive interrelations of parts. At the same time, it held together different areas of research through their representation in a common language. Last, this language sustained contact between technical and nontechnical approaches to order and control within the person, not an unimportant matter in North America where the technical subject had been funded on the promise that it would bring benefits to practical questions. This broad situation has not changed, and reference to inhibition remains common and largely unremarked in academic psychology. We may surmise that this is for the very same reasons that the term became common scientific currency in the nineteenth century. This discussion therefore concludes with an indication of the ways in which inhibition continued in the language used by psychologists after World War I.

Psychologists like Breese were not always happy with the looseness of the term, though it is striking that such criticisms did not dissuade researchers from using it. In a review of inhibition in the 1920s, it was Dodge's turn to argue that if psychologists were to use the term, then they must tie their work to investigations of inhibition's neural basis. As a psychologist, he defined inhibition as "reaction decrement," the reduction of a response by the introduction of a second stimulus in a stimulus-response couple. As a physiological psychologist, however, he believed that research on the topic should bring together the psychological with the physiological meanings of the term. As forms of inhibition, he listed "peripheral terminal inhibition, refractory phase decrement, voluntarily decreased tonus, rivalry and competition, inhibition of weaker by stronger stimuli (Heymans' Law), anode block, reciprocal inhibition of antagonistic muscles (Sherrington), protracted inhibition consequent to frequent stimulation."[171] The supposed comparability of all these phenomena suggested to him that inhibition must be a perfectly general feature, a necessary condition in the nervous system for the ordered interaction of parts within a whole. Dodge implied critically that inhibition had become a term providing merely the appearance of an explanation for the ordering of mental content. In his view, without an elucidation of inhibition's neural basis, utilizing the term to explain attention and other psychological processes just restated the problem. Perhaps his criticisms were aimed at popularizers of psychology like A. A. Roback, who made a very loose and highly normative category, which he called inhibition, fundamental to the analysis of character. "If the question of the seat of character is asked, we must look for the answer in the *direction of the fundamental condition of general inhibition and in specific phases of intelligence*."[172]

Dodge's position, which gave explanatory priority to physiological psychology, was opposed to the behaviorists, who believed that the search for explanation at the level of observable psychological events, that is, stimulus-response relations, offered better prospects.[173] Behaviorism was never a coherent school, even in the United States, but by 1930, behaviorist methods made up a very considerable research investment, focusing on animal learning. Whatever the technical complexities of learning theory, such research remained subservient to a broader vision stressing psychology's contribution to an ordering of human affairs. The president of the American Psychological Association in 1931, Walter S. Hunter, indicated as much when he characterized his discipline in the following terms: "Psychology seeks to describe and explain, to predict and control, the extrinsic behavior of the organism to an external environment which is predominantly social."[174] As in the 1890s, education remained the area where technical innovation and practical application came together most closely.

Morgan had used the term "inhibition" to describe the negative component in learning in the 1890s. This usage was continued by the neobehaviorists such as E. R. Guthrie and Clark Hull. They were familiar both with the term's physiological connotations and the variety of ways it had been used in experimental study of perception, learning, and attention. Then, in 1927, the translation of Pavlov's *Conditioned Reflexes*, which treated inhibition as a major category of independent function, gave the term particular prominence at the same time as it prompted efforts to make coherent theory out of the varieties of North American learning research. Guthrie argued that all the phenomena that Pavlov discussed as conditioning, including inhibitory conditioning, could be reanalyzed "as instances of a very simple and very familiar principle, the ancient principle of association by contiguity in time."[175] Hull's "neo-behaviorism" was a systematic attempt to rework Pavlov's ideas in terms of a rigorously positivist theory of knowledge. Inhibition was one of the terms that was central to this program, and, like everything else, it received a formal definition: "Whenever any reaction is evoked in an organism there is left a condition or state which acts as a primary negative motivation in that it has an innate capacity to produce a cessation of the activity which produced the state."[176] Through these routes, a whole generation of post-World War II North American psychologists was trained to take inhibition for granted as a key term in its technical vocabulary.

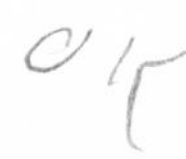

The behaviorist B. F. Skinner made a further attempt to discipline his colleagues' use of the term "inhibition" in his first major publication, *The Behavior of Organisms* (1938). He argued that there was nothing to be gained by contrasting excitation and inhibition (*pace* Sherrington), since they in fact referred to "a continuum of degrees of reflex strength," and it was simply this strength that could be specified experimentally, for example, in studies of negative reinforcement.[177] Instead, he defined a "law of inhibition," one of four dynamic laws concerning the strength of reflexes, to specify the interactive effects of simultaneously presented stimuli. He paired inhibition with "facilitation," not "excitation": "*The Law of Inhibition.* The strength of a reflex may be decreased through presentation of a second stimulus which has no other relation to the effector involved."[178]

By the 1920s, psychology was a very diverse activity indeed, even within the single national setting of the United States. Here I have illustrated the manner in which inhibition denoted the antagonistic effect of one unit of psychological analysis, whether mental or behavioral, on another. This denotation addressed long-standing questions about the ordering of mental contents, which I have illustrated in Bain's and Spencer's writings. The relational quality to which the term referred satisfied the a priori demand that the elements of an organized system oppose or arrest each other, as well as excite, facilitate, or associate with each other, in regular ways. For a psychologist like Dodge, the term was bound up with psychology's need to ground its claims in the causal processes of the nervous system. For behaviorists, the term was bound up with defining stimulus conditions. The word therefore continued to be used in a bewildering variety of local intellectual projects, from animal behavior to human attention, only some of which took account of developments in the physiology of inhibition. Inhibition did not have a specific history or career but rather, by the last quarter of the nineteenth century, was a highly malleable resource for writers concerned with physiological or psychological order. All the signs are that it was at this time that it also became an everyday descriptive word, though we would have to adopt different historical methods to trace this. The word enabled continued interaction between the content of science and public values. The form of regulative action denoted by inhibition was sometimes part of an economic and sometimes part of a hierarchical system of control, yet hierarchical systems were a striking feature of late Victorian thought—especially in the area where technical claims interacted with medical questions. To complete this picture of inhibition's place in the discourse of order, it is therefore necessary to explore further psychological theories of hierarchical control and their associated imagery.

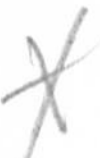

HIERARCHICAL CONTROL, EVOLUTION, AND MEDICAL PSYCHOLOGY

A hierarchy between mind and body, or a hierarchy within the body itself, was a standard feature in nineteenth-century psychological and moralistic writing. What English authors called "mental science" persisted alongside the new experimental research. Mental science was fundamentally committed to differentiating and ordering the "superior" and the "inferior" in human experience and conduct. Language represented and separated values in morphology, in physiology, in biological taxonomy, in classifying human types, in the psychology of character or mental functions, in education, in social relations, in the political economy of class, and in government. Terms that differentiated value and encoded hierarchical arrangement were shared across this terrain. In earlier chapters, I have described this language of evaluative ordering as it existed in theories about the organization of the central nervous system, going back to experimental investigations into the controlling power of "the head," and about the organization of mental content. Neurophysiological and psychological theories of inhibition developed within this framework. Once established, they then added their authority as empirical science to existing belief in ordered values.

Organizational hierarchies in physiology and psychology, supported by reference to inhibition as validated empirical knowledge, took their strongest form in medical psychology and neurology in the last third of the nineteenth century. Medical or scientific language also acquired a characteristic texture, especially in the British setting, from evolutionary theories of mind and brain. These evolutionary theories, replete with judgments separating what was valued and what was denigrated in human existence, reappeared in experimental neuroscience in the 1940s and have continued to underlie current scientific writing.

Evolutionary theory provided an extraordinarily rich language for describing every kind of hierarchy as having an embedded existence in nature.[179] Evolutionary language, like inhibitory language, had the advantage of being both scientific and public. It reinforced a directional view of time: time witnessed lower forms of existence evolving into higher forms, meaning that the most recently evolved types were the most advanced. Evolutionary theory reexpressed as temporal properties, and thereby authoritatively confirmed, evaluative differentiations already entrenched as properties of anatomical, taxonomic, and social space. Evolutionary theory was not a source of novelty in physiology and psychology by suggesting either the continuity of complex with simple structures and functions or higher dominance over lower levels. These general principles had appeared in earlier discussions. All the same, evolutionary theory articulated principles of continuity and dominance with a challenging authority and suggestiveness.

It was Spencer rather than Darwin who elaborated an evolutionary psychophysiology and whose evolutionary ideas influenced British medical psychology. As discussed above, Spencer did not use the word "inhibition," though his associationist account of mental content discussed the role played by mutual antagonism between different elements or processes. He was more original when he aligned reflex, instinctive, and intelligent actions as qualitatively comparable processes of increasing complexity and then hypothetically reconstructed the evolutionary development of each stage from its simpler predecessor. This introduced a common temporal and qualitative hierarchy into the analysis of any and every physiological or psychological process. Further, because

Spencer derived all his science from a small number of "first principles," his publications nurtured comparisons between the evolutionary hierarchy of organisms, the hierarchy of functions and structures within the organism, and the hierarchical interrelations of individuals in society.[180] His writings were thus a rich resource for comparing organization between physiological, psychological, social, and ethical levels of reality, and they facilitated expression of a language common to these levels. Spencer was also the most systematic exponent of the belief that progress, that is, directional change from lower to higher states, was the inevitable consequence of natural law, and this too invigorated the hierarchical connotations of organizational concepts.

Evolutionary theory thus confirmed and added authority to the conception of the nervous system as a linear, hierarchical organization. As Harrington's work has shown, in the second half of the nineteenth century such hierarchical conceptions, including evolutionary versions, were also often expressed in terms of the bilateral arrangement between the "dominant" left cerebral hemisphere and the "subordinate" right hemisphere.[181] (The hemispheres communicate with the opposite side of the body through the crossing of their nervous connections.) Left-right differences thus enriched and diversified the evaluative resources of psychophysiology. Relations of dominance and suppression, and occasionally of inhibition, appeared in terms of left-right as well as low-high dualities.

Medicine was the institutional setting most receptive to evolutionary psychophysiology in Britain, and it is Jackson who has particularly impressed medical psychologists, neurologists, and post-1940s neuroscientists. He successfully integrated the detailed analysis of the clinical symptoms of nervous disorders with a general theory, couched in Spencerian terms, describing the organization of nervous functions.[182] The empirical core for this integration was a clinical series exemplifying an ordered, hierarchical breakdown of nervous function. Jackson then used this knowledge to construct a theory of normal organization, and it was this theory that informed Ferrier's experimental approach to higher cortical functions.

Jackson argued that the basic sensory-motor units of nervous function were represented successively at the different levels in the central nervous system, at levels of increasing complexity and flexibility, and that these levels originated in evolutionary history. "I believe, indeed, that the very highest processes (the substrata of consciousness) are only the most multifold and complex of all sensori-motor processes, that they represent or re-represent *all* lower nervous centres, and thus the whole organism (the organism as a whole)."[183] Jackson believed that an elementary reflex was a sensory-motor act represented at a spinal level and a deliberate movement was a sensory-motor act represented at the cortical level and that these levels were hierarchically related. Evolutionary theory explained that the "higher," more complex, and in evolutionary terms most recent levels were superadded to, and overrode, "lower" levels. As a corollary, it explained why in disordered states the highest, most complex, and most recent levels were the first to be lost, reducing the ill person to a lower level of organization. "For in disease the most voluntary or most special movements, faculties, etc., suffer first and most, that is in an order the exact opposite of evolution. Therefore I call this the principle of Dissolution."[184]

Jackson also referred to this pathological process as "loss of control."[185] The phrase "loss of control" introduced order into neuropathology, for example, by arranging symptoms of epileptic attacks in a hierarchical scale.[186] At the same time, the phrase had meanings that went well beyond clinical diagnosis. Jackson was conscious of these wider connotations, and he exploited them in his attempt to communicate his neurological insights.

Jackson hardly used the word "inhibition": his only extended comment came in remarks on a paper about the concept by his pupil, Mercier.[187] "Loss of control" and "loss of inhibition," however, were synonymous. For example, while discussing postepileptic states, Jackson compared automatic muscular contractions with penile erection after a lesion in the lower spinal cord, and he then used the latter symptom as a platform for a comment on the inhibitory organization of the central nervous system.

> Thus such symptoms as foot clonus [spasm] after epileptiform seizures, and erection of the penis in cases of transverse lesion of the lower part of the cervical cord, evidently signify hyper-physiological activities from "loss of control" only.
>
> This is a complex illustration, but one worth giving as part of the evidence towards showing a series of inhibitions in the central nervous system. The nervi erigentes inhibit the arteries of the penis. But the part of the visceral column (Stilling's sacral nucleus) from which these nerves come is itself inhibited so that the penis is ordinarily flaccid. In cases of complete transverse lesion of the lower cervical cord or upper dorsal cord inhibition is subtracted from Stilling's inhibitory nucleus, whereupon it, being "let go," inhibits the arteries of the penis, they become dilated, and then the organ is turgid.[188]

In this one example, Jackson equated "loss of control," "subtraction of inhibition," and "letting go," and the example reexpressed in scientific form the most vivid and commonplace symbol of the disruptive male body, the erect penis. He also repeatedly emphasized, as I have done, that the principle of "loss of control" had long been present in the British literature on mental pathology and nervous disorder.

> I believe . . . that destruction of function of a higher centre is a removal of inhibition over a lower centre (*Principle of Loss of Control*, Anstie, Thompson Dickson), the lower centre becomes more easily dischargeable, or popularly speaking "more excitable," and especially those parts of that centre which are in activity when control is removed. So to speak, these parts become autonomous.[189]

The principle applied equally to insanity. Jackson described insanity as "double" since it had a negative side involving loss of some "higher" capacity and a positive side involving the enhancement of some "lower" capacity.

> I believe that there is a double condition in insanity, whether acute and temporary, as in epileptic mania, or chronic, as in insanity ordinarily so-called; there is a positive and a negative condition. . . . The increased action (positive state, *i.e.*, the raving, etc.) is owing to what, metaphorically speaking, is loss of control of lower centres by the highest centres, of which the function is lost or impaired (negative state, defect or loss of consciousness).[190]

This was a truism of Victorian medical psychology. But in Jackson's hands, the principle, as much a moral as a medical statement, became integrated with a technical account of physiological function. The principle was, in turn, developed in the experimental setting by Ferrier and later by Sherrington, with fundamental implications for psychological questions. Jackson, like Sechenov and Ferrier, conceived that the psychological processes of thought and memory were parallel to physiological sensory-motor processes at higher cortical levels, though with the motor element suppressed. Thus, he referred to the memory of a word or a sentence as "*suppressed articulation.*"[191] This was a technical point, though of wide significance. The broader connotations of reference to "loss of control" were most evident in writings by contemporary doctors such as Maudsley and Mercier.

Maudsley did not possess Jackson's precise diagnostic skills or theoretical ability. His historical importance rests with his critique of the custodial role played by the late Victorian asylum and his financial contribution and plans for a research institute and hospital for curable mental disorders, subsequently realized as the University of London's Institute of Psychiatry and the Maudsley Hospital.[192] His writings, which were acerbic in style and exhibited a mordant contempt for philosophical idealism and free will, have interested historians as exemplifying an evolutionary medical approach to social problems, disorder, and deviance. Maudsley's writings were also widely translated, and he was for a while perhaps the British alienist best known in continental Europe. Unlike Jackson, however, he left little intellectual legacy.

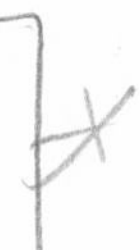

Like the medical psychologists cited by Jackson, Maudsley described insanity as illness that destroyed higher functions, releasing those based in lower nervous levels, "for it is of the essence of insanity to inhibit the higher, and to accentuate the lower qualities of a character."[193] Staunchly Victorian in manner, Maudsley identified the failure of will as the central pathological characteristic, using a single language for moral judgment and physical description.

> It cannot be too distinctly borne in mind, in relation to all cerebral disease, that the direct physical effect of debilitated nerve-energies and loosened mental organization is demoralization of will, showing itself in self-indulgence, indolence, loss of self-control, moaning self-pity, sorrowful sighings, abject weakness of will, exaggeration and even simulation of symptoms of suffering; that the failure of will and its deepening degrees means an increasing dissolution passing into disruption of the federal union of nerve-centres, whereby the present thought or feeling, losing its proper inhibitions, has unbridled sway and way.[194]

Maudsley's books, in the guise of secular, evolutionary physical science, gave new life to the ancient Christian values of the spirit and the flesh. His language clearly expressed the moral and physical denotation of the word "inhibition," referring to the higher control over lower qualities. He believed that our lower qualities, like original sin, were an ever-present power, primarily the individual's inheritance and not his or her creation, and this power resurfaced in madness. In mania, Maudsley reported,

> The higher inhibitions of thought and feeling gone, the lower passions surge to the front in turbulent welter and actuate the conduct. Sexual feeling, prone and prompt to be coarsely obtrusive, shows itself in equivocal words, in lascivious gestures and attitudes, sometimes in acts of repulsive lust. It is a strange thing to see, although it be instructive evidence of the inmost contents of human nature, what a foul and shameless fury of inflamed lust a chaste and decent woman can become when her mind is decomposed into mania.[195]

We have, he constantly emphasized, both a general evolutionary inheritance and a particular parental inheritance. This is our fate, modified only by moral training inculcating habits of inhibition. "Take away from a young child's mind the germs of those highest inhibitory functions that are presupposed by a potentiality of moral development, and you leave the natural passions and instincts free play."[196] Almost identical language was later used by A. F. Tredgold to describe a criminal type of moral defective "who is never taught to control his impulses whilst young" and whose "power of inhibition is undeveloped, with the result that his lower animal feelings have full play, and his conduct becomes vicious, immoral, and antisocial."[197] This was not abstract description but appeared in the context of discussion of the Mental Deficiency Act of 1913, which represented a concerted political attempt to find an adequate response to both idiocy, including "moral imbecility," and delinquency.

Maudsley established a reputation as a young alienist in the 1860s for the emphatic way he identified mental disorder with the breakdown of nervous function, especially in *The Physiology and Pathology of the Mind* (1867). Nevertheless, like other medical psychologists, he held together the physiology and the pathology only by general argument and not by specific detail. He may well have had in mind knowledge of physiological inhibition (e.g., of the heart) when he introduced the term "inhibition" into his writing, but the reality was that he deployed the term in entirely nontechnical ways. Indeed, his meaning is close to modern popular usage. "Inhibition" became a word meaning the opposite of excitation, and as such, it served equally well while discussing individual character, the training of children, emotional or drunken outbursts, or insane disorders. The word "inhibition" gave a physiological appearance to the psychological will.

> In order to form a conception of [the will's] probable mode of operation when it thus intervenes with effect, it is desirable to appreciate the nature of pure physiological inhibition as we observe it work to check or stop action that is entirely reflex. . . .
>
> Does it act . . . by the unsearchable path of a metaphysical volition, or by the known physical paths of physiological inhibition?[198]

Inhibition served Maudsley's purpose in attacking what he regarded as the "metaphysical" prejudices of established opinion, though his translation of will into physiological inhibition reflected little knowledge of what the latter idea had become in contemporary experimental science.

Maudsley associated inhibition with everyday ideas for explaining character and conduct in terms of mental or bodily energies. In one of the earliest Victorian psychological uses of the word, he referred to the counteraction of reasoning and will:

> Men of great reasoning powers . . . are notoriously not unfrequently incapacitated thereby from energetic action; they balance reasons so nicely that no one of them outweighs another, and they can come to no decision: with them, as with Hamlet, meditation paralyses action. In fact, the power of understanding is reflective and inhibitory, being exhibited rather in the hindrance of passion-prompted action, and in the guidance of our impulses, than in the instigation of conduct.[199]

Thus, reason was inhibitory, limiting impulsive action, making possible moral and ordered social existence.

The medical psychologists, unlike Spencer, did not elaborate deductive philosophies, and thus the comparisons they made between government and the brain might be read "simply" as metaphor. Yet metaphor is never simple. The metaphorical language evoked a rich exchange of meanings between controlling governments and controlling brains. This exchange is unmistakable in Mercier's description of neurological disorder as an army without a commander, alluding to the loss of control as riot and anarchy.[200] Clouston stated that "mental inhibition is the colonel-in-chief of the brain hierarchy."[201] These pictures of political, military, and physiological government constituted the expressive setting in which the word "inhibition" came into common use in the English language. The new psychophysiology thus perpetuated the old legal usage, in which inhibition referred to the arresting power possessed by a higher authority.

Maudsley was the first in the field. Noting that reflexes were augmented following severance of the brain and spinal cord, he concluded,

> One most necessary function of the brain is to exert an inhibitory power over the nerve centres that lie below it, just as man exercises a beneficial control over his fellow animals of a lower order of dignity; and the increased irregular activity of the lower centres surely betokens a degeneration: it is like the turbulent, aimless action of a democracy without a head.[202]

This occasioned a long paragraph on the authority of the head in the body as an expression of political relations:

> So certain and intimate is the sympathy between the individual nerve-cells in that well-organized commonwealth which the nervous system represents, that a local disturbance is soon felt more or less distinctly throughout the whole state. . . . The form of government is that of a constitutional monar-

> chy, in which every interest is duly represented through adequate channels, and in which, consequently, there is a proper subordination of parts.[203]

What Maudsley called an "adequate representation" required the mutual interaction between the different parts of the brain; he did not believe that there was a single controlling center in the nervous system. He considered "the will" to be the diffused "inhibitory action" of different associated ideas and feelings. At this point, Maudsley's comparison between the political and the psychological bodies became as confused as Spencer's, though Maudsley's political views—unlike Spencer's—did favor firm conservative authority.

Mercier, in a book and in an address to the Neurological Society of London in 1888, developed a "dynamic" view of function into a general theory that all parts of the nervous system were continuously excitatory and inhibitory. He claimed, "Every nervous centre is at all times subject to continuous control or inhibition; so that while its intrinsic tendency is ever to discharge, this tendency is continuously counteracted by an extrinsic influence which curbs it into quietude."[204] He followed Spencer in deducing what control required of the nervous system and in these terms defended the attribution of continuous inhibition to nerve centers, a claim that he feared his audience would think speculative.

> I will ask [skeptics] to remember that by the frequent use of the phrase Loss of Control (indeed I have heard an eminent alienist speak of an "outburst of loss of control"), many of them have surrendered the whole position. For control to be lost, it must first be present; and if present in some centres, why not in all? The hypothesis already exists therefore, and is already largely accepted.[205]

He suggested that this intrinsic nervous control, as well as the hierarchical arrangement of the controlling centers, was most clearly revealed in disordered regulation of muscular movements.

> The movements of walking are arranged in a hierarchy, each centre controlling and regulating those that are below, and being controlled and regulated by those that are above it. There is nothing anomalous or paradoxical in the supposition that the same centre affords both the impulses which start and accelerate, and the impulses which retard and arrest, the action of inferior centres, for we have daily illustration of a similar condition of things in every business organization.[206]

The political economy of the body, like the political economy of British society, achieved success by reconciling hierarchical arrangements with the mutual dependency of parts.

Mercier illustrated the reality of hierarchical control by reference to what happened when it was lost in insanity and nervous disorders, likening these conditions to an army whose colonel is shot or who "loses his head." This language was not one man's whimsy but evocative rhetoric grounded in a single conception of order. The loss of the head had the same effect on armies as on frogs. Jackson himself took up the language in his comments on Mercier's address, explaining a fear of anarchy:

> If the governing body of this country were destroyed suddenly, we should have two causes for lamentation; (1) The loss of services of eminent men; and (2) the anarchy of the now uncontrolled people. The loss of the governing body answers to the Dissolution in our patient (the exhaustion of the highest two "layers" of his highest centres); the anarchy answers to the no longer controlled activity of the next lower level of evolution (third "layer").[207]

We do not have to suppose that Jackson or Mercier had specific political questions in mind. They were constructing linguistic resources that were then available for use in a variety of specific settings.

In spite of substantial national and cultural differences, this discourse was not restricted to Britain, as reference to Ribot, Paulhan, and Preyer has shown. British association psychology and British neurology, for the most part, did not attract systematic attention in German research, though association did become one focus in the new experimental work. Nevertheless, German-language physiological and medical psychology shared the belief in the hierarchy of controlling levels in the central nervous system. An evolutionary perspective reinforced hierarchical notions in Wundt's work, as in Jackson's and Ferrier's, though in Wundt's case, this evolutionary theory was a biogenic law (individual development recapitulates ancestral development) little structured by Darwin or Spencer.[208] The idea that higher cortical levels controlled lower levels by inhibition as well as by excitation was widely assumed. For example, it was mentioned earlier that Meynert referred to the cortical inhibition of the subcortical mass through the excitation of sense perceptions and associated visual memories.[209]

Neurology on the European continent in the late nineteenth century was generally un-Jacksonian in approach. Most physicians followed Goltz, who had explained the symptoms in experimentally brain-damaged dogs by reference to an "irritative inhibition." He described lesions as having "an 'irritative' effect . . . expressed in positive signs and symptoms."[210] Following this interpretation, hemiplegia (partial paralysis on one side) appeared to be the positive effect of a lesion resulting in excessive reflex activity and hence rigidity. Goltz was critical about localization of function theories in general, and he therefore argued that it was the wound in the brain, rather than the destruction of a "center," that caused loss of function. He and others supported this view by citing the well-known phenomenon of surgical shock, which they believed was a form of general inhibition. "The disorders that may be observed immediately after mutilation of the cerebrum are partly related to an inhibition suffered by those parts of the brain located behind the cerebrum and owing to irritation from a cerebral wound."[211]

This view was treated more critically after 1900, and it then became untenable in the light of Sherrington's investigation into the control of reflexes and into decerebrate rigidity. World War I provided neurologists with a mass experiment in human brain damage. Synthesizing these experiences, Henry Head systematically restated Jacksonian theory, drawing on Sherrington's work to argue for its superiority over continental theory.

> It is a common experience that the manifestations of nervous disease may comprise both loss of function and some positive outburst of excessive activity. Thus, in many cases of hemiplegia, the paralysed limbs tend to be more or less rigid and the reflexes are greatly increased. This spasticity, although due to a destructive lesion, was attributed to "irritation." . . .
>
> But more than fifty years ago, Hughlings Jackson laid down the rule that destructive lesions never cause positive effects, but induce a negative condition, which permits positive symptoms to appear. This he applied to all morbid expressions of nervous activity.[212]

Jackson's theory, Head argued, permitted one to see that the symptoms of increased function in nervous disorders were not meaningless or fortuitous but "reveal to a certain degree the mode of action of the lower centres before they were dominated from above."[213] "Lower" and "before" both carried strong evolutionary connotations. Head's words perpetuated evaluative associations in the technical language of control.

> If, however, the factor eliminated by the lesion has exercised some control over the functions which still remain intact, phenomena may appear which were inhibited under normal conditions. Suppose half the scholars are absent from a class, the sum total of its vital energy is diminished, but discipline is maintained unimpaired; absence of the master, on the other hand, leads inevitably to disorder.[214]

Head thus used "inhibition" to refer to the action of the evolutionary higher "master."

Head was interested in general psychological topics. Thus, he also referred to "selective inhibition," the result of the competition between different afferent impulses, which he used to explain symptoms of altered sensitivity (symptoms that varied considerably with an individual's temperament) in nervous disorders.[215] He generalized this conclusion regarding the inhibitory interaction of stimuli from sense organs to account for the integration of stimuli in sensation. It was in this connection that W. H. R. Rivers and he conducted their ethically controversial experiment that involved sectioning a nerve in Head's forearm to study the pattern of the return of subjective sensation.[216] The physiology of inhibition, evidenced by the pathology of sensibility, enabled Head to reexpress something like the Herbartian view about the formation of mental content:

> All the incongruous impulses, generated in the various peripheral end-organs, can never affect consciousness at the same moment; some succeed in forming the basis of sensation, whilst others are inhibited and would never be recognized were it not for the fact of dissociated sensibility. During their passage through the central nervous system, they sooner or later undergo integration, carried out partly by combination into specific groups and partly by selective inhibition.[217]

By achieving integration, the human organism became more than an automaton. "If we responded constantly and inevitably to all impulses from peripheral end-organs, we should be automata, the victims of indiscriminate reactions."[218] Inhibitory processes were therefore intrinsic to the realization, through evolution, of intelligence, an argument similar to that reached independently by Morgan. The dominance exerted by the higher, integrative levels of the central nervous system over the lower, automatic levels was the physiological basis for purposive action. Integration "is carried out partly by qualitative selection, but to an even greater extent by the struggle for expression between incompatible physiological reactions. This involves permanent inhibition, under normal conditions."[219]

Head was a brilliant neurologist whose theoretical reflections brought some kind of order to the nerve and brain damage cases resulting from World War I. But Head and his contemporaries also saw that war as an outbreak of savagery. The language of lost mastery at higher levels applied equally to the wounded soldier and to the civilization for which he fought. These beliefs, that habits of civilized understanding and conduct overlay primitive instincts and urges, went back well beyond the nineteenth century, merging with Christian notions of original sin. Maudsley commented, "History shows by many lurid examples, when the checks that curb and tame the brute within the man are removed and the passions set free, how the same horrible outbreaks of lust, rapine, cruelty and bloodshed invariably and uniformly follow."[220] Evolutionary theory, however, deeply enriched the means with which to express this sensibility. It also provided the sensibility with the aura of objective authority: evolutionary rhetoric about the boundedness of the human races to their inheritance acquired mythic stature in the late nineteenth century. This was a myth that rendered intelligible the diversity and suffering in the nature of things. It reinterpreted human evil—aggression, lust, and stupidity—as the unavoidable consequences of an animal descent. The economist Walter Bagehot, developing an evolutionary social psychology in defense of constitutional democracy, referred to "the secret and repressed side of human nature."[221] T. H. Huxley, using Tennyson's words, attacked Utopian socialists who ignorantly denied "the ape and tiger" within human nature.[222] Inhibition undoubtedly carried overtones of these myths about human nature. It integrated experimental or clinical contexts and the human condition.

I use the concept of myth to refer to a socially powerful symbolic narrative about some aspect of the human condition. "Myth," in this sense, is not the opposite of "science"; indeed, as I have argued, it can be given a satisfying content by science. Thus, evolutionary myths became common in the nineteenth century, and they have indeed retained this position.

Rivers, Head's colleague in the nerve-sectioning experiment, played a major part in developing the British medical response to war neuroses. This response included acknowledgment that there were unconscious psychological processes and what Rivers called "suppression," preferring this term to "repression" as he felt it indicated better its active but unconscious nature. Rivers then used the phylogenic (or evolutionary) scheme of sensibility, which Head and he had propounded, as evidence that psychological suppression was a general feature of higher evolutionary achievement. He also adduced evidence from the way war damage had revealed previously hidden nervous functions.

> A number of processes have been found which form intermediate links connecting the suppression of highly complicated mental process at one end of the series with the suppression necessary for the perfection of reflex action at the other end of the series. . . . The suppression of conscious experience is

> only one example of a process which applies throughout the animal kingdom and is essential to the proper regulation of every form of human or animal activity.[223]

Rivers concluded that psychological suppression, the formation of unconscious mental content such as battle-induced terror, was "only one aspect of the universal physiological property of inhibition."[224] Rivers's work was one important channel through which Freudian ideas were introduced into medical, and perhaps wider, circles in Britain. This channel also suggests how easily Freud's work was assimilated to existing beliefs in the inhibitory hierarchy of psychological processes. Rivers's discussion of Freud's notion of "censorship" illustrates the point. Observing that social censorship "forms only a very small part of the total mass of inhibiting forces by which more recently developed social groups control tendencies belonging to an older social order," Rivers argued that "censorship" implied too limited a view of the suppressive or inhibitory features of dream or symptom formation.[225] It may be, therefore, that in Britain existing views about the evolutionary inheritance of hierarchical organization subsumed the particularities of Freudian ideas.

By no means all medical uses of "inhibition" in the 1920s presupposed such a systematic evolutionary perspective. Most notably, the word was common in descriptive clinical psychiatry.[226] Two German-language authorities, Emil Kraepelin and Eugen Bleuler, both used "inhibition" to describe the symptoms of depression. The word was treated as unproblematic in their textbooks and thereby became standard psychiatric vocabulary. Kraepelin wrote in relation to the manic-depressive insanities, "*Inhibition of thought* appears to form the exact opposite to flight of ideas. It is observed, more or less strongly marked, almost everywhere in depression, further in certain manic-stuporous mixed states and in forms of manic excitement related to these. The patients exhibit an incapacity, often very painfully felt by themselves, to order their own ideas aright."[227] He also described inhibition of the will and suggested experimental techniques, for example, recording hand pressure during writing, as objective measures for inhibitory symptoms.[228] In extreme cases of stupor, he concluded, the inhibition could be regarded as more or less total. Bleuler similarly used inhibition to characterize depressive conditions: "Inhibition is analogous to a slowing-up of the flow as a result of increasing viscosity of the fluid."[229]

Thus, he argued, the clinically depressed person is inhibited from making connections between ideas or in carrying out instructions and thus cannot but act lethargically. Bleuler himself noted that this psychiatric meaning of the term "inhibition" differed from that current in neurophysiology, though he assumed the usages had common roots.

Inhibition in neurophysiology or neurology conceptualized a hierarchy of functions, while usage in psychiatry described a pathological reduction of mental capacities in general. Kraepelin and Bleuler developed the latter usage, but the former was found in German-language psychiatry as well as neurology. For example, Ernst Kretschmer, now remembered for his theory of the "schizoid" type, assumed that the evolutionary hierarchy of nervous processes explained pathological symptoms. "If a higher centre is impaired or cut off from subordinate centres through shock, disease, or trauma, not only does the co-ordinated activity of the neural apparatus fail, but the subordinate centre establishes its functional independence and reveals such of its evolutionarily speaking original activities as it has retained."[230] He referred to shock causing primitive reactions to "break through" and to hysteria finding expression "through an instinctive, reflexive, or other built-in survival mechanism."[231] It must be stressed, therefore, that by the 1920s, "inhibition" had become available for use in a vast and diverse range of local contexts. But accepting this does not imply accepting that local contexts circumscribed meaning: structural features of the discourse about control remained shared.

Two important developments in the 1940s have carried this association between inhibition and evolution into modern neuroscience. Beginning in 1944, Magoun and Rhines reported that electrically stimulating the bulbar region in the brain stem produced an inhibitory effect, and they argued that this region was involved in a general way with the inhibitory control of the nervous system. This contradicted the generally accepted view that this region exercised an excitatory function.

> According to the doctrine that the nervous system is organized as a series of levels, that portion of the brain stem lying immediately above the spinal cord, and described as bulbar, has traditionally been regarded as a level contributing excitatory influences to motor outflows. . . . It has not been widely recognized that this bulbar part of the brain stem, in addition, contains a mechanism capable of exerting a general inhibitory influence on motor activity. In the experiments to be reported, this inhibitory influence has been demonstrated by observing the effect of bulbar stimulation upon reflexes, upon decerebrate rigidity and upon responses evoked from the motor cortex.[232]

This work reopened the experimental study of central inhibition, and it did so in relation to a theory that associated control with the hierarchical arrangement of organizational levels.

Such work has had significant practical consequences. The most dramatic was J. M. Delgado's technique for a surgical operation to inhibit overactive centers in the brain. Delgado argued that developing techniques to make possible physical intervention in the brain was the only way in which we might contain our innate savagery. He put forward a vision of a "psychocivilized" society in which the technology of inhibition would play a major part.

> Violence, including its extreme manifestation of war, is determined by a variety of economic and ideological factors; but we must realize that the elite who make the decisions, and even the individual who obeys orders and holds a rifle, require for their behavioural performance the existence of a series of intra-cerebral electrical signals which could be inhibited by other conflicting signals generating in areas such as the caudate nucleus [in the midbrain].[233]

He demonstrated the possibilities by operating on monkeys at Yale University, and he followed this with photographs of an angry bull brought to a dead stop by a radio impulse to an electrode implanted in its brain.

The second development was P. D. MacLean's restatement of the nineteenth-century theory picturing the brain in evolutionary, hierarchical terms, a version of neuroscience that supported the sociobiology of the 1960s and 1970s. Stimulated by a structural theory of the emotions developed in the 1930s by J. W. Papez, MacLean constructed a model for the brain that had three gross divisions, the divisions being related to one another in an order that corresponded to evolutionary development. He proposed, in effect, that humans possessed three brains: the reptilian (or visceral), the paleomammalian (or emotional), and the neomammalian (or rational).[234] Following Victorian precedent, MacLean embodied a scheme of moral qualities in the phylogenic order of the brain, providing what he claimed was an objective language with which to characterize disorder, aggression, excess emotion, and pathology as the outbreak of "the beast within." Writing for a popular audience, he thus referred to the mentally disordered patient as bringing to the doctor "the loosely leashed reptile and the poorly bridled horse."[235]

MacLean discussed inhibition in current popular language. A century after physiological and medical psychology entrenched values of moral and political order in the language of objective knowledge about organized control within the nervous system, neuroscientists, ethologists, and sociobiologists have taken up the same discourse. The nineteenth-century discourse resonated with ordinary experience and the fear that civilized progress was a tenuous achievement. In the twentieth century, after immeasurable destruction and murder, this resonance has not diminished. Ordinary words such as "inhibition"carry scientific authority, but they still remind us of original sin.

CHAPTER 5

Twentieth-Century Schools

It has been said that he who was the first to abuse his fellow-man instead of knocking out his brains without a word, laid thereby the basis of civilization.

——John Hughlings Jackson, "On affections of speech from disease of the brain"

C. S. SHERRINGTON

There was continuity between nineteenth-century and twentieth-century research on physiological inhibitory mechanisms, on inhibition between competing perceptual or behavioral elements, and on the central inhibition of lower levels by higher levels. This research continues in current neuroscience and psychology, confirming that there has been a shared way of thinking about organization and control. Modern scientists also experience this sense of continuity with the past, and they explain it in terms of empirical discovery and the cumulative understanding of the nervous system. By contrast, this history has stressed continuity at the level of both technical and everyday language and hence in modern belief and judgment about what it is to be a person in an ordered society.

To trace further this transition from the nineteenth to the twentieth century, without attempting to write the history of physiology and psychology in general, I will focus on three figures: Sherrington, Pavlov, and Freud. Everyone concedes their stature and influence: Sherrington has been the dominant voice in neurophysiology in the English-speaking world; Pavlov's work became almost synonymous with "objective psychology" for a time in the Soviet Union and other "Socialist" countries, and it has had considerable influence elsewhere; and Freud's psychoanalytic legacy, though contested by most scientists, has had far-reaching consequences for general psychological views, for therapy, and for cultural analysis. These three figures were contemporaries—Sherrington was born in 1857, Pavlov in 1849, and Freud in 1856—and each received a rigorous training as an experimental scientist and was deeply excited by neurophysiology. Last, of course, each drew on existing notions of inhibition and developed them into pivotal aspects of his theory. It is this last feature that will structure the following necessarily brief analysis and show how it is possible to understand such divergent ideas as representative of a common discourse.

The identification of "pure science" with the highest values of humanistic culture perhaps reached an apogee in the English-speaking world in the 1920s. If this was so, then Sherrington, the president of the Royal Society, personally embodied these values. His commitment to meticulous experimental research and theoretical synthesis illuminated an ideal of objective knowledge in the communal pursuit of which men and women achieved personal fulfillment and gave to society both high culture and the basis for medical advance.[1] In his hands and in the hands of the numerous and influential researchers who worked with him, vivisection and experiment revealed with unprecedented precision the structural, functional, and neuronal basis for the coordinated control of animal movement. He synthesized his views on nervous organization under the rubric of "integration."[2]

Sherrington investigated inhibition in many ways, referring to it as something that was as essential to integrative action as excitation itself. When he was awarded the Nobel Prize for Physiology or Medicine in 1932 (with E. D. Adrian), he chose as the subject for his prize address, "Inhibition as a coordinative factor."[3] He discussed inhibition as a concept essential to comprehending integration; at the same time, he attempted to understand inhibition as a mechanism at the level of the neuron or synapse. Thus, his references to inhibition did not correlate with any single factual claim or even series of such claims.

The background to the award of the Nobel Prize is oddly relevant to this. The terms of the Nobel awards stressed "discovery," and, though the exceptional quality of Sherrington's work was widely acknowledged in the first decade of the century and his synthetic achievement in *The Integrative Action of the Nervous System* (1906; 2d ed. 1961) immediately recognized, it proved difficult to say what exactly he had "discovered."

> That, in spite of the high esteem which Sherrington enjoyed, he was not awarded the prize until 1932 . . . was due to several circumstances. In the

> first investigation, in 1910, the examiner [J. E. Johansson] found that some delay was advisable; while in 1912 and 1915 he came to the conclusion that Sherrington's discovery of the reciprocal innervation of antagonistic muscles deserved a prize. In the Committee it was objected that although it had happened to be forgotten, this discovery, as Sherrington himself had stressed, had already been made in 1826, by the brothers C. and J. Bell. By the time the First World War broke out, several members of the faculty were recommending greater stringency in applying the stipulation in Nobel's will that the prize be given for a definite discovery; whereon the examiner [Johansson] felt he could not, after all, support Sherrington's candidature. After Johansson's retirement in 1927, there was a certain shift of opinion; but a few more years were to pass before the new attitude could prevail.[4]

The Nobel faculty was concerned with the symbolic rewards of endeavor, not the philosophy of knowledge, but its willingness to rank Sherrington's contribution as in some sense secondary to the work of Charles (not John) Bell in the 1820s was a remarkable act of deference to empiricist fiction. Just how much happened between that time and Sherrington's own work in the 1890s has been discussed in the previous chapters. I will therefore now look at the way Sherrington built on and transformed the nineteenth-century physiology of inhibition.

Sherrington's research terms of reference were almost entirely physiological, signifying the disciplinary and institutional separation of physiology and psychology. The world of mind was not turned by Sherrington into psychology but remained filled by humanistic learning, by commitment to the social good, and by poetry. His psychological thought was largely contained in his books written in retirement, and these books reflected humanism rather than scientific psychology, though he did give much attention to questions in sensory psychophysiology. His position on the mind-body problem made clear why there was such a division of labor:

> Reference to the brain at present affords little help to the study of the mind. . . . That is no fault of those who study the mind or of those who study the brain. It constitutes a disability common to both of them. A liaison between them is what each has been asking for. That there is a liaison neither of them doubts. The "how" of it we must think remains for science as for philosophy a riddle pressing to be read.[5]

Insofar as he was prepared to discuss mind as a biological event, Sherrington believed that evolutionary theory required belief that consciousness was an active, controlling presence: "The influence of mind on the doings of life makes mind an effective contribution to life. . . . Lloyd Morgan, the biologist, urged that 'the primary aim, object and purpose of consciousness is control.' Dame Nature seems to have taken the like view."[6] Sherrington devoted his research career to showing how the organism achieved control, but, as he stressed, this research was restricted to the level of nervous processes.

Work by Pflüger, Schiff, Goltz, Sechenov, Bernard, and Wundt, as well as many others, had established spinal reflex control as a major research topic. As Judith Swazey has shown in detail, Sherrington transformed this area in two ways. First, in a systematic study of the knee-jerk reflex, he described the specific mechanism underlying a single reflex and showed how it exhibited "integration." "The uniqueness and significance of Sherrington's concept lies in the fact that it provided the first comprehensive, experimentally documented explanation of *how* the nervous system, through the unit mechanism of reflex action, produces an 'integrated' or 'co-ordinated' motor organism."[7] Second, he synthesized existing research, so that later scientists felt that they were working within the framework that he had laid out. "Sherrington's work . . . gave unified meaning to a host of phenomena and processes previously discussed in isolation. The concept of integrative action and all that it embodied brought together in a 'final common path' many hitherto unconnected channels of neurophysiological, anatomical, and histological research."[8] As Brazier observed, "The contributions of Sherrington and his school are the basis of modern ideas of the reflex at the spinal level."[9]

One consequence of the clarity and unity that Sherrington brought to neurophysiology was that he sorted through different meanings of the word "inhibition," though this was not a specific aim. What he wrote about inhibition followed from understanding coordinated and purposeful action. He summarized the central position of inhibition in the following terms:

> The role of inhibition in the working of the central nervous system has proved to be more and more extensive and more and more fundamental as experiment has advanced in examining it. Reflex inhibition can no longer be regarded merely as a factor specially developed for dealing with the antagonism of opponent muscles acting at various hinge-joints. Its role as a coordinative factor comprises that, and goes beyond that. In the working of the central nervous machinery inhibition seems as ubiquitous and as frequent as is excitation itself. The whole quantitative grading of the operations of the spinal cord and brain appears to rest upon mutual interaction between the two central processes "excitation" and "inhibition", the one no less important than the other.[10]

Hall, Volkmann, and other early researchers on reflex control had argued that a continuous background of reflex excitation, or "tonic" state, in the central nervous system was necessary to sustain posture or the closure of sphincters.[11] It had also been assumed that different spinal levels must interact to make possible posture or movement. It was increasingly accepted that tonic and intersegmental spinal relations explained the variability and complexity of experimental results produced, for example, by following up Rosenthal's account of breathing or Sechenov's observations on central inhibition. Sherrington's research program in the 1890s translated this general physiological knowledge, as well as a host of specific and sometimes contradictory results, into knowledge of specific pathways within the spinal cord and spinal nerves responsible for the coordination of movements. Research on the dog's scratch reflex provided an experimental exemplar.[12] Parallel studies of the stretch reflex, associated with research on decerebrate rigidity in monkeys, later led to modern work on tonus, that is, the background state responsible for posture.[13]

Sherrington brought together his studies of coordination in his Silliman Lectures at Yale University, published as *The Integrative Action of the Nervous System.* He described how simple, individual reflexes, of the kind he had studied over the previous fifteen years, subserved the purposeful life of the organism as a whole. Purposeful movement was possible because of reciprocal interaction at all levels in the central nervous system. This was "integration," which he demonstrated by working up from the simplest case, the reciprocal innervation of antagonistic muscles in the knee jerk and in limb flection, which he had studied in great detail. Swazey summarized this in the following way:

> Prior to Sherrington's work four interacting factors had been isolated as the chief determinants of purposeful, coordinated spinal movements: the character of the afferent impulse, stimulus intensity, stimulus locus, and the intrinsic condition of the spinal cord. Sherrington subsequently showed that at a gross functional level the movements are effected by the reciprocal innervation of antagonistic muscles. By 1900 he had pinpointed three key mechanisms which in turn effect and affect the operations of reciprocal innervation: the muscular sense and the processes of central inhibition and facilitation.[14]

His research showed how these "key mechanisms" worked together. The result was that he described inhibition as a general feature of integrative action. He demonstrated the specific mechanism involved in the limb flection in the cat: a circular nervous pathway transmitted motor excitation to muscle, proprioception (or "muscular sense") excited afferent fibers, and these afferent fibers then caused both reflex excitation and reflex inhibition in the spinal cord. The result was the coordinated contraction of the cat's thigh muscle and the relaxation, by reflex inhibition, of its antagonistic muscle.[15] This work encouraged the belief that inhibition was part of the continuous, normal functioning of the spinal cord: "My own observations lead me to believe that *inhibito-motor* spinal reflexes occur *quite habitually and concurrently* with many of the *excito-motor*."[16] Other major examples of reciprocal inhibition were found in the movement of the eyeball and in breathing.

It is often said that Sherrington discovered reciprocal inhibition. It is a good deal more precise to say that he elucidated its specific mechanism. As he himself pointed out, his work had been "anticipated" by the anatomist Charles Bell in the 1820s, who had posited the existence of reciprocal action while studying the muscles that move the eyeball.[17] As everybody also knew, Descartes had suggested and even drawn pictures for such an antagonistic or reciprocal muscular mechanism in his posthumous *De homine* (1662).[18] None of this is surprising or says much about empirical discovery, since reciprocal action was a fairly straightforward implication of interest in regulated movement. We might say that speculation about inhibition was inherent in thought about muscular control. Sherrington himself made this point, referring to Meltzer's description of inhibition in the rhythmic movements making possible respiration and swallowing: "Of a purposeful arrangement we could expect that a nerve, the stimulation of which causes flexion, ought to contain also inhibitory fibres for the extensors."[19]

Sherrington's studies in the reciprocal action of paired muscles showed that even apparently simple and rigid reflex actions were produced by excitatory and inhibitory impulses interacting in the spinal cord. Further, he showed that reflex inhibition was minutely graded and subject to processes like facilitation in ways comparable to reflex excitation. He therefore introduced a quasi-quantitative analysis of reflex movement, treating it as the summation of simultaneous positive and negative effects of an excitation, brought about centrally through nerve connections in the spinal cord. "If we denote excitation as an end-effect by the sign *plus* (+), and inhibition as end-effect by the sign *minus* (−), such a reflex as the scratch-reflex can be termed a reflex of double-sign, for it develops excitatory end-effect and then inhibitory end-effect even during the duration of the exciting stimulus."[20] Some examples of inhibition were known to be peripheral, that is, to act via special nerves to muscle (e.g., to the muscles opening the shell of the bivalve, *Anodon*), and for a while physiologists had looked for such nerves in vertebrates. Sherrington's work, however, showed firmly that, in vertebrates, "the inhibition reflexly produced has . . . its seat in the spinal part of the reflex-arcs. It is therefore a *central* inhibition."[21]

When he began his research on reflex control in the 1880s, Sherrington too had searched for special inhibitory nerves in vertebrates. He was impressed by Biedermann's demonstration of the existence of efferent inhibitory nerves in the crayfish, as well as by the phenomenon of vagal inhibition in vertebrates. Commenting on his training with Gaskell at Cambridge, Sherrington later wrote in a letter,

> To both him and me it always seemed that the taxis [movement] of vol.[untary] muscles was impossible without inhibition. But we both expected *efferent* inhibitory nerves to them. You remember the vivid interest in Biedermann and the Astacus claw. I used to search for similar things in mammal muscle-nerve. . . . Gradually, in view of one's reflex experiments, it burst upon me that for the vol.[untary] muscles, the inhibitories play not on the muscle direct but on the spinal motor cells driving them, and in that sense are all afferent or central.[22]

This was a major insight and one that diverged substantially from Gaskell's earlier opinion. It led Sherrington to his view that control was the product of inhibition and excitation playing on the motor center of nerves to muscle.

> The state of the skeletal muscle reflects faithfully the state of its motor centre. . . . Upon that motor centre many nerve-paths converge, transmitting to it nervous impulses from various receptive points and from centres elsewhere. Of these nerve-paths some excite, others inhibit. The latter, by quelling or moderating the discharge from the motor centre, quell or moderate the contraction of the muscle. The inhibition of the skeletal muscle is therefore always reflex; and the study of skeletal inhibition falls wholly under the head of reflex action. The motor centre is a convergence point for various reflex influences competing, so to say, for dominance over the muscle.[23]

This central competition of reflex influences concluded with "*the principle of the common path*," the fact that only a single, unified impulse passed to a skeletal muscle.[24]

Research on central inhibition was also advanced by using animals in a state of "decerebrate rigidity," the rigid condition exhibited by animals after an operation to separate the cerebrum. It proved possible to study minute variations in inhibition, recorded as a degree of muscular relaxation, in animals in this state. At the same time, Sherrington studied decerebrate rigidity in its own right, and this was an important link in his thought about the relations between the spinal and higher levels of control.

Sherrington was fundamentally concerned with the integration of the organism as a whole, and he therefore investigated the relation between the spinal reflexes and the brain as well as integration at the spinal level. He dedicated *The Integrative Action of the Nervous System* to Ferrier, whose work in electrically exciting the cerebrum in the 1870s had established a means for studying experimentally the integration of cerebral and sensory-motor processes. Sherrington was also aware of the observation, going back at least to Whytt in the eighteenth century, that destroying the connection between the brain and the spinal cord appeared to enhance muscular contractions. Sherrington showed that when the operation to separate the cerebrum was performed accurately in mammals, without damage to other centers such as the one controlling respiration, it always resulted in tonic rigidity, with tremor in particular groups of skeletal muscles, and that this state lasted for about four days.[25] He argued that decerebration "released" tonic excitation, and thus he gave precise expression to the old idea that higher levels normally exercised inhibitory control over lower levels. In effect, he restated Jackson's neurological concept of "loss of control" in neurophysiological terms.[26] Head explicitly brought together these Sherringtonian and Jacksonian conceptions.[27]

Decerebrate rigidity was sharply distinguished from "spinal shock," the suspension of reflex effects immediately following severance of the cord. Many researchers followed Goltz and assumed that this well-known phenomenon was an inhibitory paralysis comparable to that produced by any brain injury. Sherrington questioned this view; he correlated the results of shock with an animal's position in the evolutionary series, and he argued that shock had permanent effects, at least in higher animals.[28] In a general way, this supported the English neurologists who interpreted symptoms with an inhibitory aspect by reference to "release of function" rather than in terms of irritation from a lesion.

Sherrington studied spinal control by experimenting on animals "simplified" by eliminating cerebral control. In undamaged animals, however, the higher levels, as well as the spinal nerves, obviously contributed to the "final common path" to muscle. Working with H. E. Hering in Liverpool, Sherrington showed that cortical stimulation in monkeys produced inhibition with a coordinated character (relaxing antagonistic muscles at the same time as contracting flexor muscles).[29] This was direct evidence that high-level processes integrated with lower-level ones, and its demonstration in monkeys suggested that mechanisms of this kind might underlie human psychological processes. Yet it was a difficult matter to couch the relevant psychological question, whether the will acted as an inhibition on movement, in experimental physiological terms. It might be supposed, for example, as Meltzer suggested, that the ability to resist the effects of tickling was explained "by the fact that either we have trained the muscle antagonistic to the movement of these reflexes, or that the involved centres have lost their sensitiveness."[30] To demonstrate the inhibitory power of volition therefore required an experiment that eliminated any possibility of antagonistic muscle action. In Meltzer's view, Sherrington achieved this with experiments on eye movement.[31]

I have stressed Sherrington's work as a physiologist: he was successively professor of physiology at the University of Liverpool (1895–1913) and Oxford University (1913–1935), and physiology was a distinct discipline and occupation.[32] Nonetheless, his overarching interest in the purposive life of the whole organism necessarily led him to consider how psychical and physical states were integrated. For example, concluding a discussion about inducing inhibition through experimental cortical excitation, he commented that "the vast role of inhibition in cerebral processes [is] evidenced by mental reactions."[33] The ambivalent physiological and psychological connotations of inhibition persisted into the heartland of neurophysiology. "Again, if there be in the working of the mind such a requirement as grading of action, and if nerve-activity have relation to mind, we can hardly escape the inference that nerve-inhibition must be a large factor in the working of the mind."[34] He also compared the excitatory and inhibitory impulses in muscular coordination to the positive and negative elements in psychological attention. Physiological and psychological descriptions alike exploited the word's capacity to denote a certain kind of relation and hence a certain kind of order.

> In higher integrations where, for instance, a visual signal comes by training to be associated to salivary flow, the key of the acquiring of the reflex and of its maintenance is attention. And that part of attention which psychologists term negative, the counterpart and constant accompaniment to positive attention, seems as surely a sign of nervous inhibition as is the relaxation of an antagonist muscle, the concomitant of the contraction of the protagonist. In the latter case the coordination concerns but a small part of the mecha-

> nism of the individual and is spinal and unconscious. In the former case it deals with practically the whole organism, is cortical and conscious. In all cases inhibition is an integrative element in the consolidation of the animal mechanism to a unity. It and excitation together compose a chord in the harmony of the healthy working of the organism.[35]

This passage beautifully expressed the power of a word like "inhibition" to re-create as the mechanistic workings of physiology the teleology and wholeness of the organized living being and thereby to preserve the potential for an integration of physiology and psychology.

Lecturing to a general audience, Sherrington extended this theme, perhaps hinting that physiological inhibition contained the seeds for the evolution of human reflective understanding. "The brain seems a thoroughfare for nerve-action passing on its way to the motor animal. It has been remarked that Life's aim is an act not a thought. To-day the dictum must be modified to admit that, often, to refrain from an act is no less an act than to commit one, because inhibition is coequally with excitation a nervous activity."[36] He did not, however, elaborate anything resembling a psychological theory. His style before a nonphysiological audience drew on classical learning and poetry rather than on a technical approach to the mind-body relation to overcome the explanatory limitations of reductionist physiology. This was exemplified in his Gifford Lectures (1937–38), published as *Man on His Nature* (1940).

Inhibition was therefore a key concept in Sherrington's analysis of integration in a large sense. His refined experimental work demonstrated the manner in which excitatory and inhibitory effects coordinated to achieve the organization of movement and posture. He also conceived, however, that there must be a higher coordination involving "psychical integration." Integration at this level was the subject of psychology: nothing Sherrington achieved at the level of neurophysiological explanation was intended to detract from the reality of psychical processes. "Psychical integration" referred to the awesome phenomenon of the unity of the self. "The full panel of the 'five-senses' is in session, and by further collaboration with the psyche, a world of subject and object for the individual is in being. The individual has attained a psychical existence. Phases and moods of mental life accrue. . . . The self is a unity."[37] He therefore stressed that biological science would ultimately require the integration of physiology and psychology.

> The formal dichotomy of the individual, however, which our description practised for the sake of analysis, results in artefacts such as are not in

> Nature. . . . For our purpose the two schematic members of the puppet pair which our method segregated require to be integrated together. Not until that is done can we have before us an approximately complete creature of the type we are considering. This integration can be thought of as the last and final integration.[38]

Sherrington made the desideratum crystal clear, but his own mind-body dualism suggested no intellectual resolution. The experimental method was brilliantly productive in elucidating reflex organization, but it left psychology utterly unintegrated. "But theoretically [the final integration] has to overcome a difficulty of no ordinary kind. It has to combine two incommensurables; it has to unite two disparate entities. . . . This is the body-mind relation; its difficulty lies in its 'how.'"[39] Sherrington did not think that theory would resolve the problem. He believed that perhaps there was hope in pursuing the experimental study of perception and specifically the integration or fusion of sensations (the subject of his last Silliman Lecture).[40]

To round out Sherrington's thought about inhibition, it is necessary to note also that he made a major contribution to understanding its physical mechanism. Earlier, I described the variety of causal explanations current at the turn of the century. Sherrington was closely associated with the research in England which analyzed summation and induction as properties of nerve conduction,[41] though he himself studied such phenomena at the level of reflex integration rather than at the level of individual nerves. In 1897, he had, indeed, introduced the term "synapse" to describe the junction between neurons, the elementary structural units of nervous conduction.[42] In a series of papers dating from the mid-1920s, Sherrington and his collaborators—"the Oxford school"—developed a theory that excitation and inhibition were distinct synaptic processes. They rejected the long-standing view that inhibition occurred as the result of a physical interference effect on the excitatory process in the neuron. They argued instead that inhibition was an occluded state of the effector mechanism at the synapse.[43] This opened up an enormously profitable line of research, leading over the next two decades to detailed accounts of the chemical nature of synaptic transmission and inhibitory occlusion.

John Eccles, who collaborated with Sherrington and who later went on to win a Nobel Prize for his work on synaptic mechanisms, stated that Sherrington "had always been emotionally attached to synaptic inhibition. Inhibition in the central nervous system was really his scientific discovery in the 1890s. Before that, there were only a few crude

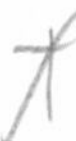

anecdotal accounts."[44] This was exaggerated, and it was only in 1925, and then in a paper that some judged too speculative, that Sherrington addressed the question directly. He then reworked what he understood by "integration" in terms of central excitatory and inhibitory states acting by summation and conflict at synaptic boundaries: movement was the outcome of summation and inhibition at synapses.[45]

The subject of inhibition acquired its most esoteric and technical form in such research. Inhibition appeared to have a precise empirical meaning in reference to the coordination of posture and movement and to the synaptic mechanisms effecting the coordination. This was not incompatible, however, with inhibition retaining its theoretical meaning as a requirement of the organism's unity of action and its connotations for wider notions of regulation. Sherrington himself was always sensitive to this wider context of meaning:

> That congeries [of vertebrate skeletal muscles], with its manifold individual pieces, some diametrically opposed to others, is so complex, and the confusion and waste of effort consequent were its component parts to obstruct each other's action would seem so foreign to Nature's usual harmonious economy, that inhibitory as well as excitatory control appears a priori almost a necessity.[46]

He was equally sensitive to the argument that a unified science of the organism required the successful integration of psychology with physiology, using such concepts as inhibition, though he disclaimed any ability to succeed in that task. Precisely this unification was claimed in the Soviet Union in 1950 as Pavlov's achievement. The next section discusses the circumstances of that Soviet claim, the difference between Sherringtonian and Pavlovian physiology, and the central position the concept of inhibition also had for Pavlov.

I. P. PAVLOV

If the 1920s in Britain saw the flowering of "pure science," exemplified by Sherringtonian neurophysiology, the 1920s in Bolshevik Russia saw the flowering of intellectual and social experimentation in science as in other areas. There were extended debates, both in philosophy and in the specific sciences, about the implications of Marxism-Leninism for achieving and implementing objective knowledge. These debates concerned the foundations of knowledge, though, at the same time, they were the vehicle for power struggles between different academic and political factions.[47] The imposition of a unified theoretical framework, grounded in dialectical materialism, occurred early in the 1930s. This was when Stalin and the party subjugated society as a whole to industrialization and "Bolshevized" all the institutions of higher education and learning. Through the 1930s and 1940s, the specific sciences became subject to the state's instrumental conception of its needs and then to the extreme exigencies of the Great Patriotic War. With the ending of the war and the shock caused by the United States developing and using nuclear weapons, the political center imposed a tightly controlled reconsideration of the foundations of each of the special sciences.

Soviet physiologists and psychologists lived through these circumstances. One significant element in the experience was the way the relation between the disciplines of physiology and psychology was always subject to scrutiny and factional maneuvering. At times, Soviet psychologists even feared that their subject would be completely subsumed under physiology. The proper scope of physiological and of psychological explanations was an ideologically sensitive matter. It was so sensitive because the relationship between physiology and psychology was crucial to the Marxist project of integrating objective knowledge about humans as material organisms with their existence as historically concrete actors. The language of dialectics provided the terms in which this goal was pursued. These circumstances sometimes fostered exciting and challenging innovations, for example, in the now influential work of L. S. Vygotsky (d. 1934). At other times, the conditions were stultifying, for example, following the three All-Union Congress decisions (1950, 1951, 1952, in physiology, psychiatry, and psychology) that the Pavlovian theory of "higher nervous activity" was the true framework for objective science.[48] These decisions, to a large extent, imposed "physiological" institutions and practices on a fragmented "psychological" discipline, though distinctive psychological practices did reemerge within a few years. What is clear at least is the contested nature of psychology's relation to physiology and the centrality of Pavlov's theories in the argument. It is therefore of more than passing historical interest that Pavlov made extensive use of inhibition.

Pavlov's contribution cannot be understood without reference to the Russian context, and his life spanned both tsarist and Bolshevik systems. Russian circumstances were different in the nineteenth century, and yet the scope of psychology and physiology was then also contested. The earlier account of Sechenov's work showed that inhibition was central to these earlier debates. His symbolic position as "the father of Russian physiology" and the associated claim that he discovered central inhibition indicate that Soviet writers have emphasized continuity in the topic of inhibition from the 1860s to the 1950s, from Sechenov to Pavlov and beyond. There is, in fact, no recent and reliable intellectual biography of Pavlov to assist our interpretation. Western scientists have sometimes discussed his work as if it had no context.[49] Soviet writers have been acutely aware that any mention of Pavlov's name has political and ideological connotations.[50]

Like so many intelligent young men of his generation, Pavlov was passionately inspired by natural science. An utter commitment to scientific methods and facts, which amounted to ruthlessness in his personal relations, dominated his long life. He had an unwavering faith in experimental natural science, in the form institutionalized in German higher learning, as a source of facts that would in themselves form the basis for humanitarian and medical progress. His judgments about the Bolshevik revolution rested on whether or not it facilitated his science. Initially contemptuous of the new "barbarians," he became perhaps the internationally most famous scientist to stay on in Soviet Russia, and the state increasingly supported his work through the 1920s. Before and after the revolution, he inspired a large number of researchers who were to play a major part in the later development of Soviet science.

Pavlov's research shifted from digestion to the study of reflexes, learning, and the higher brain at the turn of the century, when Pavlov was in middle age. He deployed the concept of inhibition in this later work, which continued until shortly before his death in 1936, in the last years principally in relation to psychiatric questions. Running through his whole career, however, from the 1870s studies on blood pressure to the early 1930s work on psychosis, was a concern with organic regulation and control. This interest made it possible for Soviet scientists to describe Pavlov's work as a major contribution to dialectical scientific thought: his focus on regulation stressed the interactive wholeness of the organism-environment relation in achieving constructive ends. It was sometimes claimed that Pavlov laid down a research program for understanding the dialectical processes of biology. The 1950s congresses made this the research program for human psychology as well. The Pavlovian scientist E. A. Asratyan wrote in 1953,

> Pavlov's data on the two fundamental antagonistic nervous processes—stimulation and inhibition—and his profound generalizations regarding them, in particular, that these processes are parts of a unified whole, that they are in a state of constant conflict and constant transition of the one to the other, and his views on the dominant role they play in the formation of

> the higher nervous activity—all these belong to the most established natural-scientific validation of the Marxist dialectical method. They are in complete accord with the Leninist concepts on the role of the struggle between opposites in the evolution, the motion of matter.[51]

The point was then made absolutely plain by juxtaposing extracts from Pavlov's and Stalin's writings. Nevertheless, there were always critics of this view, particularly those who believed that such a research program restricted understanding of the historical and cultural dimensions of the human subject.

Pavlov trained in Saint Petersburg and learned the great surgical skill that was essential to his experimental triumphs from Tsion, the professor of physiology at the Military Medical Academy from 1872 to 1875. There is some irony in Pavlov's relation to Tsion since, while the former was to become a hero of Stalinist science, the latter resigned his position in 1875 and emigrated to Paris because of his extreme reactionary views, although he was apparently the first and only Jew to be elected a full professor at the academy in the tsarist period.[52] Studying further in Germany with Ludwig and with Heidenhain from 1884 to 1886, Pavlov reported that the opening mechanism of the mussel shell included a special inhibitory nerve to the muscle responsible for closure.[53] This attracted attention as a possible model for vertebrate inhibitory mechanisms, though similar mechanisms were not in fact found. While Pavlov then turned to experimental studies of blood pressure and digestion, the interest in nerve mechanisms continued in Russia, associated with work on nerve conduction by Sechenov, V. Ia. Danilevskii, and especially Vvedenskii.

Tsion was one of the first teachers to introduce regular physiological demonstrations to students, though a commitment to experimental methods became normal in medical training during the 1870s. Pavlov owed little of his scientific commitment directly to Sechenov. Indeed, he probably had little respect for Sechenov's experimental or theoretical contribution. Pavlov acknowledged Sechenov's work only later in life and on celebratory occasions.[54] Pavlov's theory of nervous activity originated as a response to methodological contingencies in studying the control of digestive secretions, and his methods derived from Tsion rather than Sechenov. He consistently referred to Sechenov as a brilliant but speculative pioneer, not as a serious influence on his own work.

All the same, Sechenov's description of brain reflexes and central inhibition set a precedent for the "objective" language with which Pavlov described psychical processes. Pavlov recognized that Sechenov had attempted "to represent our subjective world from the standpoint of pure physiology."[55] As Daniel Todes has argued, they confronted the same general difficulty: "The problem was to bridge the gap between the general view that psychic phenomena were ultimately physiological in character and the reality that they could not yet be explained that way experimentally."[56] Both Sechenov and Pavlov therefore turned to the language of reflexes and of the interaction between excitation and inhibition. It appeared to them that the meanings of words in this language could be defined in terms of experimental variables while retaining physiological and psychological significance for the language as a whole. This language was fundamental to their attempt to construct objective psychology. Continuity between Sechenov and Pavlov existed in this abstract sense rather than in causal terms.

Russian physiologists in the late nineteenth century accommodated themselves to research rather than to the polemics for "enlightened" science that had been prominent in the 1860s. Sechenov's "Reflexes of the brain," however exciting when first published, did not suggest questions for, or guide, subsequent experimental research. When twentieth-century Soviet physiologists referred to the "Sechenov school," to cover research on nervous phenomena in the period from the 1880s to the 1920s, this must be understood as a label serving only to differentiate a group of related studies on nerve conduction from other trends and influences associated with Pavlov, V. M. Bekhterev, K. Kornilov, and others. The research known as the "Sechenov school" was institutionally located in physiology, and it interacted historically and intellectually with the Sherringtonian "school" at many points. K. S. Koshtoyants's history of Russian physiology attempted to portray work by Vvedenskii (on the refractory phase of the nerve impulse), V. Iu. Chagovets (on chemical effects on impulse strength), and A. F. Samoilov (on chemical transmission between nerve endings and muscle) as pioneering the conclusions usually attributed to Sherrington and his associates in the West.[57] In fact, the interesting historical relations and differences between Russian and Western researchers from the 1890s to the 1920s have not been studied.

The tradition of physiological experimentation on nerve conduction significantly contrasted with the research initiated by Pavlov. Pavlov's theory of "higher nervous activity" correlated gross functions in the brain with psychologically significant sensory and behavioral events, that is, with stimulus and response conditions. Pavlov referred to excitation and inhibition as the functional activity of the brain. In the

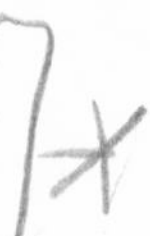

words of W. H. Gantt, an influential exponent of Pavlov's work in the West, "Pavlov thought of inhibition as an active process, and he thought of it as being able to spread and summate over the cortex."[58] Pavlov's language referred to the nervous substrata of observed correlations between sensory stimuli and physiological or behavioral responses. By contrast, the Russian neurophysiologists, here comparable with Sherrington, translated questions about excitation and inhibition into causal questions about nervous and synaptic conduction. Pavlov himself did not keep up with this literature, and by the 1920s, he was out of touch with the details of contemporary neurophysiology. The result, in the difficult material and political conditions of the 1920s as well as later, was that there was serious competition between the physiologists and Pavlov for resources and for intellectual control over research on the nervous system.

Very broadly, until the 1920s, the neurophysiologists (that is, the so-called Sechenov school) held dominant positions in academic physiology. During the 1920s, they were displaced by the so-called Pavlov school. The conception of inhibition was central to these struggles: it was an important resource for institutional conflict as well as a topic in its own right. The neurophysiologists argued that inhibition was a microphenomenon, and they accused Pavlov of not explaining inhibition at all but of misusing the term by deploying it metaphorically, generating only the semblance of an explanation for psychological events. Commentators have sometimes more particularly referred to the "Wedensky-Ukhtomsky school," based at the Institute of Physiology in Saint Petersburg/Leningrad University, which relied on research on peripheral nerve preparations to study excitation and inhibition, using these results to argue by analogy to central events.[59] Pavlov, based in the Military Medical Academy in the same city, studied the responses of animals, inferring excitation and inhibition in the brain. It was Pavlov's approach to inhibition that became dominant in Soviet science from the late 1920s until at least the early 1960s. Those who followed Pavlov, as has been explained, stated that his work genuinely elaborated a dialectical conception of the human organism. The Stalinist decision in 1950 to equate Pavlovian psychology and objective psychology entrenched an interest in Pavlovian inhibition as an orthodoxy.

The position was even more complex than this in the 1920s owing to the presence of various competing schools in psychology, each with its specific institutional interest. In Moscow, for example, Bekhterev continued his prerevolutionary rivalry with Pavlov, promulgating an eclectic program of research that claimed objectivity in ways in fact often shared by Pavlov. Bekhterev's psychology, "reflexology," also gave inhibition a very prominent place as an active process. Indeed, he described inhibition as the fundamental objective condition of subjective states: "From the objective standpoint, [subjective experiences] should be regarded as processes of inhibition or temporary blocking of correlative activity, which manifest themselves, as is well known, in weak external effects (so-called inner speech, controlled expressive movements, slight respiratory changes, vasomotor reactions, galvanic current in the skin, etc.)."[60] Thus he discussed thought as the inhibited or latent state of a reflex, with an imprecision more than a little reminiscent of Sechenov.[61] But his "school" did not outlive the 1920s.

It is therefore necessary to consider Pavlov's view of inhibition in more detail. He turned from the study of digestion to questions of higher nervous function during the years 1895 to 1901. The way in which he claimed the latter interest grew out of the former is well known. Pavlov and his colleagues showed that some of the conditions affecting salivary secretion in dogs were "psychical." For example, the sight of meat, or even a sound habitually preceding the sight of meat, led to salivation. Pavlov's collaborator A. T. Snarskii then endeavored to explain these phenomena by reference to the dog's supposed subjective sensations and desires. The methodologically rigorous Pavlov could not accept this.

> But I, putting aside fantasy and seeing the scientific barrenness of such a solution, began to seek for another exit from this difficult position. After persistent deliberation, after a considerable mental conflict, I decided finally, in regard to the so-called psychical stimulation, to remain in the role of a pure physiologist, *i.e.*, of an objective external observer and experimenter, having to do exclusively with external phenomena and their relations.[62]

As he continued, "The physiologist is obliged to abandon the subjective point of view, to endeavour to employ objective methods, and to try to introduce an appropriate terminology."[63]

Pavlov developed his theory in an extended series of lectures from 1903 to 1934 and by zealously directing the training and experiments of a close-knit and highly committed group of colleagues and students.[64] The core of the research involved exploring acquired reflexes and the influences that modified or eliminated such reflexes, that is, the laws of conditioning. He described as inhibitory anything that reduced the strength or regularity of a conditioned reflex, distinguishing three inhibitory factors, those that were external, internal, or associated with sleep. These distinctions had analogies with nineteenth-century neurophysiological studies of reflex control, but Pavlov was concerned with events that had a psychological character.

External (or "positive") inhibition referred to the disruptive effect of a new stimulus on a response.

> *External inhibition* is a complete analogue of that inhibition which was recognized long ago in the lower parts of the central nervous system when a newly arriving reflex inhibits one already present and active. It is evidently the expression of a ceaseless conflict among the different sorts of external and internal stimulations which determines which shall become at the given moment of predominant significance for the organism.[65]

"External inhibition" thus redescribed a well-known phenomenon in Pavlovian, experimental terms. Pavlov's own account built on experiments by his student M. N. Eroféeva, published in 1912, in which she induced a negative reaction to food in dogs by presenting food accompanied by an electric shock.[66] Her experiment demonstrated that innate activity could be suppressed. Continuing the experiment, she showed that the defensive reaction produced by the shock could itself be inhibited, restoring the food reflex. Sherrington, who witnessed this experiment on a visit to Saint Petersburg, reportedly commented, "Now I understand the joy with which the Christian martyrs went to the stake."[67] Eroféeva's experiments became of great theoretical and ideological importance since they appeared to demonstrate the organism's flexibility, even in relation to its innate capacities. Writing in the 1930s, Pavlov's disciple Iu. P. Frolov stated, "The central nervous system has no place for an unchanging 'hierarchy,' it has *no place for a constant, fixed mutual relation of such processes as excitation and inhibition*. . . . Theoretically speaking, we can change any centre to any degree, since all the remaining centres will have to 'efface themselves' before it."[68] Pavlov's program of research therefore appeared to be the systematic and objective study of behavioral flexibility.

Whereas external inhibition reflected the influence of an incoming excitation, internal (or "active") inhibition reflected the interaction of reflexes within the nervous system.

> *Internal inhibition* has its origin in the mutual interrelations between the new (conditioned) reflex and the old (unconditioned) reflex by means of which the conditioned reflex was formed. This type of inhibition always

> develops when the conditioned stimulus temporarily or constantly . . . is not accompanied by the unconditioned stimulus with which it was elaborated.[69]

Pavlov classified these internal inhibitions into four kinds, the first and simplest of which was "extinction," the elimination of a conditioned response by the failure of the conditioning stimulus to be followed by the unconditional stimulus (e.g., by ringing the bell the dog has learned to associate with food but then not providing the food).[70] The revival of a reflex during extinction became known as "disinhibition," and studying this phenomenon drew attention to the role that stimulus strength played in inhibitory processes. The other three kinds of internal inhibition were conditioned inhibition, inhibition of delay, and discrimination. The last type (known as "differentiation" in modern terminology) became closely associated with the study of animal perception. The relevant experimental techniques permitted research on an animal's differential response to stimuli.[71]

Pavlov's work became known to North American psychologists immediately before World War I, and in the 1920s, his "classical" conditioning technique was regarded as a major contribution to the experimental study of learning.[72] In North America, however, unlike in the Soviet Union, psychologists discussed Pavlov's laws of conditioning in relation to other learning theories rather than as a complete system in itself. They attempted to integrate Pavlov's work with research by E. L. Thorndike and the neobehaviorists, and they investigated differences between "classical" and "instrumental" conditioning. In this literature, inhibition sometimes appeared merely as a loose expression for the displacement of one learned pattern of response by another. Other psychologists argued that the concept of inhibition was unnecessary and that the extinction of a conditioned response should be regarded merely as a return to the status quo.

Pavlov did not intend to limit his research to developing a psychological theory of learning. He was committed to grounding psychology in knowledge of the brain, and hence he referred to his work as a theory of "higher nervous activity" and not as a theory of psychology.[73] Inhibition had much potential for the pursuit of this goal. The theory of higher nervous activity, however, unlike conditioning techniques, did not transfer well from the Soviet context to other settings, even though it was available in English translation from 1927.[74] Its persistence as a major focus for Soviet research into the 1960s perpetuated differences in national research styles. These differences were accentuated in the early 1950s, at the height of the cold war, when Soviet scientists claimed Pavlov's theory had achieved the dialectical integration of organism and environment.

At the same time as Sherrington and his collaborators were developing a "connectionist" approach to nervous processes, relating events to nervous arcs and the transmission of impulses along neurons and across synapses, Pavlov described nervous processes as waves of excitation and inhibition "irradiating" from nervous centers. He argued that these waves, when unimpeded, reflected and "concentrated" at their source. The English-language physiologists began to treat inhibition as a specific mechanism affecting synaptic transmission. Pavlov treated inhibition as a general activity of neurons, flowing in a wavelike manner, parallel to excitation. In the words of the English psychologist J. A. Gray, "It is not simply an interruption in the passage of neural excitation. It is a nervous process in its own right, opposite in sign to the excitatory process but equal in status."[75] Pavlov pictured waves of excitation and inhibition interacting, either to reinforce or to oppose each other. In "positive induction," the process of inhibition evoked excitation; in "negative induction," the process of excitation strengthened inhibition.[76]

Pavlov's laboratories sustained an experimental program that correlated all these "physiological" terms with the variables of "psychological" reflexes. There was a real danger that the physiological modeling was becoming so flexible that it would correlate with any kind of psychological process. The richness of the excitation-inhibition scheme for envisaging nervous regulation was leading to claims of infinite flexibility. These claims suggested a seemingly endless program of ever more refined experimental research. Given the very substantial material investment in Pavlov's work in the 1920s and its corresponding strength in personnel and institutional positions, those who had worked with Pavlov were therefore able to sustain his program for many years.

Pavlov regarded inhibition as a physiologically more fragile process than excitation. He linked this to a hierarchical, evolutionary view of inhibition as a power determining behavior. As Frolov pointed out, this had important consequences for understanding child development.

> The process of inhibition, being more delicate, also develops much later [than excitation], both in the biological sequence (the lower animals exhibit to a lesser degree than the higher) and in the course of individual development.
>
> In Pavlov's view, a child exhibits the process of inhibition to a consider-

> ably lesser degree than an adult. The child's cerebral cortex, being functionally weaker, is frequently unable to suppress the process of excitation, especially as the latter is reinforced by powerful impulses proceeding from the region of deep-seated specific instincts, the centres of which lie in the subcortical ganglia.[77]

Pavlov and Frolov therefore restated commonplaces about a child's nature. However, the restatement accompanied a powerful experimental technique for studying the questions further. It also appeared that Pavlov had made possible the study of such practical problems as "difficult" children.

Pavlov's basic concepts—excitation, inhibition, and equilibrium between nervous forces—would have been familiar to nineteenth-century physiological psychologists. This language continued to have both physical and mental meaning, to connote process rather than structure, and to link esoteric and everyday knowledge. Pavlov held that the nervous system was in a state of balance between excitation and inhibition and that this balance was constantly threatened by incoming stimuli. "We are forced to presuppose some struggle between two opposing processes, ending normally in a certain equilibrium between them, in a certain balance."[78] These processes were the irradiation of excitation and inhibition. The strength and scope of resulting movements correlated with the extent of spatial irradiation within the central nervous system: "Normal conduct is based on the elaborated delimitation of the points of excitation and of inhibition, on that magnificent mosaic in the cortex."[79] As the writer of a note in Pavlov's *Selected Works* observed, "According to Pavlov, it is precisely the relations between the excitatory and inhibitory processes, or their equilibrium, which determine all our behaviour, the normal and the pathological."[80]

Pavlov did not believe that psychology without physiology could have a separate identity or claim to be an exact science. All the same, his theory of the higher nervous centers, which supposedly grounded psychological explanation in physiological terms and thus created scientific psychology, was very speculative, and it linked only loosely to empirical knowledge about the brain. Terms like "inhibition" and "irradiation" did most of the explanatory work. Pavlov accepted that the physiological mechanism of inhibition was obscure, though he believed that it must be, like excitation, a general property of nerve cells, a point he thought established by Vvedenskii.[81] Such physiological questions, however, were not on his own research agenda. The subject for his own research, and for the "nervous" theory it supported, was set by the "psychological" phenomena of conditioning.

His work was also "psychological" and speculative in the sense that when he transferred conclusions from dogs to humans, he used everyday examples of inhibitory experiences, just as, for example, Sechenov or Brunton had done.

> For instance, in the case of games and various acts of skill, it is as difficult to abolish all sorts of superfluous movements as to acquire the necessary movements; and it is equally difficult to overcome established negative reflexes, *i.e.* inhibitions. . . . We know also how different extra stimuli inhibit and discoordinate a well-established routine of activity, and how a change in a preestablished order dislocates and renders difficult our movements, activities and the whole routine of life.[82]

As such passages made clear, reference to inhibition in Pavlovian science lost none of its nineteenth-century power to mediate between experimental science and ordinary experience and between mental processes ("to overcome") and physical events ("established reflexes").

It will be recalled that Pavlov's third major category of inhibitory factors was associated with sleep: sleep inhibition "regulates the periodic chemical metabolism of the whole organism, and especially of the nervous system."[83] He subdivided this inhibition into normal and hypnotic. Pavlov and his collaborators discussed sleep as an irradiation of inhibition through the whole cortex, presumably by a process analogous to, or even identical with, internal inhibition. Sleep inhibition supposedly spread progressively down from the cortex to the midbrain region. The variety and degrees of sleep could therefore be correlated with a lowering of brain activity, and the whole process could be studied experimentally through conditioning.[84] The general principle proved particularly suggestive in explaining hypnotic and pathological forms of sleep. For example, Pavlov explained Kircher's *experimentum mirabile*, with which he would have been familiar as a young physiologist in the 1880s, by suggesting that immobilizing the bird on its back produced cortical inhibition.[85]

> Catelepsy [fixed posture] in hypnosis is evidently an isolated inhibition of only the motor regions of the cortex, not spreading to the centres of equilibrium, and leaving free the remaining parts of the cortex. . . . Senile talkativeness and dementia too find a simple explanation in an extraordinary weakening of inhibition resulting from the feeble excitability of the cortex.[86]

In the 1930s and then particularly during the Great Patriotic War, this theory of sleep inhibition supported the extensive use of sleep therapy techniques in the Soviet Union. Psychoses and neuroses, such as those produced by combat, were treated by inducing extended periods of coma. Though this technique was tried elsewhere, it was most characteristic of Soviet psychiatry.[87]

The significance of Pavlov's work in the West, as well as in the USSR, for studying both pathology and individual differences is not widely appreciated. Yet, according to Gray, Pavlov "originated . . . the study of the biological basis of personality, and the experimental study of neurosis." Gray stated bluntly that "it is Pavlov, not Freud, who will be of lasting importance for the scientific study of both personality and neurosis."[88] This view needs to be explored.

It had been apparent to Pavlov from before World War I that differences in his dogs affected their suitability as subjects for experimental work. During the war period, these differences became a research topic in its own right, and Pavlov began to produce a typology based on characteristics that affected conditioning. This typology was designed with manifest relevance to human character. He postulated three basic dimensions to nervous processes—strength, balance, and lability—which he then used to redescribe ancient ideas of temperament.[89] "Balance" described the interaction and conflict between excitation and inhibition.

"Strength" described the correlation between the strength of a conditioned stimulus and the intensity of the conditioned response. Pavlov noted that in some animals an intense stimulus did not increase the intensity of response, and it could even lead to the weakening of the response. Terming this "transmarginal inhibition," he interpreted it as a form of protection for cortical neurons.[90] More significantly, he studied transmarginal inhibition to compare animal personalities and to classify them along a scale between strong and weak nervous systems. It was later shown that transmarginal inhibition was affected by drugs such as caffeine, and this was developed as an important analytic technique in personality studies.[91] In the last years of his life, Pavlov broadened the idea of transmarginal inhibition into a unifying explanation of hysteria and schizophrenia. He viewed such mental disturbances as simply the consequences of personality traits representing a very "weak" nervous system.[92] Pavlov's theory of the temperaments, like other character typings in the 1920s, such as Kretschmer's, was designed with pathological as much as normal subjects in mind.

Pavlov's attention shifted increasingly toward pathology after the mid-1920s. He believed that conditioning techniques, along with surgical intervention, could be used to study neuroses as well as character in dogs, and in his last work it contributed to his attempt to lay the basis for understanding human psychosis.[93] Inhibition continued to play a crucial role in this work, helping to make possible a translation of mental disorders into nervous events. All this then became a central plank in the Soviet construction of a dogmatically physicalist psychiatry during the war and in the postwar years.

It must be remembered that Pavlov had medical training. His specific interest in his dogs' neuroses, however, evolved from studies on the inhibition of unconditioned responses and the rupture in higher nervous activity that this involved. One kind of rupture appeared to be clearly analogous to psychic trauma or shock. He had a peculiar opportunity to study this after the Petrograd flood in 1924, when his dogs nearly drowned. The dogs were rescued from their cells only by pulling them underwater through low doors; different dogs reacted in different ways to the trauma.[94] A second kind of rupture was reported in 1921, in a now famous experiment by N. R. Shenger-Krestovnikova. She trained a dog to salivate in response to being shown a circle and not an ellipse, and she then exposed it to an ellipse, which the dog could discriminate from a circle only with great difficulty. The dog broke down.[95] Pavlov believed that this experimentally induced "neurosis" exemplified disturbance produced by the conflict of excitatory and inhibitory processes.

Pavlov had already begun to visit clinical wards at the end of World War I, and his support for studies of neuroses in dogs in the 1920s had strongly medical motives. He believed that his experimental research on animals was directly relevant to human illness.

> In the dog two conditions were found to produce pathological disturbances by functional interference, namely, an unusually acute clashing of the excitatory and inhibitory processes, and the influence of strong and extraordinary stimuli. In man precisely similar conditions constitute the usual causes of nervous and psychic disturbances. Different conditions productive of extreme excitation, such as intense grief or bitter insults, often lead, when the natural reactions are inhibited by the necessary restraint, to profound and prolonged loss of balance in nervous and psychic activity.[96]

Conditioning studies suggested a means by which the emotional disturbances of human life could become an object of science. Frolov wrote, "Pavlov succeeded in his latest work in building a firm bridge between the modern physiological laboratory and the modern neurological clinic."[97] It is likely, however, that the language that formed the structure of this bridge would have appeared familiar to Victorian psychiatrists. An everyday language of shock, disturbed balance, conflict between excitation and inhibition, and so on, preceded experimental research. Everyday psychology remained as the framework in terms of which Pavlov approached nervous organization and its disruption. The work on neurotic dogs after the Petrograd flood was a perfect symbol for the construction of esoteric knowledge out of shared experience.

Pavlov's work suggested forms of therapy as well as an understanding of mental disorder. He proposed "that a gradual development of internal inhibition in the cortex should be used for re-establishment of the balance of normal conditions in cases of an unbalanced nervous system."[98] This was the language describing order common throughout Victorian medical psychology, but in Pavlovian theory, it referred to techniques for building internal inhibition into the activity of experimental dogs or mentally ill patients. In practice, Pavlov himself recommended bromides or sleep to strengthen inhibition or restore the balance between excitation and inhibition in the cortex.[99] These were certainly therapies used by Soviet psychiatrists in the 1940s. Pavlov himself did not recognize the therapeutic potential of counterconditioning techniques, such as those initiated by Eroféeva in 1912, though behavior therapy was to be founded on his work.

Pavlov's legacy excited Russian, British, and North American psychiatrists alike during World War II, especially as his techniques appeared to be applicable to the treatment of war neuroses, and a number of psychiatrists experimented with conditioning.[100] This was an important route for the revival of Western interest in Pavlov's research. Learning theory, indebted both to Pavlov and to work in the United States in the 1930s, became an important source of ideas for treating the neuroses. Joseph Wolpe, for example, elaborated a therapy based on what he called "reciprocal inhibition," the extinction of undesirable behavior through forming new habits by conditioning.[101] Twentieth-century therapists, as well as their Victorian predecessors, have believed in the mental competition for limited resources of energy. Therapy, following this psychoeconomic model, became a normative intervention to control the distribution of those resources.

The German psychologist H. J. Eysenck, who had emigrated to Britain where he became a major influence over many years, sought to integrate Pavlov's studies on the variation among dogs with an experimental approach to human personality. Initially, he attempted to analyze personality quantitatively, bringing together earlier typologies, notably, the introversion-extraversion polarity derived from C. G. Jung, with the mathematical analysis of individual differences.[102] Working in association with the Maudsley Hospital in London, he was especially concerned to correlate personality and the incidence of neurosis. He considered that a predominance of excitation (and lack of self-control) fostered extraversion, while a predominance of inhibition (and tendency to self-control) fostered introversion. During the 1950s, scornful of the "untestable" claims put forward by psychoanalysts, he turned to behaviorist psychology, particularly Pavlov, for experimental inspiration in studying personality and in finding therapy for personality disorders. This led Eysenck to consider Pavlov's typology.[103] Thus, Eysenck recycled notions of inhibition taken from the American behaviorists, such as Hull, and from Pavlov's more physiological work. He kept in touch with parallel Soviet personality studies, particularly by B. M. Teplov, and inhibition retained its position as a central descriptive term in both British and Soviet work. Subsequently, Eysenck ventured to ground his conceptions of personality in physical processes, to "find biological causes underlying the psychological concepts of emotion, excitation, and inhibition which formed the building stones of my earlier effort."[104] Drawing on the conventional picture of hierarchical arrangements in the nervous system, he redescribed personality in relation to the degree to which higher brain levels were aroused and hence repressively active over lower levels. Greater arousal, he argued, enhanced inhibition, while decrease of higher-level activity released excitation.[105] Thus, introversion correlated with intense levels of "higher" activity, that is, thought rather than action.

Pavlov's lectures applying conditioning to psychiatry were known to Russians in the 1930s and appeared in English translation in 1941. By addressing questions of manifest psychological and pathological relevance, while yet appearing to ground psychology and pathology in objective brain science, he achieved a combination that was extremely attractive to researchers on both sides of what became divided Europe. He restated inhibition as a fundamental concept in brain science, and in so doing, he restated in a richly suggestive manner the nineteenth-century language that related internal individual control to external social forces. The therapy that used conditioning to induce inhibition of some behavioral trait brought Victorian moral language into a technically more refined age.

SIGMUND FREUD

Sherrington and Pavlov both won Nobel Prizes and the lasting respect of the scientific community for their experimental research. This cannot be said for Freud. Whatever Freud's status among academic psycholo-

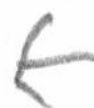

gists, however, common opinion closely associates his work with the achievements of psychology. The divergence of "scientific psychology" from anything resembling psychoanalysis, counterposed to the fascination that both social scientists and ordinary people express about psychoanalytic explanations, is a remarkable comment on our fragmented culture. Current representations of experience, conduct, and culture, outside of natural-scientific communities, refract an endless variety of Freudian themes. Many of these themes refer to inhibition.

Freud's work is central to debates about what counts as scientific knowledge and whether any approach that is not natural science contributes to objectivity about the human subject. These issues reappear in disagreement among historians about the sense in which Freud constructed psychoanalysis as a scientific project. The debate over whether Freud promoted biology or *Geisteswissenschaft* (hermeneutic or interpretive "human science") cannot be resolved only by empirical historical research, since it involves different viewpoints about the nature of explanation. The most specific point at issue concerns language, especially the meanings of words in German and the change of meaning that translation into English may have involved.[106] That it is possible to devote a book to the meaning of just one word, "inhibition," broadly supports the view that these debates about Freud's language have a fundamental character. Discussions about the meanings of words are about what sort of human science we want as well as about the claims of historical actors.

"Inhibition" was not a major term or organizing concept in Freud's writings. He developed his early psychoanalytic ideas after a training in neuroanatomy and neurology, and he thus took for granted physiological ideas of functional interaction, hierarchical control, and inhibition. At the same time, he used "Hemmung" in an everyday fashion, referring to the suppressing influence one part of the personality exercised over another.[107] Elements from both sources, the technical and the everyday, came together in his approach to psychopathology, notably, in the theory of defense, which incorporated his notion of repression. This mixture of the technical and the common remained characteristic of Freud's writing, and this, no doubt, in part explains the extraordinary impact it has had. It follows, however, that discussing inhibition is not the best way to provide a systematic exposition of Freud's work. Nonetheless, Freud's use of "inhibition" does exemplify my theme that the word was central to the discourse of control integrating physiological and psychological science and technical and popular modes of representing human action.

Historians and biographers have examined Freud's early scientific and clinical career in great detail, describing his slow construction of psychoanalytic practice and a theory of the neuroses in the early 1890s. Kenneth Levin, in particular, has tied this period of Freud's life to the Viennese medical, especially neuropathological, context.[108] As a result, we are able to see Freud as a member of the scientific community whose dimensions I have been mapping with reference to inhibition.

In the period after his return from studying with the neurologist J.-M. Charcot, in Paris (1885–86), Freud worked with patients presenting both distinct neurological symptoms and less clear-cut neurotic ones. His studies of the former resulted in the monograph, *Zur Auffassung der Aphasien* (1891), in which he used Jackson's ideas of nervous hierarchy and dissolution to criticize the attribution of speech disorders to localized lesions, which was the dominant view in the German-speaking world and fiercely asserted by Freud's one-time superior, Meynert, and elaborated by Meynert's protégé, Wernicke.[109] Jackson and Freud believed that the retrogression to "lower" modes of nervous activity, which had been so much remarked by all writers on neuropathology, should be explained in functional rather than anatomical terms, that is, they believed that the "release of function" occurred within the cortex and not simply by elimination of cortical control over subcortical centers.

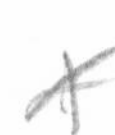

At about the same time, Freud was endeavoring to make sense of his experiences with hypnotism and hysteria in patients, some of whom he initially shared with Breuer. As Levin noted, it was common to discuss hypnotism as a release of inhibition.[110] Breuer used inhibition to describe the hysterical muteness of his patient, Anna O., a muteness she overcame in her spontaneously produced somnambulistic states. It appeared to Breuer that his patient was unwilling or unable to talk about something: "When I guessed this and obliged her to talk about it, the inhibition, which had made any other kind of utterance impossible as well, disappeared."[111] Breuer reflected theoretically on this experience, metaphorically interpreting what he supposed were the dynamic physiological energies of the nervous system.[112] Inhibition referred to a blocking memory or nervous energy creating hysterical symptoms. Freud, who collaborated with Breuer in the *Studies of Hysteria* (1893–1895), made Breuer's observation the starting point for the theory of repression and the dynamic unconscious.

Breuer and Freud used inhibition as a psychological term while discussing hysterical symptoms, and their usage suggests that a psychological meaning was unexceptional. It was not their primary interest to discuss whether or not psychological inhibition corresponded with any particular physiological process, though since they were trained in scientific medicine, the potential physiological meaning of inhibition was apparent to them. They were interested in comparing the general knowledge that individuals inhibited thoughts and impulses and the specific medical claim that hysterical patients inhibited memories to an extent and in a way that was pathological.

> Can it be a matter of chance that attacks in young people . . . take the form of ravings and abusive language? This is no more the case, I think, than the familiar fact that the hysterical deliria of nuns revel in blasphemies and erotic pictures. In this we suspect a connection which allows us a deep insight into the mechanism of hysterical states. There emerges in hysterical deliria material in the shape of ideas and impulsions to action which the subject in his healthy state has rejected and inhibited—has often inhibited by a great psychical effort.[113]

Freud's effort to compare what was known to be normal and what clinical experience revealed as pathological became the theory of defense.

Freud thus took for granted a general psychology involving the suppression of impulses. "How does a person with a healthy ideational life deal with antithetic ideas against an intention? With the powerful self-confidence of health, he suppresses and inhibits them so far as possible, and excludes them from his associations."[114] In hysterical patients, he argued, this suppression resulted in an unacceptable cost: what had been suppressed ("repressed") proved so active that it found an expressive outlet in physical symptoms. He surmised that the repressed content, which could not achieve conscious expression precisely because of the painful quality of the experience that led to the repression in the first place, returned as symptoms. What required explanation in the medical context was therefore not so much inhibition but the conditions in which repressions were successful or unsuccessful. Freud's early answer leaned on contemporary ideas about dissociated or split consciousness. He thus stated that in hysteria, "the distressing antithetic idea, which seems to be inhibited, is removed from association with the intention and continues to exist as a disconnected idea, often unconsciously to the patient himself."[115] Soon thereafter, Freud suggested that repression was a specially strong inhibition of ideas that were completely incompatible with conscious life. This was associated with his description of "resistance," the patients' inability or unwillingness to acknowledge that they did indeed have such suppressed memories. He also began to extend the notion of repression to account for more than hysterical neurotic symptoms, and this generalized approach to psychopathology became the theory of defense.[116] As he developed this theory in the period after 1894, he restored the comparison between normal inhibition and pathological repression, and he constructed a general psychological theory based on the avoidance of unpleasure, the dynamics of conscious and unconscious life, and the individual's developing sexuality.

Freud was a bold and deeply ambitious thinker who aimed to construct a general psychology. The empirical materials for this task came principally from his work as a specialist in nervous or neurotic illness. Such materials, however, did not provide Freud with the assumptions that structured the way he translated particular symptoms into general theory. Freud was well aware of this, and, accordingly, he made several attempts to state and define his assumptions, first in the famous theoretical chapter 7 of *The Interpretation of Dreams* (1900) and then in the papers on what he called "metapsychology." These theoretical writings show that his thought was deeply embued with nineteenth-century conceptions about nervous and mental processes of the kind discussed earlier in this book: causal determinism, explanation by dynamic forces, an economic model of energy, and a structural, developmental, and hierarchical approach to functional interaction.

These assumptions were reviewed in the 1950s by David Rapaport, in the context of the American Psychological Association's search for a way to compare psychological theories. Rapaport, himself an analyst, was set the task of stating Freudian theory in such a way that it could be compared with the current North American claimants to natural-scientific psychology. This led him to recognize that Freud had the viewpoint of a neurophysiologist trained in the 1870s and 1880s. Rapaport distinguished "topographic," "dynamic," "economic," "genetic," and "Jacksonian" (or hierarchical) models in this viewpoint, though these models were not sharply distinguished from one another in Freud's own writing.[117] Freud's starting point, and the continuing framework for his thinking, was a cluster of assumptions concerning the dynamic interaction between different elements of nervous or psychic energy and the way in which this interaction was ordered in spatial, developmental, and evolutionary terms. Freud said simply that "we shall be obliged to set up a number of fresh hypotheses which touch tentatively upon the structure of the apparatus of the mind and upon the play of forces operating in it."[118] In carrying through this program, Freud's expression was replete with references to energy, flow, damming up, diversion, cathexis (or energization of a system), and other words indicating the way in which competitive forces produced order. The power of complex metaphors was especially evident in the treatment he gave unconscious and conscious processes in *The Interpretation of Dreams.* He was aware that he had discussed the relationship between unconscious and conscious thoughts in possibly misleading spatial terms: images "of a preconscious thought being repressed or driven out and then taken over by the unconscious . . . [are] derived from a set of ideas relating to a struggle for a piece of ground."[119] Attempting to escape this metaphor, however, he jumped straight into another, replacing spatial by dynamic language, while preserving the imagery of physical competitiveness.

> Let us replace these [spatial] metaphors by something that seems to correspond better to the real state of affairs, and let us say instead that some particular mental grouping has had a cathexis of energy attached to it or withdrawn from it, so that the structure in question has come under the sway of a particular agency or been withdrawn from it. What we are doing here is once again to replace a topographical way of representing things by a dynamic one.[120]

This was a creative muddling of physical and mental categories that served his study of psychic systems.

The publication of Freud's discarded "Project for a scientific psychology" (written in 1895), which also occurred in the 1950s, drew further attention to psychoanalysis's intellectual debt to physiological science. This debt is not best described in terms of "influences," as was once done, but in terms of Freud's education in a scientific culture that equipped him, like his contemporaries, with certain models and conceptual resources.[121] For example, the "economic" model, which pictured psychic life as the distribution of limited resources and described energy flowing along lines of least resistance, was common property and not a specific influence on Freud. Freud gave a new direction to the common viewpoint, representing the instinctual forces in complex, dynamic interaction with the forces of social reality. According to Rapaport, in Freud's economic model, "the primary process operates with drive energies, and its regulative principle is the tendency toward tension reduction (pleasure principle)."[122] However, this economic model was not "patterned on the principle of conservation [of energy]"[123] expressed by Helmholtz, since the economic way of thinking about human conduct set the terms in which nonphysicists understood physical principles in the first place. Similarly, when Freud referred to one psychic force suppressing or inhibiting another, he was exploiting for his own purposes the conceptual resources of a common scientific culture. As Rapaport wrote, "In Freud's theory, inhibition of lower levels by higher ones served as the model for the conceptualization of conflict. Thus inhibition became a dynamic event: the result of a clash of forces."[124] None of this detracts from the creative way Freud developed these resources, but it does suggest a central reason why Freud's psychology fed back into common understanding. The dynamic and economic models, with their rich metaphorical and evaluative connotations, set both psychoanalysis and neurophysiology in a common culture. When the technical knowledge became "popularized," it was in the terms that had set the tasks for scientific study in the first place, namely, the terms of order and control.

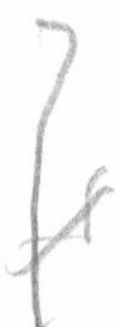

The fact that Herbart's philosophy occupied a central place in the Austrian school curriculum and that a professor of philosophy in Vienna, Robert Zimmermann, described himself as a Herbartian has suggested a Herbartian influence on Freud's belief that ideas may be inhibitory. The previous chapters, however, add weight to Levin's judgment that reference to inhibition was "pervasive" and that "there were also other extremely important sources for the same concept."[125] To pick out Herbart's "influence" involves pulling out just one thread. There was more common ground between Freud's view of inhibition and current psychophysiology and neuropathology than between his account and Herbart's discussion of dynamics. Further, while Freud was familiar with Griesinger's psychiatric text and with the ideas on attention put forward by his friend, Obersteiner, both of which reflected Herbartian notions, this is no reason to single them out as the particular sources for a way of thought that was commonplace.[126] Levin's history of the theory of defense stresses instead interaction between French writers, such as Pierre Janet, the theory of the dissociation of consciousness, and Freud's clinical observations, and this account is persuasive.

Freud referred to repression and resistance as psychological processes in his early published papers on hysteria and defense, and this commitment to a psychological level of explanation dominated all his later work as well as the public reception of his views. In a few intense weeks in 1895, however, he wrote, though he did not publish or even later discuss, the now famous "Project for a scientific psychology," which attempted to represent his psychological ideas in terms of the function of neurons. This incomplete essay (first published in 1950) revealed—as I have mentioned—the extent to which neurophysiological concepts and models informed Freud's creative theorizing.[127] The "Project" was in fact an extremely condensed and speculative, if perhaps brilliant, piece of "brain mythology." As such, it showed Freud integrating neurophysiological ideas of inhibition, generally available psychological beliefs, again including inhibition, and his clinical material.

Freud considered the neuronal basis for mental events as the possession of quantity of excitation (the "cathexis") by three different kinds of neurons. Neuronal interconnections and communication by excitation, inhibition, and facilitation thus structured the discharge of cathexis. He defined the discharge of cathexis as the state of pleasure, this state being the purpose of neurophysiological/psychological function. In turn, he defined the ego as "the totality of the ψ cathexes [cathexes in mnemic neurons, not altered by each new excitation], at the given time, in which a permanent component is distinguished from a changing one."[128] Thus characterizing the ego provided Freud with the means to describe a division between "primary processes" and "secondary processes." The former were the unimpeded discharges of excitation, whether originating externally or internally; this was, in effect, uninhibited discharge. The latter modified or inhibited the former, and the means to achieve this came with the formation of the ego: "those processes . . . which represent a moderation of the foregoing [primary processes], are described as *psychical secondary processes*."[129]

The division between primary and secondary processes—and the inhibitory relationship between them—was fundamentally important to Freud's general psychology. He argued that ω neurons, associated with consciousness, furnished a distinction between a perception (cathexes in ϕ neurons), and thus "it is probably the ω neurons which furnish . . . the *indication of reality*."[130] The indication of reality mediated the interaction between physiological needs and actual circumstances. This ensured that the pursuit of pleasure was driven not only by primary processes but also by secondary processes that imposed a recognition of reality and hence made it possible actually to avoid unpleasure. As Freud concluded his definition of the psychical secondary processes, "It will be seen that the necessary precondition of the latter is a correct employment of the *indications of reality*, which is only possible when there is inhibition by the ego."[131] Alternatively, "if there is inhibition by a cathected ego, the indications of ω discharge become quite generally *indications of reality*, which ψ learns, biologically, to make use of."[132]

At this point in his argument, Freud pictured a possible physiological mechanism for inhibition by the cathected ego. The details were arbitrary constructs, but, as was shown earlier, causal explanations for inhibitory mechanisms were rife at this time, and Freud's ideas were therefore relatively conventional speculation. He drew and annotated a network of neurons, so that the cathexis of one branch, which was part of the ego, facilitated the discharge of an excited neuron in a direction away from the neuron's connection with those neurons responsible for a motor or other effect. "A *side-cathexis* [in the ego] thus acts as *an inhibition of the course of* [quantity of excitation]. . . . Therefore, if an ego exists, it must *inhibit* psychical primary processes."[133]

The way in which Freud enmeshed physiological and psychological language in constructing a theory was more important than the details of the mechanism. The "Project" illustrates vividly the value of "inhibition" as a word that merged physiological and psychological meaning. The term acquired significance as a means for representing control in avoiding unpleasure, and that representation was then embedded in both a general psychophysiology and a specific theory of the neurons. Subsequently, Freud dropped the attempt to express his theories in physiological language. Indeed, accounts of the "Project" have exaggerated the role played by neurophysiological as opposed to psychological concepts and data: even in this essay, Freud relied on an everyday psychology of inhibition as a source of experience about what it was that required explanation. Thus, in a section on emotional disturbances, he observed that "it is quite an everyday experience that the generation of affect [i.e., emotion] inhibits passage of thought, and in various ways."[134] In these circumstances, he believed, the ego failed to inhibit primary processes. "The affective process approximates to the uninhibited primary process."[135] Physiological language was not essential to such descriptions; nevertheless, in the period when he was creating psychoanalytic theory, physiology did provide Freud with an authoritative and highly suggestive resource with which to systematize psychopathology.

Freud's thought developed rapidly after 1895 to encompass a theory of sexuality, his self-analysis and the interpretation of dreams, and jokes and verbal play of every kind. He sustained the most minute analysis into what people commonly thought of as trivial events alongside the attempt to formulate the most general assumptions of metapsychology. The general theory continued to represent dynamic and economic notions that had ambivalent physiological and psychological connotations. This was notable in the treatment of the primary and secondary processes at the end of *The Interpretation of Dreams*, a treatment strongly reflecting the earlier "Project." Discussing the unknown mechanism underlying the ability of experience and memory to influence the pursuit of primary pleasure, Freud observed,

> All that I insist upon is the idea that the activity of the *first* ψ-system [the primary process] is directed towards securing the *free discharge* of the quantities of excitation, while the *second* system [the secondary process], by means of the cathexes emanating from it, succeeds in *inhibiting* this discharge and in transforming the cathexis into a quiescent one, no doubt with a simultaneous raising of its level.[136]

Thus, Freud equated inhibition with the basic mechanism producing psychical repression. The secondary process functioned by inhibiting unpleasure, by imposing experience and memory on the unbridled pursuit of pleasure by the primary process. Thus, the activation or cathexis of the secondary process "implies a simultaneous inhibition of the discharge of excitation."[137] Inhibition was intrinsic to the secondary process, the process that, as Freud believed, mediated a person's primitive urges in the social world.

He also believed that the inhibitory relation between secondary and primary processes was temporal as well as structural.

> But this much is a fact: the primary processes are present in the mental apparatus from the first, while it is only during the course of life that the secondary processes unfold, and come to inhibit and overlay the primary ones; it may even be that their complete domination is not attained until the prime of life. In consequence of the belated appearance of the secondary processes, the core of our being, consisting of unconscious wishful impulses, remains inaccessible to the understanding and inhibition of the preconscious.[138]

Freud characterized what it was to be human in terms of inherited urges that were to some degree modified and contained by development, both individual and evolutionary, working through inhibition, but always retaining the power to dominate psychic existence. This was to prove a powerful and appealing re-creation of an ancient theme.

Inhibition remained a common term in Freud's writing, used in relation to a variety of activities such as work, feeling, or sexual aims, but it had no special prominence or technical significance. He thus used the word much as his contemporaries used it in relation to common psychological experience. His technical discussion about the economics of psychic control developed as part of the theory of defense. This, in its turn, in the period following World War I, became attached to a much more elaborated theory of the instincts. The possible exception to inhibition's marginalization as a technical concept in Freud's later work was the study, *Inhibitions, Symptoms and Anxiety* (1926). This work has usually been regarded as a not entirely successful attempt to explain anxiety, involving a further review of repression and defense.

Freud's main purpose was to understand anxiety, and in this 1926 study, he introduced his belief that "the *affect* of anxiety . . . came, not from the process of repression, not from the libidinal cathexes of the repressed impulses, but from the repressing agency itself."[139] He prefaced his main discussion, however, with comments on the relation between inhibition as a "function," that is, a normal psychic activity, and as a "symptom," that is, a sign of a pathological process.

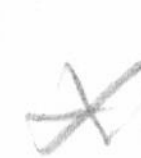

> Linguistic usage, then, employs the word *inhibition* when there is a simple lowering of function, and *symptom* when a function has undergone some unusual change or when a new phenomenon has arisen out of it. Very often it seems to be quite an arbitrary matter whether we emphasize the positive side of a pathological process and call its outcome a symptom, or its negative side and call its outcome an inhibition.[140]

Freud might also have noticed the further ambiguity that inhibition could refer both to a process and to the product of that process—"inhibitions." Thus inhibition was a process in the ego ("inhibition is the expression of a *restriction of an ego-function*"), while "inhibitions obviously represent a relinquishment of a function" and were thus symptoms requiring analysis.[141] When Freud described "inhibitions," he had in mind cases such as those involving denial of the sexual function or a disinclination to eat. His purpose, of course, was to go below the surface of inhibition (or inhibitions), which he assumed was familiar to his readers, to the psychic mechanisms involved.

While Freud considered that all inhibition was a restriction of ego function, he distinguished between specific inhibition, in which the ego avoided conflict with the id (or instincts) or with the superego (or conscience), and generalized inhibition, in which there was a general decrease in available psychic energy.

> When the ego is involved in a particularly difficult psychical task, as occurs in mourning, or when there is some tremendous suppression of affect or when a continual flood of sexual phantasies has to be kept down, it loses so much of the energy at its disposal that it has to cut down the expenditure of it at many points at once. It is in the position of a speculator whose money has become tied up in his various enterprises. . . .

> As regards inhibitions, then, we may say in conclusion that they are restrictions of the functions of the ego which have been either imposed as a measure of precaution or brought about as a result of an impoverishment of energy.[142]

Exploring the mechanism that underlay these processes, whether in normal function or in pathological symptom formation, required a restatement of defense and repression in the light of Freud's structural theory of the id, the ego, and the superego. This restatement may be considered to be Freud's distinctive psychological explanation for the mechanism of inhibition. 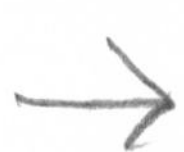 Anxiety was a characteristic result of inhibitory activity, and Freud thus treated anxiety as an affective symptom, not as part of the mechanism, though he also understood that anxiety, which, for example, accompanies coitus interruptus, may set repression going.

Freud and other analysts were naturally especially concerned with the particulars of symptom formation in different neuroses. At the same time, they had a zealous conviction that psychoanalysis, by comprehending the human condition, would influence the future of civilization. Freud constantly moved in his writing from detailed technical discussions to arguments with the most general implications. Further, despite his disavowals, these arguments were deeply evaluative. He wrote keenly for a general as well as for a psychoanalytic audience. Inhibition was a valuable term in this connection, since it was a familiar part of the vocabulary of personal control, character development, and the representation of higher values in a person's life, and at the same time, it aptly conveyed an analytic sense of repression (or repressed products). It appears likely that an existing discourse of inhibitory control provided Freud with a ready audience and that his work then greatly reinforced and enriched that discourse.

Freud's earliest pronouncements about repression and civilization came in his response to Christian von Ehrenfels, the Prague professor who had boldly criticized marriage in 1907. Freud accepted unquestioningly that modern civilization had produced an actual increase in nervous illness and "that the injurious influence of civilization reduces itself in the main to the harmful suppression of the sexual life."[143] He believed that his theory of sexual development, which explained that the sexual instinct did not initially serve reproductive functions at all but was directed toward autoerotic satisfaction, could illuminate this process. The key point, he thought, was to recognize that sexual energy could be turned to diverse uses.

> It places extraordinarily large amounts of force at the disposal of civilized activity, and it does this in virtue of its especially marked characteristic of being able to displace its aim without materially diminishing its intensity. This capacity to exchange its original sexual aim for another one, which is no longer sexual but which is psychically related to the first aim, is called the capacity for *sublimation*.[144]

Referring to the maturing of sexual development from autoerotism to object love, Freud argued that "a part of the sexual excitation which is provided by the subject's own body is inhibited as being unserviceable for the reproductive function and in favourable cases is brought to sublimation."[145] In unfavorable cases, the suppression of the sexual excitation was either incompletely carried through, producing perversions, or required so much energy that nothing was left for creative work. In the latter case, as Freud observed, people "are, as it were, inwardly inhibited and outwardly paralysed."[146] It was this, he believed, not physiological inferiority, that explained women's lack of intellectual accomplishment: "I think that the undoubted intellectual inferiority of so many women can rather be traced back to the inhibition of thought necessitated by sexual suppression."[147]

Freud's writing, in such passages, illustrated and presumably in some sense influenced the characteristic usage of inhibition in twentieth-century language. Inhibition tended to refer to the fact and not to the mechanism suppressing an agency opposed to conscious ends, and most commonly of all, it referred to suppressing instinct—with the clear implication that the instinct was arrested but not destroyed. These views continued to be present, though amplified by extensive metapsychological reflection, in Freud's later work. Thus, in 1926, discussing obsessional neuroses, he commented on "with what tenacity the ego clings to its relations to reality and to consciousness, employing all its intellectual faculties to that end—and indeed how the very process of thinking becomes hypercathected and erotized."[148] And thus, the inhibitory function may take on the form of pathological repression. While rejecting the view that inhibition involved a simple opposition between conscious life and instinctual impulse, Freud provided ample reinforcements for this conventional image of subjective conflict. Writing in a way that was reminiscent of a nineteenth-century mental pathologist like Maudsley, Freud dwelled pessimistically on the likely outcome of repressions: "If the ego succeeds in protecting itself from a dangerous instinctual impulse, through, for instance, the process of repression, it has certainly

inhibited and damaged the particular part of the id concerned; but it has at the same time given it some independence and has renounced some of its own sovereignty."[149] Inhibition thus appeared simultaneously as a condition for achieving civilized relations and, through this achievement, as a condition that removed instinct or repressed material to a realm in which it was no longer accessible to control.

This was the theme of Freud's polemic, *Civilization and Its Discontents* (1930), which retains its position as a reference point in the critical analysis of modern cultural and moral life. Abandoning religion as a childhood illusion of mankind, Freud stubbornly detailed the consequences of accepting that "what decides the purpose of life is simply the programme of the pleasure principle."[150] The vicissitudes of this pursuit, sustained in the face of sexual and destructive instincts and the material conditions of existence—and above all, of even modestly civilized existence—accounted, he argued, both for suffering and for achievement, the latter not being realizable without the former. Drawing together his theories of defense, sexual development, and the sublimation of instinctual energies, he drove home the fundamental principle that "civilization is built up upon a renunciation of instinct" and that "this 'cultural frustration' dominates the large field of social relationships between human beings."[151] The possibility of a social existence depended on successfully sublimating erotic love. Love for family, and what was claimed as love for humanity, was "aim-inhibited love": "Love with an inhibited aim was in fact originally fully sensual love, and it is so still in man's unconscious."[152] Thus, Freud did not hesitate to attribute to inhibition all the crucial processes through which control in the individual rendered possible order with a social character. "Aim-inhibited love [leads] to 'friendships' which become valuable from a cultural standpoint because they escape some of the limitations of genital love, as, for instance, its exclusiveness."[153]

During and after Austria's terrible experiences in the war of 1914–1918, Freud concluded that there must be an instinctive aggressive force in the psyche, independent at its source from the sexual forces he had previously emphasized. Freud imagined this force to be inherently destructive, assuming the form of what he called "the death instinct," which "operated silently within the organism towards its dissolution."[154] In part, in *Beyond the Pleasure Principle* (1920), Freud was undoubtedly seeking an expression for the killing called war. He was also endeavoring to think through his earlier presuppositions about the primitive forces driving the organism. Last, he was trying to comprehend the refractory nature of many symptoms, notably, "the compulsion to repeat" in illnesses such as traumatic neuroses (including so-called shell shock). Reflecting on his assumption that the pleasure principle was to be explained causally as a reduction of tension, he defined instinct as "*an urge inherent in organic life to restore an earlier state of things* which the living entity has been obliged to abandon under the pressure of external disturbing forces."[155] If the aim of life was tension reduction, then, it appeared to Freud, "*the aim of all life is death.*" This claim went far beyond the clinical setting, and Freud acknowledged that "we must therefore turn to biology in order to test the validity of the belief."[156] The biological evidence to which he turned once again portrayed organic processes as the balance of forces, exemplified by reproduction giving life, on the one hand, and foreshadowing death, on the other. Assembling his biological evidence, he cited Ewald Hering's general physiology, which had argued that life consisted fundamentally of two complementary but opposite continuously active processes, assimilation and dissimilation. This physiology had also featured in turn-of-the-century discussions of the mechanism of inhibition.[157] This was badly dated evidence for an argument in 1920, but it did reveal the kind of natural-scientific thought that informed Freud's most general presumptions about the psyche.

Freud believed that the death instinct was always in fact alloyed with sexual forces, and sexual development caused destructiveness to be directed outward as aggression as well as inward in complex ways, especially through the formation of guilt. As a consequence, the inhibitory processes that formed other-directed love and that sublimated sexual love as friendship and even just plain cooperation were the means of taming not only sexuality but destructiveness itself. Though Freud referred to "the antithesis between civilization and sexuality," it was sexuality, when successfully aim inhibited, that provided the power to control the threat of annihilation from within and that thus ultimately rendered civilization possible. But "in order for these aims to be fulfilled, a restriction upon sexual life is unavoidable."[158] Significantly, Freud also expressed himself rather loosely, referring, as so many other writers had done, to barbarism as a failure of inhibition to control innate aggression.

> In circumstances that are favourable to ["this cruel aggressiveness"], when the mental counter-forces which ordinarily inhibit are out of action, it also manifests itself spontaneously and reveals man as a savage beast to whom consideration towards his own kind is something alien. Anyone who calls to

> mind the atrocities committed during the racial migrations or the invasions of the Huns . . . or even, indeed, the horrors of the recent World War—anyone who calls these things to mind will have to bow humbly before the truth of this view.[159]

The attempt to contain aggression thus consumed society's energies and explained the extraordinary moral injunctions with which people attempted to bound their lives. "Hence, therefore, the use of methods to incite people into identifications and aim-inhibited relationships of love, hence the restriction upon sexual life, and hence too the ideal's commandment to love one's neighbour as oneself—a commandment which is really justified by the fact that nothing else runs so strongly counter to the original nature of man."[160]

In passages such as this, Freud's usage brought the language of inhibition back full circle, via medical psychology and neurophysiology, to refer again to containing fallen nature. He offered a secular eschatology, a meditation on innate sin, but without the possibility of redemption. Where faith in redemption had once inspired hope in the spiritual future, knowledge about the means of inhibition and sublimation now offered a tenuous grasp over the material present. "The instinct of destruction, moderated and tamed, and, as it were, inhibited in its aim, must, when it is directed towards objects, provide the ego with the satisfaction of its vital needs and with control over nature."[161]

Freud explained how moral culture and social tradition interacted with the individual's maturation to achieve inhibition. During the course of the individual's development, moral culture became internalized as the superego, which, "in the form of 'conscience,' is ready to put into action against the ego the same harsh aggressiveness that the ego would have liked to satisfy upon other, extraneous individuals."[162] Drawing on his metapsychological deductions and his experience of psychopathology, Freud elaborated an influential theory of guilt, stressing its necessary but also damaging effects on the ego's aims. Guilt, he argued, was the subjective consequence of sustaining a moral culture. "Civilization, therefore, obtains mastery over the individual's dangerous desire for aggression by weakening and disarming it and by setting up an agency within him to watch over it, like a garrison in a conquered city."[163] In these circumstances, "the price we pay for our advance in civilization is a loss of happiness through the heightening of the sense of guilt."[164]

Freud's approach to these issues also incorporated the assumption that individual development, that is, the containment and sublimation of the instincts, repeated human history as it had developed from savagery to civilization.[165] Thus, inhibition was at one and the same time both a collective and an individual achievement, an ancient accomplishment that has been endlessly repeated. The choice of the word "inhibition" was a reminder that the accomplishment was constantly at risk, collectively and individually, since it conveyed belief that the disruptive powers were contained or diverted but never destroyed. Viewed from this perspective, Freud's work, similarly with neurobiology from the 1940s, reinforced yet further commonplace belief in the necessary repressiveness of civilized existence and the corresponding willingness to describe both individual and collective violence as the reemergence of natural forces.[166] Nevertheless, from a different perspective, the work of Freud and other analysts on the psychic mechanisms of inhibition developed a new means to restore to reason a critique of the dominance of "natural instincts" in human affairs. Understanding what had previously been unknown perhaps created the means, in the form of collective rational insight, to regulate inhibition with minimum damage and suffering. The exploration of this ambivalent legacy has sustained reference to inhibition in the years since 1945.

The analysis in this section has remained close to Freud's own writing. This has enabled what he wrote to emerge as part of a discourse about the regulated person shared with Sherrington and Pavlov. This should not seem strange or remarkable: they shared training in physiology and shared technical and everyday concepts describing inhibitory control. Freud's writing, however, has fed back into nonspecialist language to a unique degree. Further exploration into inhibition in the twentieth century would therefore have to encompass the public's assimilation of psychoanalysis.

The word "inhibition" is now a popular rather than a technical term. Barry Richards has suggested that a popular receptivity to Freud followed from psychoanalysis's capacity to make coherent sense out of incoherence in modern experience.[167] On this view, Freud is crucial to our understanding of modernity. Other writers, notably Philip Rieff, have interpreted Freud as a figure offering therapy in place of redemption, the source for a moral vision in an age that has lost a vision of Christ.[168] In yet another approach, taken by Christopher Lasch, psychoanalytic language suggests terms with which to understand a culture seemingly unable to value anything other than individual subjectivity and thereby destructive of values themselves.[169] As such broad arguments make clear, Freud has inspired critique rather than historical studies about "popularized" psychoanalysis, however much the latter work would contribute resources for the former. Freud's assimilation into common language has undoubtedly been an active process, structured by meanings already in place in the nineteenth century. Further, his significance is associated with the general rise to prominence of psychology as a group of academic and applied disciplines but more especially as the discursive medium through which we conduct social life.[170] As I have suggested, the manner in which the late twentieth century represents psychological practices to itself draws on the language of ordered relations that acquired authority in the nineteenth century.

Scientific work discussed organized activity, which constituted something of value, as a consequence of ordered relations in body and mind. In turn, the values of organized social existence entered into how the body was understood. Further, we may suggest, though to support the claim would require a different historical study, bodily activity itself also expressed meanings in common with what was understood about its function. Posture, habit, "gut feelings," or inhibition embodied value, internalizing meaning. Bodily life, we may presume, is as much a part of the discourse as the systematic language that describes that life.

When Freud described inhibition as a condition of civilized existence, he described how the order that makes society possible became an order within the person. As that social order also distributes and differentiates power, so the bodily order also distributes and differentiates power. Thus, Freud provided richly suggestive terms for assimilating the personal to the political, or the political to the personal, and this has been the cornerstone for social critiques drawing on the Freudian legacy. Herbert Marcuse opened his book, *Eros and Civilization* (1955), by stating simply, "Sigmund Freud's proposition that civilization is based on the permanent subjugation of the human instincts has been taken for granted."[171] Beginning after World War I, when Marxists responded to the failure of workers in Central Europe to act "objectively" in their own revolutionary interest, an eminent left Freudian tradition has identified social power in internalized values.[172] Inhibition, though more particularly repression, has acquired a richly resonant political meaning in the life of the physical body as much as in the political body.[173] This is evident even in everyday exchanges with little political intent. I have tried to show that these meanings have a history and that this history encompasses natural science.

CHAPTER 6

Reflections

Avons-nous donc enfin le dernier mot de ces questions? Hélas! non.

———François Magendie, *Leçons sur les fonctions et les maladies du système nerveux*

It seems to me that you are solving a problem which goes beyond the limits of physiology in too simple a way. Physiology has realized its problem with fortitude, breaking man down into endless actions and counteractions and reducing him to a crossing, a vortex of reflex acts. Let it now permit sociology to restore him as a whole. Sociology will wrest man from the anatomical theater and return him to history.

———Alexandre Herzen, writing to his son, Alexander, in July-August 1868, quoted in K. S. Koshtoyants, *Essays on the History of Physiology in Russia*

Narratives must end. To be sure, each strand in the story continues in current physiological and psychological science, just as each strand leads off into larger historical questions. A natural scientist might therefore expect the story to end more concretely in present knowledge. A social scientist, by contrast, might wish to learn about the political economy of inhibition in industrial society or of disinhibition in post-industrial society. These endings, however, are not my own, since this has been a *history*. Presumably nobody unsympathetic to the purposes of history will have read to the end of a book such as this. As history, it has construed the meaning of inhibition by describing contexts of use in scientific and nonscientific communities. Such history is a form of knowledge in its own right, not subordinate to either natural or social science.

This is not "the history of ideas," since no historical sense can be made of such a project. As Quentin Skinner argued, "There is . . . an underlying conceptual confusion in any attempt to focus on an idea itself as an appropriate unit of historical investigation."

> The appropriate, and famous, formula . . . is rather that we should study not the meanings of the words, but their use. For the given idea cannot ultimately be said in this sense to *have* any meaning that can take the form of a set of words which can then be excogitated and traced out over time. Rather the meaning of the idea must *be* its uses to refer in various ways.[1]

Bearing this in mind and wishing to focus on the content of scientific knowledge, I have written about language as a system of meaning. The Renaissance historian William J. Bouwsma noted that so-called intellectual history was exhibiting "an increasing concern with the location, the description, and perhaps the explanation of what passes for meaning in a variety of historical situations."[2] The language of inhibition expresses what controlled and organized relations have meant within the body, between mind and body, or between a person and society. This book describes these uses of the word "inhibition": this is what the word has meant.

Keith Michael Baker has argued that history's special business is "to reconstitute the context (or, more usually, the plurality of contexts) in which [a historical] phenomenon takes on meaning as human action."[3] What still confuses many people is the claim that the same practice could be central to the history of "science." I have argued, by exemplification rather than theoretically, that this is indeed so. The language of control was a language shared among social, moral, psychological, and physiological contexts. History here therefore argues against the still dominant natural-scientific view that scientific language shuts out normative meaning, the view most firmly expressed in philosophies of science drawing a categorical distinction between factual and value statements. This narrative has rejected that distinction, thereby restoring to scientific language its full range of reference in historical experience.

It is common to refer to the subject matter of narratives such as this as a "discourse." I intend the word to denote the presence of a common language or other system of representations, each term of which articulates with every other term across a broad but specifiable time and place. It indicates that this language constitutes an integrated world of meanings, encompassing knowledge claims, evaluative presumptions, and codes of practice. More forcibly, a discourse includes a particular normative criterion of what it is for a claim or a quality to count as knowledge or as a value. It thus identifies the framework in terms of which descriptive and evaluative claims, and action and power based therein, acquire an appearance of naturalness and inevitability. To describe the discourse of control, as I have done in a limited way for inhibition within the individual person, is to describe the linguistic conditions for modern Western views on what this control is or could be.

There are well-known problems associated with making discourse the subject of historical work.[4] First, it undoubtedly fosters description rather than explanation, *if* by the latter is meant the assimilation of knowledge, or knowledge-based practices, to material, social, and political conditions. Historians who think of what they do as a contribution to social science, as that has generally been understood in the empiricist English-speaking world, seek explanations in this sense. From that point of view, a focus on meaning may appear to presuppose epistemological idealism, assigning conditions of knowing or meaning logical priority over material conditions. This point was also raised against structuralist theories. What is therefore needed is an effort to transcend this dichotomy of material and knowledge conditions by recognizing that the material and the ideal are mutually constitutive in discourse. But the historian will note in particular that what is perceived to be material (or social or political), and hence explanatory in the orthodox social science sense, is itself part of a system of representations whose meaning is open to historical study.

Second, many historians consider that they have a special responsibility to explain *change*. By contrast, concentration on discourses tends to bring out a static continuity in experience. The description of inhibition, for example, is subject to circularity, presupposing and establishing continuity between early-nineteenth-century theories of character and twentieth-century physiological psychology. It is nevertheless possible to identify the *changing contexts* in which each elaboration of the discourse occurred. If the demand were made that change should be the prime question, then the history would have to be about the detailed lives of particular individuals, institutions, and practices. The explanation of change is a subject for micro-historical or micro-sociological analysis, as in the case studies presented by the historical sociologists of science. Change in scientific knowledge occurs as the result of day-to-day negotiations of a kind that I have generally not sought to describe. There is, I have supposed, something to be said about significance and meaning in knowledge, that is, about the reasons, as well as the causes, for its production.

Third, discourses can appear to be monolithic entities permitting no position external to them from which they can be criticized, let alone overthrown. If a discourse contains its own norms regarding truth and values, and if it encompasses all modes of representing experience, then there can be no purchase for alternative visions. The discourse of regulation, however, has never had this monolithic character. At no time was it either entirely coherent or comprehensive. Thus, inconsistencies in empirical data, divergences in training between scientific groups, or dialogue between specialist and generalist writers all sustained conditions for criticism within the discourse.

Fourth, debates about discursive analysis are tied up with rejection of the authorial subject and intentionality, while the overwhelming majority of English-speaking historians turn, at least in part, to the purposive acts of individual persons in explaining events. I have not questioned the liberal humanist values behind such history. Indeed, constant reference to the meaning that statements had implicates the intentionality of persons. Nevertheless, the stress on discourse indicates that more weight has been placed on the communal nature of language and on the way it conveys a message going well beyond the conscious intentions of any one individual. It may well be, at some abstract level, that I have adopted an eclectic practice; but, writing as a historian, it is the intelligibility of the narrative rather than the coherence of abstract propositions which comes first.

These criticisms do, of course, suggest historical as well as philosophical questions that I have not addressed and to which I do not pretend to know the answers. How was regulation conceived in the eighteenth century, and did a new discourse originate at the beginning of the nineteenth century? Were other ways of framing knowledge about regulation, perhaps excluding inhibition, possible in other circumstances? Has inhibition lost its Victorian resonance as Western countries approach the end of the twentieth century in conditions of material surplus? To what extent has inhibition literally become embodied—as postural expression, as gender relations, or as pathology?

This book has taken only a first step. Readers without a specialist interest in the history of science, for example, might wish that it had pursued inhibition into literature or into the political economy of society. There are two related responses to this. The first is simply to observe that published history of physiology or psychology is in no state to provide authoritative resources for larger ambitions. Anyone who has puzzled about the extraordinarily complex development of the brain sciences, let alone the relation of brain to mind, will have sympathy with this view. The existing histories are partial, often unreliable, and always incomplete. I have therefore not hesitated to use my theme as a device for introducing some historical clarity into this area. Even with this relatively restricted theme, it has still been necessary to locate the brain sciences in relation to a great range of other topics—philosophical, medical, and moral.

The second response concerns the unique authority that natural-scientific knowledge commands in modern Western culture. It is not the historian's part to defer to the scientist's understanding of what now constitutes objective knowledge of nature. Objectivity, too, has its history. But the historian of science does want to write history about that knowledge of nature for which the value of truth is claimed. History must comprehend the elaborate, detailed, and precise content of modern science if it is to stand any chance of explaining what it is that sustains science's authority. Hence the preceding chapters have taken time to explore the content of scientific knowledge, even if this is at the expense of other areas of culture.

The history of meaning is not hampered by prior categories as to what is "scientific" and what is "social" and by the consequent problem of describing the causal relation ("influence") between the two realms. It has therefore been possible to describe "inhibition" as a conceptual vehicle for integrating scientific and everyday meanings. It has been an empirical, historical matter to describe the variety of ways in which meanings have passed between different contexts of use. This has frequently been a subtle and complex process. Efforts to correlate gross elements of a scientific world view (e.g., holism) with large-scale social groupings (e.g., a conservative class) have foundered on exceptions and qualifications. Investigators of the social relations of science therefore find it more profitable to describe claims about nature as resources available for social negotiation or conflict. "Resources" are drawn on as reason and opportunity suggest; they do not dictate a strategy. I have not discussed the social relations of physiological or psychological knowledge by correlating, for example, hierarchical conceptions of nervous organization with the interests of a hierarchical class society. Sometimes, indeed, the Victorians did construct this correlation in the crudest way, opposing the heads of the upper classes to the hands of the lower. More often, however, the correlation was constructed indirectly by small groups negotiating over specialized interests (typically, the status of experimental results). Insofar as individuals or groups expressed wider social values in their work—and I have tried to show that they did—they did so within the framework of the standards, conventions, and linguistic resources of occupational practice.

Scientific language frames the concepts that are a condition of possibility for the existence of certain kinds of knowledge. Such framing, however, obviously occurs in specific institutional contexts, and these may be narrowly specialized with a highly restricted entry. At the same time, and without contradiction or denying its suitability for scientific usage, language crosses into domains wider than any specialized scientific community. A specialized community may reconstruct language for a particular narrow purpose, but it does not thereby empty language of its wider meaning.

Scientific communication now has strikingly distinctive characteristics. Scientific texts therefore require special techniques of interpretation. As Gyorgy Markus has argued, it was natural-scientific communities in the nineteenth century that achieved clear normative frameworks for expressing a "depersonalized objectivity" in scientific texts and for constructing specific, restricted expectations concerning relations among author, text, and reader. "Natural science as the cultural genre which *we* know, as the familiar form of institutionalized discursive activities, is the product of a nineteenth-century development in which the cognitive structure, institutional organization, cultural forms of objectivation and its global function have changed together."[5] This has undoubtedly reduced, sometimes to vanishing point, the meaning of these texts for the wider culture. The meaning of a research paper in neurophysiology must be understood in reference to the community in which it appeared and to which it was addressed. It does not seem to me, however, that this in principle excludes scientific texts from having meanings in relation to a wider culture, though it may in practice do so. It is an empirical and historical matter to trace the exclusivity of language and meaning to particular communities and to decide just how exclusive it in fact is. I have interpreted meaning in the light of such contingencies rather than in the light of an idealized epistemology of science or assumptions about the hermetically sealed nature of scientific communities.

Inhibition is therefore a history of the relation, as embodied in language, between specialized claims about nature and social values. There has indeed been a common discourse over the last two centuries or so for the science and the morality of control within the individual person and in political economy. The vocabulary of this discourse has been put to use in an endless variety of ways and for an endless variety of purposes.

I have given priority to describing the discourse in the areas of research where physiology and psychology met. The concept of inhibition was a sine qua non of scientific knowledge of the organized nervous system, the substratum of mind. It was also integral to psychological analysis of the organized mind, the function of brain. It was a concept with special value since it denoted a process of control that could be represented as a physiological or psychological event or left conveniently ambivalent. More richly yet, the language of inhibition integrated scientific and lay visions of control and thereby retained a seductive potential for those writers who desired a human science speaking to and for general as well as specialized audiences. Even within technical scientific writing, the language of inhibition proved attractive in the difficult task of formulating neurophysiological concepts capable of characterizing the physical basis of mind. These concepts had somehow to represent mind or intelligent action supervening as control over automatic functions. As Peter Amacher commented, "At some point in their description of physical processes [neuroscientists] are forced to fall back on something which has most of the attributes of an intelligent being and which is located somewhere in the upper parts of the nervous system."[6] Reference to inhibition was a key resource mediating this intelligent "something" in the physical world.

It was necessary to clarify developments in understanding the brain and mind in the century between 1830 and 1930 to make possible any wider argument. This detail about science was also part of a rhetorical strategy. No one should underestimate the continuing strength of the belief that science constructs knowledge that is strictly separable, by virtue of its empirical rationality, from other human endeavors. Obviously, science is different in many respects, and studies of argumentation in science have shown how. All the same, science—even the indubitably "real" or "hard" science of neurophysiology—shared a discourse with wider domains that encompassed the psychology, the morality, and the economy of organized control. It was necessary to include some detail on neurophysiology to make this point. Some readers will feel I labor the issue. Other readers, scientists perhaps, will remain attached to the faith that when all is said and done, science can be distinguished as autonomously rational discourse. I can only ask members of this church to draw the line separating the "scientific" from the "nonscientific" meanings of inhibition in the earlier chapters. The boundaries that can in fact be drawn are those delimiting occupational groups with the power to require language to be used in particular ways. Even the most prestigious of these groups, such as Sherrington's at Oxford, or the most authoritarian, such as Pavlov's in Leningrad, drew on and enriched what was finally a common discourse of inhibition.

These chapters allude frequently to the richness of the language of inhibition in mediating between physiological and psychological explanation and between technical and lay understanding of human action. It is evident, I think, that we cannot say that inhibition "really" denoted one thing, while it only connoted others. Nor can we say that one phenomenon exhibiting inhibitory control (the action of the will, perhaps) uniquely established a metaphor for the description of others. Sometimes, undoubtedly, metaphor was at work, as with Jackson's and Mercier's fondness for likening the cerebrum to an army commander. Even then, however, it was not simply the case that one social phenomenon stimulated the metaphorical expression of scientific knowledge. Rather, there was a set of discursive resources, linked by descriptive and normative connotations, permitting almost limitless creative expression. There were, of course, certain recurrent expressive patterns, conventions that indicated shared values concerning the mind controlling the body, the rational intelligence controlling the emotions, and the individual person contributing to social order. The possibility of metaphorical expression became attenuated as specialized scientific communities developed aspects of the discourse into an elaborate body of knowledge about regulation in the body. Peculiarly rigorous techniques of experimental observation, supported by the refinement of an esoteric language, increasingly isolated scientists from the wider society. Even so, the need to tie together the physiology of regulation and psychological life led scientists to revert repeatedly to a language that bridged specialist and lay communities. Sherrington did so when he considered the whole, cortical and conscious, integration of the organism. Freud did so throughout his psychoanalytic writings, creating an approach to regulation that proved accessible to a wider audience in a way denied to physiological writing.

A very interesting question about metaphor was raised by Sechenov when he posited a center for inhibition in the brain on the grounds that we all experience the power of the will to repress automatic movements, as when we regulate our response to pain or tickling. It was indeed common to argue that knowledge of psychological control required physiological inhibition. More generally, major models of brain function, like those constructed by Ferrier or Meynert, for example, translated psychological categories into physiological structures. We may ask whether anything other than metaphor lay behind this translation. Critics of model building ("brain mythology") like Head believed that clinical or experimental data had an authority unmatchable by psychological metaphor. By contrast, James's biographer, Ralph Barton Perry, quoted James's belief that our subjective psychology necessarily equipped brain physiology with its key notions.[7] Some thirty years earlier, John Stuart Mill had observed that knowledge derived through introspective analysis "is in a considerably more advanced state than the portion of physiology which corresponds to it."[8] Thus, the question as to whether psychology could or should be a source of notions for brain research, or whether this source was problematic metaphor, was unresolved.

Reference to "metaphor" may not be adequate to describe the transfer of meaning between the areas of interest relevant to the history of inhibition. Instead, we might refer to a network of mutually constitutive meanings. The notion of a "network" derives from Mary Hesse. Her critical analyses of the possibility of independent observation statements and her demonstration that models (or metaphor) had more than heuristic functions in scientific theory contributed to a rejection of philosophies opposing society and nature as sources of knowledge.[9] A network, then, is a system of interlocked predicates informed by society and its values as well as nature and its facts. Characterizing predicates as "observational" or "theoretical" is a matter for social negotiation, though the result of this negotiation may be the achievement of stable patterns. Such stability is dependent on satisfying *both* correspondence and coherence conditions. As David Bloor has observed,

> It is perfectly possible for systems of knowledge to reflect society and be addressed to the natural world at the same time. Put simply, the answer to the problem is that the social message comprises one of the coherence conditions, whilst the negotiability of the network provides the resources for reconciling those demands with the input of experience [the correspondence conditions]. The idea that knowledge is a channel which can convey two signals at once requires us to drop the assumption that nature and society are polar opposites.[10]

From this perspective, the social value of the self-regulated person—someone with a "good character"—was a coherence condition for any scientific theory of mental or bodily control. Scientific theory, to be intelligible, had to show how the workings of nature made possible normative controlling actions in the lives of human subjects. At the same time, and in a manner that was profoundly complementary, the scientific interrogation of nature fashioned the construction of knowledge, thus satisfying the correspondence conditions for authoritative knowledge.

The body, subjectively perceived and objectively presented, is the richest of symbols for social values. Mary Douglas referred to "the two bodies"—self and society.[11] The individual and the collective body live as terms within a common language expressive of relations between parts and a whole. The history of inhibition is one concrete example of this language in Western society. It also exemplifies her dictum that "there is a continual exchange of meanings between the two kinds of bodily experience so that each reinforces the categories of the other."[12] This "exchange of meanings" occurred between subjective perception (e.g., the controlling will) and social relations (e.g., the army commander), and this exchange informed the construction of science. Esoteric neurophysiology, as well as everyday psychological descriptions, exchanged meaning between social and bodily experience. Assuredly, as the history of physiological inhibition shows, that exchange came to be indirect, the outcome of a complex historical process involving the differentiation of communities and occupations. Unless there is an understanding of this historical process, it will appear that the connection between inhibition in modern neurophysiology and inhibition as a social value is nonexistent. That appearance of "nonexistence" is a historically contingent outcome. It also serves the interests of parties whose authority is invested in compartmentalizing knowledge of nature and social existence. Sometimes, however, the exchange of meaning between science and society is direct and unabashed, as in MacLean's and Delgado's discussions of the human emotional brain.

This book is about the individual and not the social body, except insofar as the meanings of the latter were represented in knowledge of the former. It is also a history of knowledge about the controlled body and not a history of subjective experience or emotional expression regarding the body. It would be a different though complementary task to describe the literal embodiment of knowledge and values. Undoubtedly, reference to inhibition resonates with modern subjective psychological and bodily experience. We are therefore left with questions. Have the complex sciences of the organized person reconstructed subjective awareness of what it is to be so organized? Does the notion of a "well-regulated" person refer to the same thing in the late twentieth century as it did a century earlier? How far has inhibition come to define the possibility of self-control and even self-identity? How has inhibition changed in conjunction with class and gender? What does it mean to be uninhibited?

It has been claimed that nineteenth-century society placed an unparalleled stress on the body as "the arena of *self*-control."[13] The language of inhibition indeed articulated this stress and corresponding subjectivity. Living the life of a repressed body seemed central to Victorian virtue. Such repression has been traced more generally by Norbert Elias in his account of "the civilizing process," linking bodily manners to the development of orderly political life. "Physical clashes, wars and feuds diminish [in the transition from medieval to early modern society]. . . . But at the same time the battlefield is, in a sense, moved within. Part of the tensions and passions that were earlier directly released in the struggle of man and man, must now be worked out within the human being."[14] If indeed bodily repression achieved its apotheosis during the nineteenth century, then this appears of a piece with the extent and prominence of physiological and psychological accounts of inhibition. Such accounts appealed as the authoritative means to represent the regulated body and the ordered person, themselves often conflated, as the condition of civilization.

Elias linked the capacity to reflect rationally on nature with the establishment of affective controls. This view was anticipated by nineteenth-century psychological theory (propounded, for example, by Sechenov or Morgan) making thought conditional on inhibited reflexes. Elias charted the development of internalized affective controls by studying the history of external manners, just as Sechenov studied inhibition in modified reflexes. He then described a reciprocal relationship between these affective controls, which distanced the person from his or her body, and the achievement of intellectual distance, that is, objectivity, in the study of external nature.

> Scientific modes of thought cannot be developed and become generally accepted unless people renounce their primary, unreflecting, and spontaneous attempt to understand all their experience in terms of its purpose and meaning for themselves. The development that led to more adequate knowledge and increasing control of nature was therefore, considered from one aspect, also a development toward greater self-control by men.[15]

In turn, Elias claimed, internal and external distancing processes fostered the individual's separation from society and the subjective experience of that separation as a personal individuality. "What is encapsulated are the restrained instinctual and affective impulses denied direct access to the motor apparatus. They appear in self-perception as what is hidden from all others, and often as the true self, the core of individuality."[16] The argument has the potential to turn the history of inhibition through a full circle. The embodiment of repression made possible the objectivity characteristic of natural science. That embodiment altered subjectivity, and subjective inhibition and objective knowledge of inhibition then established themselves through reciprocal exchanges of meaning. Finally, objective and apparently autonomous science gave authority to a particular vision of the individual's subjective being and social presence.

Early mentions of inhibition referred to descriptions of character, the dynamics of mental content, and the physiological control of bodily functions. Inhibition appeared in two schemes of dynamic relation, a hierarchical one emphasizing the top-down arrest of spontaneously active processes and an interactive one emphasizing the mutual moderation of equivalent processes. Herbart's statics and dynamics of mental content expressed a different logic and exploited a different metaphor from J. C. Bucknill's reference to woman's tenuous repression of "the subterranean fires." Different notions of regulation therefore contributed to the consolidation of inhibition, though it was the hierarchical schemes that most directly incorporated traditional values of the relation between mind and body. The projection of hierarchies onto nature made possible the insertion of value—intelligence, judgment, choice, thought—into the workings of the human mechanism. Inhibition made possible, in Todes's words, the "asymmetry between stimulus and response . . . that distinguished psychic phenomena from simple reflex actions" and therefore made room for traditional values in a scientific world.[17]

This stress on the mind-body hierarchy as the vehicle for moral values may not do justice to a historical dimension relevant to interactive schemes of dynamic regulation. I refer to control engineering, the technology of self-regulating machinery, with a history from mill machinery to James Watt's governor for the steam engine to the feedback loops of electronic circuits. The logic of regulation in this area concerns the distribution of energy within a closed system. We may assume that there was a more or less close relationship between an industrializing economy, dependent on control technology as well as productive technology, and the sciences of the mental and bodily economy.[18] Early industrialization prompted efforts to regulate machinery and workers alike as part of the production process. Further, as social historians have shown, ideals of ordered labor were extended outward to encompass leisure and society generally.[19]

The relationship between industrial society and the sciences of organic control was perhaps most evident in the United States in the present century. In the period between the world wars, the American physiologists L. J. Henderson and Walter B. Cannon drew considerable scientific and public attention to the formidable and often exquisite self-regulatory capacities of organisms. Cannon and Henderson portrayed life as the achievement of stability under varying conditions. Cannon called the body's ability to alter its own activity to compensate for externally induced change organic homeostasis. Thus, for example, the dilation of peripheral blood capillaries changes with changes in temperature, ensuring that the organism maintains a constant body heat. The ability of the body to regulate itself—which Cannon made famous as "the wisdom of the body"—depends on structures integrating nervous and hormonal information.[20] Such integration is, in essence, a process of balancing forces to preserve a stable condition. Henderson's research, which reached similar general conclusions, focused on the maintenance of the properties of the blood as a physicochemical system. This followed his earlier work on understanding the physical constitution—"the fitness"—of the environment that made life possible.

Cannon and Henderson also shared both a prospective and a retrospective vision of the centrality of physiological regulation. The prospective vision saw in organic stability a model for the ordering of society, an ordering that would reduce the excessive swings of economic and political forces that had created disorder and suffering in the twentieth century. Both looked to market forces to create self-regulation within capitalist society. Cannon wanted to supplement these forces with a permanent regulatory bureaucracy that he compared to the nervous system within the body. Henderson, by contrast, sought for ways to enhance those individual sentiments that, he argued, were the means to sustain society in equilibrium. In both views, it was the rationality of control within the individual organism that suggested the strategy to achieve social rationality. Their message, which appeared to utilize scientific knowledge to address questions of social disorder, resonated widely among professional people in the 1930s.

The retrospective vision portrayed the physiology of regulation as a working out of the classic insights of Bernard. Cannon and Henderson discovered in Bernard's concept of the internal environment their own idea of physiological constancy. Beyond Bernard, they found inspiration in the ancient belief in the healing power of nature: "The idea that disease is cured by natural powers, by a *vis medicatrix naturae*... implies the existence of agencies which are ready to operate correctively when the normal state of the organism is upset."[21] In their accounts, the healing power of nature, the stability of the internal physiological environment, and the general homeostatic mechanisms of the body all fostered the realization that stable organization was the condition for maintaining life—and, by what was more than analogy, society, too. Cybernetics and systems thinking subsequently confirmed the generality and productiveness of this focus on organization and control, whether at the level of machines, organisms, or societies.

This brief excursion into the twentieth-century sciences of organization and control indicates something of the breadth and complexity of the subject, of which the history of inhibition is only part. As a matter of historical fact, theories of regulation from Bernard to Cannon, Henderson, Wiener, and von Bertalanffy did not use the word "inhibition." These scientists described regulation in terms of the equilibration of forces, or the equilibration of information, and they chose language other than that of inhibition to describe the arrest of one force by another. But, in abstract terms, they described dynamic relations that other writers, working in different settings, represented as inhibition.

Nineteenth-century writers, from Herbart to Spencer to Freud, also perceived a common logic in the dynamics of physical systems and those regulating the person. Such writers envisaged the body or the person (once again, the interchangeability of these categories is noteworthy) as a conservative energy system. Spencer went so far as to conceive every relationship, the mental and social included, as a redistribution of energy, and he believed that relationships could therefore ultimately be deduced from the newly formulated laws of thermodynamics. By the mid-twentieth century, the paradigm of the closed energy system was giving way to one based on communication theory, which separated control information from the energy driving a system.[22]

Even in the nineteenth century, Watt's "governor" and later refinements appeared as an analogy in physiological and psychological literature. In the 1860s, the physicist James Clerk Maxwell presented a paper on the theory of the governor (differentiating a "moderator"), which much later attracted the attention of Wiener.[23] A variety of self-regulating devices were well known by this time. Thirty years earlier, Charles Babbage had systematically considered the technical and economic significance of regulating power in the new factory system. His point, that power had economic virtue insofar as it was regulated power, was well brought out by Bagehot in the 1860s in his complacent, conventional view of the superiority of English character.

> The English not only possess better machines for moving nature, but are themselves better machines. Mr. Babbage taught us years ago that one great use of machinery was not to augment the force of man, but to register and regulate the power of man; and this in a thousand ways civilized man can do, and is ready to do, better and more precisely than the barbarian.[24]

Thus, the technological and economic transformation of Europe perhaps also transformed sensibility in relation to regulation. But this aspect of the discourse on inhibition is, as yet, largely unexamined.

The meanings and contexts of use that linked even one term, "inhibition," were therefore complex and diverse. Christian imagery, governors and government, political and bodily economy, physiological or psychological experiment all played a part. Such complexities cannot be described simply as the play of metaphor. Metaphors were commonplace, but the ground or source of metaphor was sometimes the biological body, sometimes society, sometimes a phenomenologically derived account of being. It was not possible, in the last resort, to draw a firm distinction between what inhibition denoted and what it connoted. There was no ground independent of the web of metaphorical meanings. Each description of inhibition was a sign or representation within a common discourse. Meaning derived from the sign's articulation within the whole "picture." No one signification had absolute truth. Within natural science, inhibition came to signify regulative processes embedded in natural reality and known through observation and experiment. But the historical evidence is that science developed as a set of signs constructed through training, technique, and convention.

The history of science is a history of profound attempts to represent the world as order. Nineteenth-century physiological and evolutionary science included humankind within the ordered world of scientific knowledge, with implications that continue to bewilder—witness seemingly unresolvable debates about responsibility or the mind-body relation. It has been all too easy, for advocates and critics of science alike, to view scientific knowledge and religion as autonomous endeavors, forced into confrontation with each other by nineteenth-century science. Modern historiography, however, substantially rejects this conflict thesis, and it has instead described extensive and diverse interconnections.[25] A related conclusion follows from this history of regulation, since it has shown that the evaluation of human conduct was constitutive in comprehending the bodily or mental conditions making organized activity possible. Physiology was not in conflict with ethics. If physiological science provoked a "crisis" about what it was to be human, this was as much a crisis of coherence within science as between science and the wider culture. A science of human action did not develop without serious incoherence about fundamentals—concerning mind and body and values and facts. Theories of inhibition served to elide some of these difficulties.

Turgenev's famous portrait of the nihilist, Bazarov, in *Fathers and Sons* (1861) captured the moment when the new experimental physiology of frogs laid claim to human nature. Bazarov, like his nonfictional counterparts, believed that his research achieved an objectivity transcending the world of human values. Nevertheless, when scientists constructed a neurophysiology of frogs, they had in mind and they represented in language principles of order deeply informed by the human sphere. Those who also wished to be psychologists, like Sechenov, James, and Freud, restored the connection as an explicit part of the scientific enterprise. Others, such as Vvedenskii or Eckhard, eschewed nonphysiological statements but without thereby constructing a language that had no psychological reference. Even rigorous twentieth-century experimentalists like Sherrington and Pavlov, when they tried to talk about the broader implications of scientific understanding, indicated the difficulties faced by a physiology cut off from psychology. Concepts like inhibition, which characterized process and organization rather than mind or matter, suggested a way out.

Reference to organization, in the frog or the human, implied reference to the environment or to society. Terms such as "inhibition" therefore necessarily implicated thought and judgment about how the individual interacted with society and, indeed, made social order possible. Organization at the social level assumed the capacities of people, capacities bound up in the West with a Christian culture—the regulation of the flesh by the spirit and the value of individual grace, autonomy, and responsibility. By the nineteenth century, political economy and a burgeoning industry and technology stressed the value of the self-regulated individual. Physiology represented this stress in theories of bodily regulation. It "embodied" the imputed contribution of the individual to social order within the individual. Through its minutely precise practice of experimental research, it reconstructed this embodiment as empirical knowledge. Empirical knowledge, in its turn, generated authority for claims about human nature and social progress.

Notes

1: THE HISTORY OF INHIBITION

1. For an overview and exemplification of the body as a form of political discourse, see Outram, *The Body and the French Revolution.* For nineteenth-century case studies, see Gallagher and Laqueur, eds., *The Making of the Modern Body.*

2. Smith-Rosenberg, *Disorderly Conduct.* Women were also often associated with madness: Showalter, *The Female Malady.*

3. Walter Bagehot, among English writers, exemplified this social psychology of political order: Bagehot, *Physics and Politics.* For the ethos of reform politics, see Harrison, *Peaceable Kingdom*, 378–443.

4. Jordanova, *Sexual Visions*, 20–23. For an exploration of these resources in relation to criminal law, see R. Smith, *Trial by Medicine.*

5. Mercier, *The Nervous System and the Mind*, 141. Mercier took his conception of the body politic from Spencer: "The social organism."

6. Freud, *Civilization and Its Discontents*, 122. This argument was taken up, e.g., by Norbert Elias in his account of "the civilizing process"; see esp., Elias, *The Civilizing Process: State Formation and Civilization*, 229–247.

7. Genesis III: 14.

8. R. Williams, *Keywords*, 12.

9. E.g., Collins, *Changing Order*; Mulkay, *Science and the Sociology of Knowledge.* For this sociological approach applied to the history of the brain sciences, see Star, *Regions of the Mind.*

10. See Beer, *Darwin's Plots*, chap. 2; Danziger, "Generative metaphor"; Figlio, "The metaphor of organization"; Jordanova, ed., *Languages of Nature.*

11. Brunton, "On the nature of inhibition," 419. This was cited as the "classic" definition in the most comprehensive review of the subject: Diamond, Balvin, and Diamond, *Inhibition and Choice*, 7.

12. Canguilhem, "The development of the concept of biological regulation." Adolph (1961: 749) concluded that the term was "domiciled" by Hermann Lotze in 1842 (contemporaneously with ideas relating physiological metabolism to the conservation of energy). For the technological dimension, see below, chap. 6.

13. This was the title in translation of the famous book by J. O. de La Mettrie, *L'homme machine* (first publ. 1747): *Man a Machine.*

14. Grimm and Grimm, *Deutsches Wörterbuch*, 4: cols. 983–985. For usage in philosophical writing, see Ritter, ed., *Historisches Wörterbuch*, cols. 1054–1056.

15. Littré, *Dictionnaire de la langue français*, 4: 991. When first published in 1863–1872, Littré cited only a jurisprudential use, equivalent to a prohibition. Robert (1963, 4:4) attributed the physiological use to C.-É. Brown-Séquard (see below, chap. 4), indicating that the psychological use followed from this.

16. Cortelazzo and Zolli, *Dizionario . . . italiana*, 3: 596.

17. The question of the Russian equivalent of inhibition was mentioned by W. Horsley Gantt, who worked with Pavlov on the latter's theory of cortical processes: Gantt, "Pavlov," 181. The transliterated word in question is *tormozhenie.*

18. On evolution, from divergent perspectives, see Kohn, ed., *The Darwinian Heritage*; R. J. Richards, *Darwin and the Emergence of Evolutionary Theories*; Stocking, *Victorian Anthropology*; Young, *Darwin's Metaphor.*

19. This process has been described as "the naturalization of values." Relevant studies include Haraway, *Primate Visions*, and Young, "The historiographic and ideological contexts of the nineteenth-century debate on man's place in nature."

20. This question is pursued further below, chap. 6.

21. As Steven Shapin has argued, much history of science has become implicitly if not explicitly highly sociological: Shapin, "History of science and its sociological reconstructions." See also Barnes and Shapin, eds., *Natural Order.* For a clear and concise statement of the sociology of scientific knowledge, see B. Barnes, "On the conventional character of knowledge and cognition." I discuss further my claims for intellectual history, below, chap. 6. The level of detail needed to reconstruct the causal production of knowledge was exemplified in Rudwick, *The Great Devonian Controversy*; for an example in the brain sciences, see Star, *Regions of the Mind.*

22. E.g., Dodge, "The problem of inhibition." The problem, of course, is not unique to inhibition. For an analysis of the meanings of "stimulus," see Gundlach, *Reiz—Zur Verwendung.*

23. I use "biology" in a conventional sense that has been questioned: Caron, "'Biology' in the life sciences." Caron argued that existing histories have not succeeded in identifying biology as a nineteenth-century discipline (except in a very limited way). Even if this were to be accepted, my point, linking inhibition to structure-function relations, would still hold.

24. Bichat opened his best-known work with the famous definition, "La vie est l'ensemble des fonctions qui resistent a la mort": Bichat, *Recherches phys-*

iologiques, 43. See Lesch, *Science and Medicine in France*, 50–79. Bernard's views developed between 1857 and his death in 1878: Bernard, *Leçons sur les phénomènes de la vie*, 113–124; Coleman, "The cognitive basis of the discipline"; Grmek, "Évolution des conceptions de Claude Bernard sur le milieu intérieur"; Cannon, *Wisdom of the Body*. See Cross and Albury, "Walter B. Cannon, L. J. Henderson, and the organic analogy." On "organization" and biology, see Jacob, *The Logic of Living Systems*; and Schiller, *La notion d'organisation*.

25. Von Bertalanffy, *General Systems Theory*. For his own views of his historical context, see ibid., 8–15, 95–100. For a critical review of the background to systems thinking, see Phillips, *Holistic Thought in Social Science*.

26. N. Wiener, *Cybernetics*. Interestingly enough, Rosenbleuth first made public Wiener's and his own ideas on cybernetics at a conference on inhibition, sponsored by the Josiah Macy, Jr., Foundation. I have not traced details of this conference.

27. Rosenbleuth, Wiener, and Bigelow, "Behavior, purpose and teleology."

28. E.g., Diamond, Balvin, and Diamond, *Inhibition and Choice*; Fearing, *Reflex Action*; Cofer and Appley, *Motivation*, 147–157.

29. E.g., Koshtoyants, *Essays on the History of Physiology in Russia*; Iaroshevskii, *Psychologie im 20. Jahrhundert*, 88–93.

30. Diamond, Balvin, and Diamond, *Inhibition and Choice*, 69.

31. Neuburger, *The Historical Development of Experimental Brain and Spinal Cord Physiology before Flourens*, 289. This insight was developed in relation to British psychophysiology in Clark, "'The data of alienism,'" 115–122.

32. Riese, "Principle of integration," 309.

33. Clarke and Jacyna, *Nineteenth-Century Origins of Neuroscientific Concepts*; Riese and Hoff, "History of . . . cerebral localization"; Young, *Mind, Brain, and Adaptation*.

34. Morgan, *Animal Life and Intelligence*, 461.

35. Clark, "'The data of alienism,'" 119.

36. Fearing, *Reflex Action*, vii.

37. Boakes, *From Darwin to Behaviourism*, 109.

38. Fearing, *Reflex Action*, 187. Fearing was not always reliable; thus, he dated the experimental demonstration of vagal inhibition to 1846 rather than 1845.

39. Dodge, "The problem of inhibition," and "Theories of inhibition."

40. Eckhard, "Beiträge zur Geschichte der Experimentalphysiologie des Nervensystems."

41. Aphorisms, Sect. II, 46. Latin quoted in Sherrington, "The spinal cord," 838. English from Lloyd, ed., *Hippocratic Writings*, 212.

42. Mercier, "Inhibition," (1888*a*), 370. Mercier was paraphrasing Voltaire's famous remark about God, in "Épitres. XCVI. A l'auteur des trois imposteurs" (1771), line 22, in Voltaire, *Oeuvres complètes*, 727.

43. Barnes and Edge, eds., *Science in Context*, 13–34; Ravetz, *Scientific Knowledge and Its Social Problems*, 245–249; Zloczower, *Career Opportunities*.

44. Diamond, Balvin, and Diamond, *Inhibition and Choice*, 11.

45. Ibid., 9.

46. Anstie, *Stimulants and Narcotics*, 80–81; quoted in Diamond, Balvin, and Diamond, *Inhibition and Choice*, 33–34. J. Hughlings Jackson cited Anstie frequently: Jackson, "On temporary mental disorders," 123; "Remarks on dissolution of the nervous system," 6; "Evolution and dissolution," 58–59, 67–68.

47. Brazier, "The historical development of neurophysiology," 36–40, 50–52.

48. Brazier, *A History of Neurophysiology in the 17th and 18th Centuries*, and *A History of Neurophysiology in the 19th Century*.

49. Clarke and O'Malley, *The Human Brain and Spinal Cord*, v, 361–382.

50. Clarke and Jacyna, *Nineteenth-Century Origins of Neuroscientific Concepts*. Other studies, which have a biographical orientation, include Haymaker and Schiller, eds., *The Founders of Neurology*; and Rothschuh, ed., *Von Boerhaave bis Berger*.

51. Jeannerod, *The Brain Machine*, 35, quoting M. Merleau-Ponty. Cf. Meijer, *The Hierarchy Debate*.

52. Jeannerod, *The Brain Machine*, 39. Jeannerod misleadingly stated that "the influence of Sechenov is obvious." I attempt to look historically at this conclusion.

53. Graham, Lepenies, and Weingart, eds., *Functions and Uses of Disciplinary Histories*; Lemaine et al., eds., *Perspectives on the Emergence of Scientific Disciplines*.

54. Canguilhem, *La formation du concept de réflexe aux XVIIe et XVIIIe siècles*, and "Le concept de réflexe au XIXe siècle"; Harrington, *Medicine, Mind, and the Double Brain*; Young, *Mind, Brain, and Adaptation*.

55. For reflections on this question, see Danziger, "Toward a conceptual framework"; G. Richards, "Of what is the history of psychology a history?"; R. Smith, "Does the history of psychology have a subject?"; Sonntag, "'Zeitlose Dokumente der Seele.'"

56. E. G. Boring's history did not so much portray a break with philosophy as it portrayed theoretical psychology as an implicit strand in Western thought, rendered scientific by the application of experimental methods derived from physiology: Boring, *A History of Experimental Psychology*. For the context of Boring's work, see O'Donnell, "The crisis of experimentalism in the 1920s."

57. Young, "Scholarship and the history of the behavioural sciences"; *Mind, Brain, and Adaptation*; "The role of psychology in the nineteenth-century evolutionary debate." Robert J. Richards, by contrast, has interpreted the history of evolutionary psychology in terms of an evolutionary ethics and epistemology: R. J. Richards, *Darwin and the Emergence of Evolutionary Theories*.

58. Ash and Woodward, eds., *Psychology in Twentieth-Century Thought and Society*; O'Donnell, *The Origins of Behaviorism*.

59. The first draft of my book was complete before the appearance of the major study by David Joravsky, *Russian Psychology*. Other secondary sources are discussed below, chap. 3 and chap. 5.

60. Arens, *Structures of Knowing*.

2: CONDUCT, LOSS OF CONTROL, AND MENTAL ORGANIZATION

1. Gay, *The Bourgeois Experience Victoria to Freud.* Vol. 1: *Education of the Senses,* 157.

2. J. Barlow, *The Connection Between Physiology and Intellectual Philosophy,* 58.

3. J. Barlow, *On Man's Power Over Himself to Prevent or Control Insanity,* 15.

4. Houghton, *The Victorian Frame of Mind 1830–1870,* 233, quoting John Henry Newman, *Discourses Addressed to Mixed Congregations* (first publ. 1849).

5. Prichard, *On the Different Forms of Insanity,* 135.

6. Houghton, *The Victorian Frame of Mind,* 235, quoting A. J. C. Hare, *The Years with Mother.*

7. Ibid. Hare's upbringing was described at greater length in M. Barnes, *Augustus Hare,* 31–36, 43–52.

8. Bailey, *Leisure and Class in Victorian England*; Cooter, *The Cultural Meaning of Popular Science*; Russell, *Science and Social Change 1700–1900,* 151–173; Shapin and Barnes, "Science, nature and control."

9. Shapin and Barnes, "Head and hand." Shapin and Barnes's description of the rhetorical resources of "head" and "hand" was particularly suggestive, and it was not dependent on their interpretation (which has been questioned) of adult education in this period. For wider debate about the explanatory limits of social control arguments, see Cohen and Scull, eds., *Social Control and the State*; and Rose, *Governing the Soul.*

10. Blackstone, *Commentaries on the Laws of England,* 1: 165.

11. Shapin and Barnes, "Head and hand," 233, quoting A. Ure, *The Philosophy of Manufactures* (first publ. 1835).

12. R. Williams, *Keywords,* 67. On the late-eighteenth-century physiology of the *sensorium commune,* see Figlio, "Theories of perception and the physiology of mind in the late eighteenth century."

13. Cooter, "The power of the body," 77. See also idem, *The Cultural Meaning of Popular Science.*

14. Carpenter, *Principles of Human Physiology* (1st ed.), 152. For the later development of studies on reflex action and sphincter control, see Eckhard, "Beiträge zur Geschichte der Experimentalphysiologie des Nervensystems," 178–183.

15. E.g., Jordanova, *Sexual Visions*; Russett, *Sexual Science.*

16. Burstyn, *Victorian Education and the Ideal of Womanhood.* For the general fear of woman, see Gay, *The Bourgeois Experience,* 169–225. For broader social issues, see Mort, *Dangerous Sexualities.*

17. For a review with extensive references, see Clark, "Morbid introspection." See also Gay, *The Bourgeois Experience,* 294–318.

18. Maudsley, "Sex in mind and in education," 467. The literature on masturbation, it should be noted, well recognized the activity in women. On the spermatic economy, see Barker-Benfield, *The Horrors of the Half-known Life,*

175–188; Haller and Haller, *The Physician and Sexuality in Victorian America*, 195–225.

19. E.g., Clouston, *Clinical Lectures on Mental Diseases*, 490–500. Insanity is discussed below.

20. See Foucault, *The History of Sexuality*; Gay, *The Bourgeois Experience*; Weeks, *Sex, Politics and Society*. For a Victorian forcibly acknowledging sexuality, see Maudsley, *The Physiology and Pathology of Mind*, 238, 240, 273–278, 285–286.

21. Spencer, "The social organism," 415. See Russett, *Sexual Science*, 104–129.

22. Shuttleworth, "Female circulation."

23. Spencer, "A theory of population," 496–501. See Peel, *Herbert Spencer*, 137–139, and Stocking, *Victorian Anthropology*, 227–228, discussing the inverse relation between instinct and reason.

24. Spencer, "The social organism." In response to Huxley (1871), who pointed out that the organic analogy suggested that centralized power had an important role, Spencer (1871) refined his analysis—but at the expense of consistency. For other social/organic views in the nineteenth century, see Haines, "The inter-relations between social, biological, and medical thought, 1750–1850"; Sturdy, "Biology as social theory"; Weindling, "Theories of the cell state in Imperial Germany."

25. Stephen, *A General View of the Criminal Law of England*, 77.

26. Carpenter, *Principles of Mental Physiology*, 6.

27. Casper, *A Handbook of the Practice of Forensic Medicine*, 4: 204.

28. On radical uses of science, dubbed materialism by critics, see Desmond, *The Politics of Evolution*. Cf. the tsarist opposition to Sechenov's work discussed below, chap. 3.

29. R. Smith, *Trial by Medicine*.

30. Danziger, "Mid-nineteenth-century British psycho-physiology"; Jacyna, "The physiology of mind"; idem, "Somatic theories of mind"; R. Smith, "The background of physiological psychology."

31. On sympathy, especially the role attributed to the nervous system, see Lawrence, "The nervous system and society."

32. Combe, *The Constitution of Man*; Cooter, *The Cultural Meaning of Popular Science*, 101–133.

33. Cooter, "Phrenology and British alienists"; Young, *Mind, Brain, and Adaptation*.

34. Peel, *Herbert Spencer*; R. J. Richards, *Darwin and the Emergence of Evolutionary Theories*, 243–294; Stocking, *Victorian Anthropology*, 128–137, 140–143; Young, *Mind, Brain, and Adaptation*, 150–196.

35. Shapin, "Homo phrenologicus," 59–60; Cooter, *The Cultural Meaning of Popular Science*, 110–117.

36. R. D. French, "Some problems and sources in the foundations of modern physiology"; Geison, *Michael Foster and the Cambridge School of Physiology*, 13–47. For physiology in general, see Rothschuh, *History of Physiology*. The growth of experimental physiology was also intimately connected with medical interests in Continental Europe: Coleman and Holmes, eds., *The Investigative Enterprise*.

37. Carpenter, *Principles of Human Physiology* (1st ed.); Todd, "Nervous system"; Todd and Bowman, *The Physiological Anatomy and Physiology of Man*.

38. Clarke and Jacyna, *Nineteenth-Century Origins of Neuroscientific Concepts*, 29–57.

39. Neuburger, *The Historical Development of Experimental Brain and Spinal Cord Physiology before Flourens*.

40. Clarke and Jacyna, *Nineteenth-Century Origins of Neuroscientific Concepts*, 244–256, 267–285; Young, *Mind, Brain, and Adaptation*, 55–74.

41. Flourens, *Recherches expérimentales . . . du système nerveux*, 242–243. This edition included revised and extended versions of the original memoirs of 1822 and 1823.

42. Flourens, *Examen de la phrenologie*. The book was dedicated to the memory of Descartes, whose philosophy Flourens opposed to the "materialism" of Gall.

43. Persistent criticism of Flourens came from Dr. J.-B. Bouillaud, who argued for the presence of a localized speech center in the cerebrum but whose views were dismissed until the 1860s: Harrington, *Medicine, Mind, and the Double Brain*, 35–51; Young, *Mind, Brain, and Adaptation*, 134–149. Young (ibid., 111–113) drew attention to the discussion of sensory-motor functions in the midbrain region in Todd and Bowman, *The Physiological Anatomy and Physiology of Man*, 1: 347–358; and Carpenter, *Principles of Human Physiology* (1st ed.), 228–230.

44. Legallois, *Expériences sur le principe de la vie*, 35–62, 138–141; Flourens, *Recherches expérimentales . . . du système nerveux*, 196–204. See Clarke and Jacyna, *Nineteenth-Century Origins of Neuroscientific Concepts*, 245–247. Legallois (op. cit., x) also reported that decapitation produced feebler movements, the phenomenon later interpreted as "spinal shock" (see below, chap. 5).

45. Magendie, "Expériences sur les fonctions des racines des nerfs rachidiens"; idem, "Expériences sur les fonctions des racines des nerfs qui naissent de la moelle épinière." See Cranefield, *The Way In and the Way Out*, 11–13; Lesch, *Science and Medicine in France*, chap. 8.

46. Meynert, "On the collaboration of parts of the brain," 166, quoted in Young, *Mind, Brain, and Adaptation*, 80. Meynert simplistically attributed the law to Charles Bell.

47. Ibid., 83.

48. Holland, *Chapters on Mental Physiology*, 109.

49. Carpenter, *Principles of Human Physiology* (4th ed.), 850–861.

50. Maudsley, *The Physiology and Pathology of Mind*, 306.

51. Holland, *Chapters on Mental Physiology*, 90. See Danziger, "Mid-nineteenth-century British psycho-physiology"; Jacyna, "The physiology of mind"; R. Smith, "The background of physiological psychology."

52. Bennett, *The Mesmeric Mania of 1851*; Carpenter, "Electrobiology and mesmerism"; Wood, *What Is Mesmerism?*

53. Braid, *Neurypnology*, xviii.

54. Ibid., 22–23, 75–76. Braid became fascinated by the psychological reality of mesmeric phenomena, and he introduced the word "hypnotism" to coun-

ter the vital fluid or spiritualist connotations of "mesmerism." See Ellenberger, *The Discovery of the Unconscious*, 82.

55. Carpenter, "On the influence of suggestion"; idem, *Principles of Human Physiology* (4th ed.), 828. Thomas Laycock, similarly, had earlier extended the idea of reflex action to the higher brain to explain hysterical automatisms: Laycock, "On the reflex functions of the brain."

56. Carpenter, *Principles of Mental Physiology*, 25. On hypnotism, see ibid., 601–626.

57. For the social history of drink, more especially opposition to drink, see Harrison, *Drink and the Victorians*.

58. Darwin, *Zoonomia*, 1: 242–243.

59. Carpenter, *On the Use and Abuse of Alcoholic Liquors, in Health and Disease*; idem, *Principles of Mental Physiology*, 636–637, 649–653.

60. Cf. Berridge and Edwards, *Opium and the People*.

61. Spencer, *The Principles of Psychology*, 1: 611.

62. Brodie, *Psychological Inquiries*, 102.

63. Pinel, *A Treatise on Insanity*, 63.

64. Mayo, *Medical Testimony and Evidence in Cases of Insanity*, 47. For the context of moral treatment, see Bynum, "Rationales for therapy"; Donnelly, *Managing the Mind*; Scull, "Moral treatment reconsidered."

65. Bucknill and Tuke, *A Manual of Psychological Medicine*, 323.

66. J. Barlow, *On Man's Power Over Himself*, 6.

67. Ibid., 23.

68. Ibid., 45. For an exploration of the role of psychophysiological ideas of the will in fiction, see Shuttleworth, *George Eliot and Nineteenth-Century Science*, 185–190. She drew attention to Victorian use of Plato's metaphor (1961: 246ff.) of the soul as a charioteer controlling opposed horses.

69. Berman, *Social Change and Scientific Organization*.

70. For an overview of late Victorian psychiatry, see Shortt, *Victorian Lunacy*. For practices concerning mental abnormality and the constitution of psychology as a discipline, see Rose, *The Psychological Complex*.

71. Bradley, "The vulgar notion of responsibility," 48.

72. Browne, "Notes on homicidal insanity," 205. For mid-nineteenth-century cases of violence by lunatics, see R. Smith, *Trial by Medicine*; idem, "Defining murder and madness."

73. E.g., Tuke, *Prichard and Symonds in Especial Relation to Mental Science*, 83–86; Mercier, "Inhibition."

74. Bucknill and Tuke, *A Manual of Psychological Medicine*, 238, quoting James Reid, "On the causes, symptoms, and treatment of puerperal insanity" (1848).

75. Bucknill and Tuke, *A Manual of Psychological Medicine*, 273. The reference was to Pope's "Moral essays. Epistle II. To a lady" (1735), l. 216, in Pope, *The Poems of Alexander Pope*, 567.

76. Cf. Jackson, "Notes on the physiology and pathology of language," 123; idem, "On the nature of duality of the brain," 134–138; idem, "On affections of speech from disease of the brain," 181.

77. Maudsley, *The Physiology and Pathology of Mind*, 174. The reasons for

this shift to a physiological language have been attributed to medical occupational pressure to demonstrate a specialized expertise; see Clark, "The rejection of psychological approaches"; Jacyna, "Somatic theories of mind"; Scull, *Museums of Madness*, 158–171; R. Smith, *Trial by Medicine*, 40–56.

78. Kant, *Anthropology from a Pragmatic Point of View*, 43 (§ 26). In German: Kant, *Anthropologie*, 165–166.

79. Ringer, *The Decline of the German Mandarins*.

80. Marx, "A re-evaluation of the mentalists in early 19th century German psychiatry"; Verwey, *Psychiatry in an Anthropological and Biomedical Context*. Heinroth's reference to "sin" in his discussion of mental illness aroused particular criticism. In the setting of *Naturphilosophie*, however, he intended to describe something that (in our terms) was at least as naturalistic as it was theological.

81. For Heinroth as medicolegist, see Marx, "J. C. A. Heinroth on psychiatry and law."

82. Heinroth, *Lehrbuch der Störungen des Seelenlebens*; trans. as Heinroth, *Textbook of Disturbances of Mental Life or Disturbances of the Soul and Their Treatment*, with an introduction by George Mora.

83. Heinroth, *Lehrbuch der Störungen des Seelenlebens*, 1: 380–381, para. 253; trans. in idem, *Textbook of Disturbances of Mental Life*, 1: 220–221.

84. Marx, "Wilhelm Griesinger and the history of psychiatry."

85. These terms were of secondary significance compared to the overarching concept of anthropology, see Verwey, *Psychiatry in an Anthropological and Biomedical Context*, 1–36.

86. Griesinger, *Die Pathologie und Therapie der psychishen Krankheiten*. The same combination of languages was evident in the second edition (1861), trans. as Griesinger, *Mental Pathology and Therapeutics*. For Herbart and Griesinger, see Verwey, *Psychiatry in an Anthropological and Biomedical Context*, 117–138. Herbart's work is discussed below.

87. Griesinger, "Ueber psychische Reflexactionen," 77; trans. in Verwey, *Psychiatry in an Anthropological and Biomedical Context*, 105. See Marx, "Wilhelm Griesinger and the history of psychiatry," 519n. Clarke and Jacyna (1987: 133–138) placed in morphological context Griesinger's extension of reflex action to higher levels. For the wider psychiatric setting, see Doerner, *Madmen and the Bourgeoisie*, 272–290.

88. Griesinger, "Ueber psychische Reflexactionen," 99–100. Cf. idem, *Mental Pathology and Therapeutics*, 75–76, on the increase and diminution of reflex action in diseased conditions. For Budge, see below, chap. 3.

89. Griesinger, "Ueber psychische Reflexactionen," 99.

90. Ibid., 103.

91. For Zeller, see Verwey, *Psychiatry in an Anthropological and Biomedical Context*, 140–151. Griesinger gained his clinical experience with the insane under Zeller in 1840–1842.

92. Griesinger, "Ueber psychische Reflexactionen," 106. Cf. idem, "Neue Beiträge zur Physiologie und Pathologie des Gehirns"; idem, *Die Pathologie und Therapie*. Griesinger did not use the language of inhibition so directly in these later discussions.

93. Griesinger, *Mental Pathology and Therapeutics*, 40. See ibid., 42–53, on the importance of "limitation" for the development of firm character.

94. Bynum and Porter, *Brunonianism in Britain and Europe*; Canguilhem, "John Brown's system"; Risse, "The Brownian system of medicine." For the nineteenth-century view of pathology as quantitative variation, see Canguilhem, *The Normal and the Pathological*, 47–89.

95. Salter, *On Asthma*, 178. See Gabbay, "Asthma attacked?"

96. Salter, *On Asthma*, 25–28, 177–187.

97. Carter, *On the Pathology and Treatment of Hysteria*, 93, 21–22. See Kane and Carlson, "A different drummer"; Micale, "Hysteria and its historiography," 77–79.

98. Carter, *On the Pathology and Treatment of Hysteria*, 47. Cf. Maudsley's view (1867: 153–154) of the control of emotion by reflective inhibition.

99. Carter, *On the Pathology and Treatment of Hysteria*, 61–66.

100. Eisler, "Hemmung." See also Baldwin, ed., "Mental inhibition."

101. Warren, *A History of the Association Psychology*.

102. On the Kantian context of Herbart's and Beneke's work, see Arens, *Structures of Knowing*, 84–104; Brandt, *Friedrick Eduard Beneke*; Leary, "The philosophical development of psychology in Germany." The association psychology was contrasted unfavorably with the German tradition in Stout, "The Herbartian psychology"; idem, "Herbart compared with English psychologists and with Beneke"; idem, "The psychological work of Herbart's disciples." British idealists argued that presentations were constituted through the differentiation of an original unity (also an assumption in the German tradition). This contrasted with the analytic priority given to sensations or "ideas" in the British tradition. Cf. Ward, "Psychology," 45–46.

103. Ribot, *German Psychology of To-day*, 24. Cf. Leary, "The historical foundations of Herbart's mathematization of psychology."

104. Herbart, *Psychologie als Wissenschaft*," vol. 1 when first published. The synthetic part contained the major sections, "Grundlinien der Statik des Geistes" and "Grundlinien der Mechanik des Geistes." Cf. idem, "Von den Vorstellungen als Kräften," in *Lehrbuch zur Psychologie*, 369–386; trans. as Herbart, *A Text-book in Psychology*, 9–35. (References to the German edition subsequently cited in parentheses after the English edition; there were substantial differences of arrangement.)

105. Dunkel, *Herbart and Herbartianism*, 135. On the Herbartian approach to consciousness and the interaction of presentations by mutual "arrest," see Stout, "The Herbartian psychology," 325–332, 484–486. Both the "statics" and the "mechanics" of mind depended on quantifying the effects of summation and inhibition. For the latter, see Herbart, *Psychologie als Wissenschaft*, 5: pars. 41–51, 74–76.

106. Herbart, *A Text-book in Psychology*, 141 (393).

107. Ibid., 157 (403).

108. Verwey, *Psychiatry in an Anthropological and Biomedical Context*, 123–130.

109. Herbart, *A Text-book in Psychology*, 38 (310).

110. Dunkel, *Herbart and Herbartianism*, 139–194. The significance of pedagogy for establishing a subject of psychology was discussed in Jaeger and Staeuble, *Gesellschaftliche Genese der Psychologie*, 180–202.

111. Herbart, *Psychologie als Wissenschaft*, 6: 24. See also idem, "Ueber einige Beziehungen zwischen Psychologie und Staatswissenschaft."

112. Herbart, *A Text-book in Psychology*, 110 (356). Cf. idem, *Psychologie als Wissenschaft*, 6: 319–328.

113. Griesinger was not a materialist, a position excluded by his theory of knowledge: Verwey, *Psychiatry in an Anthropological and Biomedical Context*, 107–117, 135–138. On the wider reference to unconscious forces, see Ellenberger, *The Discovery of the Unconscious*.

114. Verwey, *Psychiatry in an Anthropological and Biomedical Context*, 130–131.

115. Beneke, *Psychologische Skizzen*; idem, *Erziehungs- und Unterrichtslehre*; idem, *Psychologie als Wissenschaft*.

116. Stout, "Herbart compared with English psychologists and with Beneke," 22. See Beneke, *Psychologische Skizzen*, 1: 418–482; Brandt, *Friedrick Eduard Beneke*, 95–101.

117. Drobisch, *Empirische Psychologie*, 338–385. See Dunkel, *Herbart and Herbartianism*, 10–13. Waitz, *Lehrbuch der Psychologie als Naturwissenschaft*, 73–79, 95–105, 136–159. Waitz later linked this psychology to anthropology and *Völkerpsychologie*: Ribot, *German Psychology of To-day*, 52–67. W. Volkmann, *Lehrbuch der Psychologie vom Standpunkte des Realismus*, 1: 338–385 (historical review), and 2: 329–338, 421–426.

118. Stout, "The psychological work of Herbart's disciples," 357.

119. Drobisch, *Erste Grundlehren der mathematischen Psychologie*, 22, 25–63.

120. Lotze, *Microcosmus*, 1: 198.

3: INHIBITION IN NEUROPHYSIOLOGY

1. In general, see Clarke and Jacyna, *Nineteenth-Century Origins of Neuroscientific Concepts*; R. Smith, "The background of physiological psychology"; Woodward and Ash, eds., *The Problematic Science*; Young, *Mind, Brain, and Adaptation*. The histories of neurophysiology and vivisection have been intimately connected; for the latter question, see Rupke, ed., *Vivisection in Historical Perspective*.

2. On the commitment to experimental physiology, see Coleman and Holmes, eds., *The Investigative Enterprise*; Rothschuh, *History of Physiology*; R. S. Turner, "The growth of professorial research in Prussia"; Turner, Kerwin, and Woolwine, "Careers and creativity in nineteenth-century physiology"; Zloczower, *Career Opportunities*.

3. The phrase is from Gillispie, *Edge of Objectivity*, though he did not use nineteenth-century physiology to illustrate his thesis.

4. The basic source for the mid-nineteenth century remains Eckhard, "Beiträge zur Geschichte der Experimentalphysiologie des Nervensystems," which

was used extensively and uncritically in Fearing, *Reflex Action*. See also Gault, "A sketch of the history of reflex action"; Stirling, "On the reflex function of the spinal cord."

5. Hall, *Memoirs on the Nervous System*, containing (1) a reprint of his 1832 paper to the Royal Society which the Society published in 1833, "On the reflex function of the medulla oblongata and medulla spinalis"; (2) "On the true spinal marrow, and the excito-motory system of nerves," read before the Royal Society in 1837 but refused publication. See also idem, *Synopsis of the Diastaltic Nervous System*; Clarke and Jacyna, *Nineteenth-Century Origins of Neuroscientific Concepts*, 114–124. On the relation of Hall's work to eighteenth-century studies, see Canguilhem, *La formation du concept de réflexe aux XVIIe et XVIIIe siècles*, 132–154; Fearing, *Reflex Action*, 122–145; Lawrence, "The nervous system and society." For the immediate context of Hall's ideas in debates about "sympathy," see Leys, "Background to the reflex controversy." For the political context of Hall's work, see Desmond, *The Politics of Evolution*, 124–134.

6. J. Müller, *Handbuch der Physiologie*, 1: 688–701. For the various editions of Müller's *Handbuch*, see Clarke and Jacyna, *Nineteenth-Century Origins of Neuroscientific Concepts*, 470–471. On Müller's place in the institutionalization of experimental physiology, see Rothschuh, *History of Physiology*, 59 ff.; *D.S.B.*, "Müller, Johannes."

7. Hall, *Memoirs on the Nervous System*, v–xiv. For Hall's German influence, see Eckhard, "Beiträge zur Geschichte der Experimentalphysiologie des Nervensystems," 53–78. Müller's English translator, W. Baly, added footnotes regarding Hall's claims: J. Müller, *Elements of Physiology*, 1: 768–772.

8. Hall, *Memoirs on the Nervous System*, Memoir II.

9. Hall, "Memoirs on some principles of pathology in the nervous system," 205; reprinted in idem, *On the Diseases and Derangements of the Nervous System*, 207–268 (quote on 216). See Spillane, *The Doctrine of the Nerves*, 249–256.

10. Hall, *Memoirs on the Nervous System*, Memoir I.

11. W. F. Barlow, "The influence of volition," 572.

12. Romberg, *A Manual of the Nervous Diseases of Man*, 2: 78. See Todd, "Nervous system," 720z (on increased reflex excitability in hemiplegia) and 722e–i (on increased reflex excitability with decrease in the will); Spillane, *The Doctrine of the Nerves*, 265–266, 284–285, 294.

13. Romberg, *A Manual of the Nervous Diseases of Man*, 2: 81–99.

14. Hall, *Memoirs on the Nervous System*, Memoir II, 73, 93–94; idem, *On the Diseases and Derangements of the Nervous System*, 76–78.

15. Hall, *Memoirs on the Nervous System*, Memoir II, 73.

16. Ibid., 73–74.

17. Schäfer, "The cerebral cortex," 712. See also Ferrier, *The Functions of the Brain* (1st ed.), 17–19.

18. Hall, *On the Diseases and Derangements of the Nervous System*, 290.

19. Ibid., 97.

20. Ibid., 29.

21. J. Müller, *Handbuch der Physiologie*, 1: 700.

22. Ibid., 716–720. On sympathy and integration, see Riese, *A History of Neurology*, 127–139. For the context of Müller's thought, see Clarke and Jacyna, *Nineteenth-Century Origins of Neuroscientific Concepts*, 346–370.

23. J. Müller, *Handbuch der Physiologie*, 1: 721. Baly (J. Müller, *Elements of Physiology*, 1: 738–739) used the words "impede" and "arrest" but not "inhibition" in translating (and altering) this and related passages.

24. J. Müller, *Elements of Physiology*, 2: 1335, 1345. Cf. idem, *Handbuch der Physiologie*, 2: 506–507, 516–517.

25. J. Müller, *Elements of Physiology*, 2: 934. Cf. idem, *Handbuch der Physiologie*, 2: 92–93.

26. Carpenter, *Principles of Human Physiology* (1st ed.), 132. See Clarke and Jacyna, *Nineteenth-Century Origins of Neuroscientific Concepts*, 139–141. For Carpenter's philosophy of mind, see Jacyna, "The physiology of mind"; R. Smith, "The human significance of biology."

27. Neuburger, *The Historical Development of Experimental Brain and Spinal Cord Physiology before Flourens*, chaps. 9, 10.

28. Canguilhem, *La formation du concept de réflexe aux XVII*[e] *et XVIII*[e] *siècles*, 101–107; Fearing, *Reflex Action*, 74–83.

29. Sherrington, "The spinal cord," 837–838. Cf. Eckhard, "Beiträge zur Geschichte der Experimentalphysiologie des Nervensystems," 42–47.

30. Whytt, *The Works*, 260–261 (also 303–304) (in "Observations on the sensibility and irritability of the parts of men and other animals," reprint of 3d ed., 1766), and 500–501 (in "Observations on the nature, causes, and cure of those disorders which are commonly called nervous, hypochondric, hysteric," reprint of 3d ed., 1767). For the larger significance of Whytt's work for psychological concepts, see Danziger, "Origins of the schema of stimulated motion." For his life and work, see R. K. French, *Robert Whytt, the Soul and Medicine*.

31. Whytt, *The Works*, 291.

32. Eckhard, "Beiträge zur Geschichte der Experimentalphysiologie des Nervensystems," 44.

33. Ibid., 99–100. For a description of "spinal shock" without reference to inhibition, see A. W. Volkmann, "Ueber Reflexbewegungen," 17–18.

34. Sherrington, "The spinal cord," 846. Cf. idem, "Experiments in examination of the peripheral distribution . . . of the posterior roots"; reprinted in part in Sherrington, *Selected Writings of Sir Charles Sherrington*, 120–154. See also below, chap. 5.

35. A. W. Volkmann, "Von dem Baue und den Verrichtungen der Knopfnerven," 85–88; idem, "Ueber die Bewenskraft derjenigen Experimente," 370 (this page, as published, was numbered wrong). Cf. Hoff, "The history of vagal inhibition," 468–469; Käbin, *Die Medizinische Forschung und Lehre an der Universität Dorpat/Tartu*, 78–81.

36. A. W. Volkmann, "Ueber Reflexbewegungen," 31.

37. Ibid., 32.

38. Ibid., 33.

39. Flourens, *Recherches expérimentales . . . du système nerveux*, 38, trans. (of identical passage in 1st ed.) in Clarke and O'Malley, *The Human Brain and*

Spinal Cord, 658. See Clarke and Jacyna, *Nineteenth-Century Origins of Neuroscientific Concepts*, 285–302.

40. Budge, *Neue Untersuchungen über das Nervensystem*, 1: 62.

41. Ibid., 72.

42. Olmsted, *Charles-Édouard Brown-Séquard*, 35–40.

43. Carpenter, *Principles of Mental Physiology*; Holland, *Chapters on Mental Physiology*. Cf. Clark, "'The data of alienism'"; Danziger, "Mid-nineteenth-century British psycho-physiology"; Jacyna, "The physiology of mind"; R. Smith, "The background of physiological psychology."

44. The experiment was reported in an Italian journal in 1845 (which I have not seen) and then in Weber and Weber, "Expériences physiologiques." For the role of E. F. W. rather than E. H. Weber and the almost simultaneous and related experiments by J. L. Budge, see Hoff, "The history of vagal inhibition," 470–471; Milne Edwards, *Leçons sur la physiologie*, 120–168.

45. Weber, "Muskelbewegung," 47.

46. Ibid., slightly altered from trans. in Clarke and O'Malley, *The Human Brain and Spinal Cord*, 352.

47. Weber, "Muskelbewegung," 42–48.

48. Hoff, "The history of vagal inhibition"; Geison, *Michael Foster and the Cambridge School of Physiology*, Pt. 3. For an earlier summary by the central physiologist involved, see Gaskell, "The contraction of cardiac muscle."

49. On the development of this important piece of apparatus, which the Webers applied to physiological questions in the 1830s, see Hoff, "The history of vagal inhibition," 469–470. It was illustrated in Weber, "Muskelbewegung," 11.

50. A. W. Volkmann, "Beiträg zur nähern Kenntniss der motorischen Nervenwirkungen," 425. Volkmann's article (1844) for Rudolph Wagner's standard *Handwörterbuch* referred to "Hemmung" (without distinguishing the notion in any specific way) while discussing the control needed for a continuous excitation to produce a movement or to explain how more extensive movements resulted from a stronger stimulus. He also referred (534) to the inhibition of brain activity in sleep and associated states.

51. Hoff, "The history of vagal inhibition," 478.

52. Weber, "Muskelbewegung," 46, trans. in Hoff, "The history of vagal inhibition," 478.

53. Hoff, "The history of vagal inhibition," 478.

54. For overviews and bibliographies, arguing for inhibition as a basic physiological phenomenon, see H. E. Hering, "Die intracentralen Hemmungsvorgänge"; Meltzer, "Inhibition."

55. For the background to the involuntary nervous system, especially Bichat's separation of the *vie animale* and the *vie organique* with their corresponding nervous systems, see Clarke and Jacyna, *Nineteenth-Century Origins of Neuroscientific Concepts*, chap. 7.

56. Pflüger, *Ueber das Hemmungs-Nervensystem*, 1–16; *D.S.B.*, "Pflüger, Eduard." Pflüger announced his results to the Prussian Academy of Sciences in Berlin in 1855, but I have not seen this. He saw his work as building on the earlier research of C. Eckhard and G. Valentin on the electrical excitation of nerves and on Müller's discussion of the sympathetic nerve.

57. Pflüger, "Experimentalbeitrag zur Theorie der Hemmungnerven," 13. For the subsequent study of inhibitory regulatory control of the gut, see Meltzer, "Inhibition," 662–663; Starling, "The nervous and muscular mechanisms of the digestive tract."

58. Goltz, "Vagus und Herz," 31, trans. in Hoff, "The history of vagal inhibition," 478–479. Goltz made this remark while criticizing Rosenthal's theory of the regulation of breathing (see below). It appeared to Goltz that there was a danger of a reductio ad absurdum in each function being assigned an inhibitory nerve.

59. Lister, "Preliminary account of an inquiry into the functions of the visceral nerves"; reprinted in idem, *Collected Papers*, 1: 87–98. I have seen no reference in English in the nineteenth century to psychological or physiological inhibition before this date.

60. Quoted in Godlee, *Lord Lister*, 297. See D. W. Taylor, "The life and teaching of William Sharpey," 142–143.

61. Cf. Lister, *Collected Papers*, 1: xvi–xvii.

62. Lister, "Preliminary account of an inquiry into the functions of the visceral nerves," 367.

63. Ibid., 372.

64. Ibid., 378.

65. *D.S.B.*, "Schiff, Moritz"; Guarnieri, "Moritz Schiff."

66. Schiff, *Lehrbuch der Physiologie des Menschen*, 187–192; idem, "Physiologie der sogenannten 'Hemmungsnerven'"; idem "Zur Physiologie des Nervensystems." The debate was related to Lister's work in *British and Foreign Medico-chirurgical Review*, "Review of physiology."

67. Schiff, *Lehrbuch der Physiologie des Menschen*, 199–202. Pflüger (1859) offered his own interpretation of these results. According to Olmsted (1946: 163–165), Brown-Séquard also explained the increase of reflex action following sectioning of the cord in terms of the augmentation of the excitation to action by the part that normally would have flowed to the brain. But I have not seen Brown-Séquard's 1855 publication with these conclusions.

68. Sechenov, *Autobiographical Notes*, 106.

69. Bernard set his own work in context in *De la physiologie générale*; on nervous regulation and the *milieu intérieur*, see 32–47 (and nn. 30–48). On Bernard's biology, see Coleman, "The cognitive basis of the discipline"; Grmek, "Évolution des conceptions de Claude Bernard sur le milieu intérieur"; Lesch, *Science and Medicine in France*, 197–224; Schiller, *Claude Bernard et les problèmes scientifiques*; *D.S.B.*, "Bernard, Claude."

70. Bernard, *Leçons sur la physiologie et la pathologie du système nerveux*, 2: 473. See also idem, "Expériences sur les fonctions . . . du grand sympathique," continued as "Sur les effets . . . du grand sympathique"; Budge and Waller, *Neue Untersuchungen über das Nervensystem*. The role of spinal centers in sympathetic reflex actions had often been discussed (with speculation on vasoconstrictor and vasodilator effects): Milne Edwards, *Leçons sur la physiologie*, 199–205; Eckhard, "Beiträge zur Geschichte der Experimentalphysiologie des Nervensystems," 62–78. For the later development of this work, see ibid., 91–99, 164–171. It was also observed that stimulating the nerve supply to the heart

and aorta evoked reflex inhibition of the arterial ring musculature: Tsion and Ludwig, "Die Reflexe eines der sensiblen Nerven"; reprinted in Tsion, *Gesammelte physiologischen Arbeiten*, 38–54. See Geison, *Michael Foster and the Cambridge School of Physiology*, 344; Schröer, *Carl Ludwig*, 156–162.

71. Bernard, "L'influence du grand sympathique . . . sur la calorification"; idem, "De l'influence du système nerveux . . . sur la chaleur animale"; idem, "Recherches expérimentales sur le grand sympathique"; idem, *Leçons sur la physiologie et la pathologie du système nerveux*, 2: 474–520. Cf. Olmsted and Olmsted, *Claude Bernard and the Experimental Method in Science*, 81–83.

72. Bernard, "De l'influence de deux ordres de nerfs," 251. See also idem, "Sur les variations de couleur dans le sang veineux"; idem, *Leçons sur la physiologie et la pathologie du système nerveux*, 2: 146–173; Olmsted and Olmsted, *Claude Bernard*, 103–105.

73. Brown-Séquard, *Course of Lectures on the Physiology . . . of the Central Nervous System*, 139–177; Olmsted, *Brown-Séquard.*

74. Bernard, *Leçons sur la chaleur animale*, 232–233.

75. Eckhard, "Über die Erection des Penis"; idem, "Untersuchungen über die erection des Penis beim Hunde."

76. Rosenthal, *Die Athembewegungen*, 21–47. J. Traube (1848) had observed vagal inhibition of respiration and Rosenthal (1861) described the superior laryngeal nerve as having an inhibitory function associated with the diaphragm. Rosenthal's view that breathing involved specific inhibitory fibers was criticized in Goltz, "Vagus und Herz," 29–31; and Schiff, "Kritisch und Polemisches zur Physiologie des Nervensystems."

77. Rosenthal, *Die Athembewegungen*, 256. For Legallois, see above, chap. 2.

78. E. Hering, "Die Selbsteuerung der Athmung"; Breuer, "Die Selbsteuerung der Athmung." See Starling, "The nervous and muscular mechanism of the respiratory movements."

79. Kronecker and Meltzer, "Der Schluckmechanismus." Sherrington considered this work on swallowing to be an important anticipation of reciprocal inhibition (see below, chap. 5); Sherrington, *The Integrative Action of the Nervous System*, 100. On the background history of swallowing, see Eckhard, "Beiträge zur Geschichte der Experimentalphysiologie des Nervensystems," 172–175.

80. Meltzer, "Inhibition," 663.

81. Eulenburg and Landois, "Die Hemmungsneurose."

82. Sherrington, "The spinal cord," 887.

83. Bernard, "Du rôle des actions réflexes paralysantes," 511–512.

84. Schiff, *Leçons sur la physiologie de la digestion*, 1: 212–308 (Leçons 10–12).

85. Biedermann, "Beiträge zur allgemeinen Nerven- und Muskelphysiologie" (1887, 1888); Pavlov, "Wie die Muschel ihre Schaale öffnet." See below, chap 5.

86. On the 1840s group, see Rothschuh, *History of Physiology*, 204–242; Verwey, *Psychiatry in an Anthropological and Biomedical Context*, 52–71.

87. Cranefield, "The organic physics of 1847." See also Schröer, *Carl Ludwig*.

88. Especially in Germany: Gregory, *Scientific Materialism in Nineteenth-Century Germany*; Kelly, *Descent of Darwin*; Verwey, *Psychiatry in an Anthropological and Biomedical Context*, 71–76.

89. Bernard, *An Introduction to the Study of Experimental Medicine*, 87–94.

90. Canguilhem, "Le concept de réflexe au XIXe siècle," 300.

91. Hoff, "The history of vagal inhibition," 477.

92. Fearing, *Reflex Action*, 191; Brazier, "The historical development of neurophysiology," 52–53.

93. Sherrington, "The spinal cord," 838.

94. Vyrubov in Sechenov, *Études psychologiques*, ii.

95. Iaroshevskii, *Ivan Sechenov* (a translation of a book for a popular scientific series, based on his Russian biography of 1968, which I have not seen); idem, "I. M. Sechenov—the founder of objective psychology"; idem, "The logic of scientific development." Cf. Koshtoyants, "I. Sechenov"; idem, *Essays on the History of Physiology in Russia*; Shaternikov, "The life of I. M. Sechenov." For Sechenov and the political context, see Joravsky, *Russian Psychology*, 53–70, 92–104, 125–134; Todes, "From radicalism to scientific convention"; Vucinich, *Science in Russian Culture*, 119–129. For an illustration of the "colonization" of Sechenov to demonstrate the Russian origins of brain research, see Beritashvili, "Central inhibition." See also Brožek, "The psychology and physiology of behavior"; idem, "Soviet historiography of psychology."

96. Sechenov, *Autobiographical Notes*, 52.

97. Ibid., 51–52. For his psychological reading, see below.

98. Iaroshevskii, "The logic of scientific development," 235–236. Todes ("From radicalism to scientific convention," 496) qualified the term "school," since Sechenov did not lead a coherent group working on a single problem.

99. Sechenov, *Autobiographical Notes*, 105–111, on 106.

100. Sechenov, "Physiologische Studien über die Hemmungsmechanismen"; trans. (by himself?) in idem, "Études physiologiques sur les centres modérateurs." His results were also announced in a note Bernard presented to the Académie des Sciences: Sechenov, "Sous les modérateurs des mouvements réflexes." His work appears to have attracted little attention in France. In his much cited text, A. Vulpian (1866: 438–449) criticized Sechenov's inhibitory center theory, suggesting instead that the increase of reflex actions after decapitation was caused by all the excitation to a reflex passing into movement, whereas some excitation normally diverted to the head. This reflected Herzen's criticisms of Sechenov (see below) and the views of Schiff. Vulpian repeated these views in an encyclopedic survey of spinal cord function: Vulpian, "Moelle épinière," 481–484.

101. Iaroshevskii, "I. M. Sechenov—the founder of objective psychology," 100.

102. Translated as "Les actions réflexes du cerveau" in Sechenov, *Études psychologiques*, 1–174. This translation was made from a book published in

Russian in 1873 (which I have not seen), which included two programmatic essays for the development of psychology as well as "Reflexes of the brain"; see below. In Joravsky's view (1989: 103), "the [French] book sank into instant oblivion"; this appears correct.

103. There have been two translations into English; they differ in detail but not in substantial meaning. (1) Sechenov, "Reflexes of the brain," which appeared originally in a 1935 volume of Sechenov's *Selected Works* presented to delegates to the XVth International Physiological Congress in Moscow. The 1935 volume was reprinted in 1968, and I cite from this. (2) Sechenov, *Selected Physiological and Psychological Works*, including "Reflexes of the brain," 31–139. This was a translation of vol. 1 of the two-volume Russian selected works (1952–1956). This version was also published separately as Sechenov, *Reflexes of the Brain*. This English edition was stimulated by another congress: Purpura and Waelsch, "Brain reflexes." I have not seen either of the Russian versions published in 1863 or 1866 (the latter was revised and updated), nor am I aware of any discussion of the reliability of the existing English-language translations or interpretations. Differences between the translations and the use of twentieth-century language suggest that neither was particularly accurate.

104. The passage on central inhibition was translated in Sechenov, *Selected Physiological and Psychological Works*, 516–522. See also Sechenov, *Autobiographical Notes*, 119–121.

105. Todes, "From radicalism to scientific convention," 113–122. According to Todes, Sechenov thought of his essay as a contribution to radical polemics, since it defended N. G. Chernyshevskii's "anthropological principle in philosophy." Sechenov's Soviet biographers have been keen to emphasize his links with radical materialism; see, e.g., Koshtoyants, "I. Sechenov," 9–13. In his autobiography, written about 1904, Sechenov (1965*a*: 110) was silent about his relations with *Contemporary*.

106. Sechenov's *Autobiographical Notes* quoted in the editor's notes to Sechenov, *Selected Physiological and Psychological Works*, 580. The version in Sechenov, *Autobiographical Notes*, 110, leaves out the reference to the editor of the *Medical Herald*'s own views.

107. For censorship of scientific works, see Todes, "From radicalism to scientific convention," chap. 2; idem, "Biological psychology and the tsarist censor." On the "Westernizing" of Russian medicine, see Frieden, *Russian Physicians in an Era of Reform*.

108. Iaroshevskii, "I. M. Sechenov—the founder of objective psychology," 79.

109. Quoted in Todes, "From radicalism to scientific convention," 116.

110. Quoted in Shaternikov, "The life of I. M. Sechenov," xxii, from the handwritten sentences in the copy Sechenov presented to his partner and future wife, M. A. Bokova, who was a translator with medical qualifications.

111. Editor's note to Sechenov, *Selected Physiological and Psychological Works*, 581. There was also a lively debate in response to Sechenov's articles: "Observations on Mr. Kavelin's book" (Russian 1871; trans. in Sechenov [1960*a*], 140–178); "Who must investigate the problems of psychology" (Russian 1873). Sechenov attacked the liberal lawyer K. D. Kavelin, who had

argued that a theory of the freedom of the will was essential to modernizing the social order and that psychology should not be reduced to physiology. Cf. Todes, "From radicalism to scientific convention," 192–204, 219–233, 271–281.

112. Sechenov, *Autobiographical Notes*, 158–159. In 1874, I. R. Tarkanov (who had been Sechenov's student) published a defense of Sechenov's idea of localized inhibitory centers, arguing that positive and negative currents to the brain had opposite effects on the speed of reflex actions. Cf. Todes, "From radicalism to scientific convention," 307. I have not seen the paper in Russian. This was an indication of the future direction of interest, focusing on causal mechanisms of inhibition; see below, chap. 4. See also Sechenov, "Galvanische Erscheinungen."

113. Sechenov, *Autobiographical Notes*, 109. See Iaroshevskii, "I. M. Sechenov—the founder of objective psychology," 73–88.

114. Sechenov, *Autobiographical Notes*, 109, quoting his own 1860 thesis. See Todes, "From radicalism to scientific convention," 242–248.

115. Iaroshevskii, "The logic of scientific development," 242. This approach contrasted with the earlier account given by K. S. Koshtoyants, which traced an anticipation of Sechenov's results to A. A. Sokolovskii at Kazan in 1858 and related both Sokolovskii's and Sechenov's work to unpublished research by Ludwig: Koshtoyants, *Essays on the History of Physiology in Russia*, 127–129.

116. Türck, "Ueber den Zustand der Sensibilität," 190. Cf. Eckhard, "Beiträge zur Geschichte der Experimentalphysiologie des Nervensystems," 78–81. Sechenov (1875*a* and 1875*b*) later defended this technique against criticisms from I. Tsion.

117. Sechenov, "Physiologische Studien über die Hemmungsmechanismen," 169, trans. in Clarke and O'Malley, *The Human Brain and Spinal Cord*, 365. Sechenov italicized the whole passage.

118. Sechenov, "Physiologische Studien über die Hemmungsmechanismen," 171–173.

119. For overviews, see Eckhard, "Beiträge zur Geschichte der Experimentalphysiologie des Nervensystems," 86–89, 99–120; H. E. Hering, "Die intracentralen Hemmungsvorgänge," 513–516. Sechenov (1965*a*: 119–120) reported that he described these continuing experiments in his Russian-language *Physiology of the Nervous System* (1866), chaps. 3 and 4, but I have not seen this. His research papers were published in German as well as Russian (I have not seen the latter): Sechenov, "Weiteres über die Reflexhemmungen"; idem, "Über die elektrische und chemische Reizung"; Sechenov and Pashutin, *Neue Versuche am Hirn und Rückenmark*.

120. Matkevich, "Ueber die Wirkung des Alkohols, Strychnins und Opiums auf die reflexhemmenden Mechanismen."

121. A. Danilevskii, "Untersuchungen zur Physiologie des Centralnervensystems."

122. Iaroshevskii, "The logic of scientific development," 239. A comparable dynamic and integrated view of nervous energies was developed in England by G. H. Lewes: Lewes, *The Physical Basis of Mind*, 288–304.

123. Schiff, *Lehrbuch der Physiologie des Menschen*, 199–202. Herzen, *Expériences sur les centres modérateurs*, 4–6, 41–44. For Herzen's background, see Carr, *Romantic Exiles*, 152, 244, 269–270.

124. Herzen, *Expériences sur les centres modérateurs*, 29.

125. Ibid., 37.

126. Ibid., 61.

127. Sechenov and Pashutin, *Neue Versuche am Hirn und Rückenmark*. (Publication also noticed in *Centralblatt für die medicinischen Wissenschaften*, no. 50 [1865], 789–793.) Sechenov had tried an electrical (galvanic) stimulus in 1862, but his results were unclear. The effect of a continuous current on reflexes was also studied in Sechenov, "Über die elektrische und chemische Reizung," and by Tarkanov. Cf. Eckhard, "Beiträge zur Geschichte der Experimentalphysiologie des Nervensystems," 86–89.

128. Simonov, "Die Hemmungsmechanismen der Säugethiere"; J. G. M'Kendrick, "On the inhibitory or restraining action," 734. M'Kendrick, a Scottish physiologist, did nevertheless claim (ibid., 734–736) to have demonstrated a direct inhibitory effect of the brain on spinal reflex actions in pigeons. Significantly, he coupled this experimental demonstration with knowledge of the will's controlling power over the response to tickling.

129. Sechenov, "Weiteres über die Reflexhemmungen"; idem, "Über die elektrische und chemische Reizung." See also idem, *Autobiographical Notes*, 123–124.

130. Suslova, "Beiträge zur Physiologie der Lymphherzen." For Sechenov's defense of comparison between inhibition of lymph hearts and inhibition elsewhere, see Sechenov, "Zur Frage über die Reflexhemmungen." See Eckhard, "Beiträge zur Geschichte der Experimentalphysiologie des Nervensystems," 112, 183–186; Todes, "From radicalism to scientific convention," 266–271. Rothschuh (1973: 236) described the physiological institute at Graz as "virtually being a Russian colony." It has been conventional to describe Suslova as the first woman in Europe to gain a full medical degree (there being some vagueness about what constituted a degree): Koblitz, "Science, women, and the Russian intelligentsia."

131. See letters from Sechenov to M. A. Bokova, in Koshtoyants, *Essays on the History of Physiology in Russia*, 130–135.

132. Tsion, "Über die Fortpflanzungsgeschwindigkeit der Erregung," reprinted in idem, *Gesammelte physiologischen Arbeiten*, 210–232; idem, "Zur Hemmungstheorie," reprinted in *Gesammelte physiologischen Arbeiten*, 232–238. For the "interference" theory, introduced in 1870, see below, chap. 4. Sechenov responded in "Notiz die reflexhemmenden Mechanismen" (1875*a* and 1875*b*).

133. Iaroshevskii, "The logic of scientific development," 241–242.

134. Sechenov, *Autobiographical Notes*, 107–108. See Weber, "Muskelbewegung," 47 (cited above). Sechenov knew that his mentor, Ludwig, was skeptical about many current claims to knowledge of central nervous function. See Schröer, *Carl Ludwig*, 189–193.

135. Sechenov, *Autobiographical Notes*, 109.

136. Iaroshevskii, "I. M. Sechenov—the founder of objective psychology,"

83–84. This interpretation, and the Soviet historiography it exemplified, has been attacked strongly in Joravsky, *Russian Psychology*, 125–134. Joravsky argued that Sechenov was indeed motivated by a search for scientific psychology but that his research on inhibition, which quickly lost its clear focus and results, caused him to abandon the physiological approach to psychology. This argument was aimed at the heart of the Soviet claim to have pioneered and even established "objective" psychology (i.e., a psychology transcending mind-body dualisms).

137. Sechenov, "Reflexes of the brain," 335–336.

138. Ibid., 334.

139. Ibid., 322.

140. Ibid., 264.

141. Ibid., 270.

142. Ibid., 271.

143. Ibid.

144. Ibid., 275.

145. Ibid., 276. As this chapter has suggested, Sechenov's account does not justify Iaroshevskii's claim (1968: 87) that "Sechenov for the first time gave a deterministic interpretation of self-regulation."

146. Sechenov, "Reflexes of the brain," 290–291.

147. Ibid., 291.

148. Ibid., 292–317 (par. 11). Sechenov's account built on German sensory physiology and only incidentally on eighteenth-century sensationalism. It did not derive any specific content from the "association psychology" that Amacher (1964) identified as the main influence on the extension of the reflex theory to all levels of the brain. Sechenov himself wrote (1935*a*: 335), "I must confess that I have built up all these hypotheses without being well acquainted with psychological literature. I have only studied the Beneke system, and that in my school years. The works of the same author have given me a general knowledge of the theories of the French school of sensualists." Sechenov bought Beneke's *Psychologische Skizzen* and *Erziehungs- und Unterrichtslehre*, books that were written for a nonacademic audience. Sechenov appreciated the fundamentally nonsensualist basis of Beneke's psychology when he claimed (1965*a*: 52) that, for Beneke, "the whole picture of psychological life came out of the primary forces of the soul." Sechenov informed Helmholtz in 1859 that he read English, but I know of no evidence that he read English psychological writers at this time: ibid., 90. For Beneke, see above, chap. 2.

149. Sechenov, "Reflexes of the brain," 317.

150. Ibid., 320. Iaroshevskii (1968: 91) argued that Sechenov's account of inhibition laid the basis in reflex theory for a mechanism of learning, by describing the basis of selective response in the nervous system.

151. Sechenov, "Reflexes of the brain," 320–321.

152. Sechenov, *Selected Physiological and Psychological Works*, 479–485; idem, *Autobiographical Notes*, 167–170.

153. Sechenov, "Reflexes of the brain," 334.

154. Cf. Todes, "From radicalism to scientific convention," 331–355, 368–370, 377–388.

155. Ibid., 270, quoting from a letter to M. A. Bokova. It was at this time that he read extensively in psychological literature.

156. Sechenov, "Who must investigate the problems of psychology," 350. For the context, see Koshtoyants, *Essays on the History of Physiology in Russia*, 168–173.

157. Sechenov, "Who must investigate the problems of psychology," 346–347.

158. Ibid., 356.

159. Koshtoyants, *Essays on the History of Physiology in Russia*, 166–168; Todes, "From radicalism to scientific convention," 267–270. He also read Herbart at this time. Sechenov elaborated his psychology in several later works, especially "Elements of thought" (first published 1878, revised 1903). Cf. idem, *Études psychologiques*, "Notions générales sur l'étude de la psychologie," chap. 3, "Histoire de l'évolution psychique." Sechenov's developmental psychology was ontogenetic rather than phylogenetic (in this regard, more like Bain than Spencer).

4: INHIBITION AND THE RELATIONS BETWEEN PHYSIOLOGY AND PSYCHOLOGY, 1870–1930

1. Foster, *A Text Book of Physiology*, 125, 487.

2. Goltz, *Beiträge zur Lehre von den Functionen der Nervencentren*, 39–51. The idea of "summation" was also elaborated in Freusberg, "Reflexbewegungen beim Hunde"; Wundt, *Grundzüge der physiologischen Psychologie* (1st ed.), 175. See Eckhard, "Beiträge zur Geschichte der Experimentalphysiologie des Nervensystems," 113–114.

3. Goltz, *Beiträge zur Lehre von den Functionen der Nervencentren*, 44, trans. in Gault, "A sketch of the history of reflex action," 535. Further experimental support for this rule was provided by Nothnagel, "Bewegungshemmende Mechanismen."

4. Goltz also described the croak reflex, the croaking response of a frog to a gentle stroke on its back, which was much more easily evoked in a decerebrate animal: Goltz, *Beiträge zur Lehre von den Functionen der Nervencentren*, 1–20 (first publ. 1865). The reflex could be inhibited by simultaneously pricking the frog's leg: ibid., 42–46. Lewisson (1869) observed that strong compression of the neck of a frog produced reflex inhibition and considered that inhibition must therefore be a general rather than a localized function of the nervous system.

5. Goltz, "Vagus und Herz," 10–16. This experiment was known as the *Klopversuch* (tap experiment). Clinical evidence in support of the peripheral origin of inhibition was given in Nothnagel, "Beobachtungen über Reflexhemmung."

6. Goltz and Freusberg, "Ueber die Functionen des Lendenmarks des Hundes"; followed by Freusberg, "Reflexbewegungen beim Hunde." These papers made possible the comparison of inhibition in warm- and cold-blooded animals. For Eckhard, see above, chap. 3.

7. Goltz, *Beiträge zur Lehre von den Functionen der Nervencentren*, 42.

8. H. E. Hering, "Die intracentralen Hemmungsvorgänge," 515.

9. See Eckhard, "Beiträge zur Geschichte der Experimentalphysiologie des Nervensystems," 108–120; Meltzer, "Inhibition," 699–700.

10. Langendorff, "Ueber Reflexhemmung," 112–115.

11. Freusberg, "Ueber die Erregung und Hemmung der Thätigkeit."

12. Fritsch and Hitzig, "Ueber die elektrische Erregbarkeit des Grosshirns," trans. in part in idem, "On the electrical excitability of the cerebrum"; Ferrier, "Experimental researches in cerebral physiology and pathology." See Young, *Mind, Brain, and Adaptation*, 224–248.

13. Ferrier, *The Functions of the Brain* (1st ed.), 19. For Wundt, see below; for Schiff and Herzen see above, chap. 3. For "summation," Stirling, "On the reflex function of the spinal cord," 1099–1107.

14. Ferrier, *The Functions of the Brain* (1st ed.), 18.

15. Ibid., 282. Ferrier was not the first in Britain to link inhibition, volition, and Sechenov's idea of brain inhibitory centers: Rutherford, "Lectures on experimental physiology," 566.

16. Ferrier, *The Functions of the Brain* (1st ed.), 17–18.

17. Ibid., 287.

18. Ibid., 282.

19. Ibid., 283.

20. Ferrier, *The Functions of the Brain* (2d ed.), 424–468.

21. Ferrier, *The Functions of the Brain* (1st ed.), 284. Ferrier cited the English physiologists Laycock and Carpenter for having anticipated the view that attention interrupted the flow of sensation into motion. Cf. Carpenter, *Principles of Human Physiology* (4th ed.), 806–807, 815–818, 823–824. It is not apparent to me if and where Laycock stated this in any direct way. The psychology of attention is discussed below.

22. Ferrier, *The Functions of the Brain* (1st ed.), 285. He continued in the 2d ed. (436–438) to describe thought as suppressed speech. See Young, *Mind, Brain, and Adaptation*, 240–243.

23. Ferrier, *The Functions of the Brain* (1st ed.), 286.

24. Ibid., 18, 287–288.

25. Ibid., 288.

26. Cf. Wundt, *Untersuchungen zur Mechanik der Nerven und Nervencentren*. For Wundt's career prior to his call to the Leipzig chair of philosophy in 1875, see Diamond, "Wundt before Leipzig"; van Hoorn and Verhave, "Wundt's changing conceptions."

27. Wundt's *Grundzüge* was initially published in several parts in 1873 and 1874 and then in a single volume in 1874. On Wundt's program for a distinct subject of psychology, see Danziger, "Wundt's theory of behavior and volition"; Woodward, "Wundt's program for the new psychology."

28. Wundt, *Grundzüge der physiologischen Psychologie* (1st ed.), 174–175.

29. Wundt, *Untersuchungen zur Mechanik der Nerven und Nervencentren*, 2: chap. 3.

30. Wundt, *Grundzüge der physiologischen Psychologie* (5th ed.), 1: 86–87, trans. in idem, *Principles of Physiological Psychology*, 92. (Page of translation subsequently cited in parentheses after the German.)

31. Wundt, *Grundzüge der physiologischen Psychologie* (1st ed.), 175.

32. Langendorff, "Ueber Reflexhemmung."

33. Wundt, *Untersuchungen zur Mechanik der Nerven und Nervencentren*, 2: 99–102; idem, *Grundzüge der physiologischen Psychologie* (5th ed.), 1: 85–87 (91–93).

34. Dodge, "Theories of inhibition," 109. Cf. Wundt, *Grundzüge der physiologischen Psychologie* (5th ed.), 1: 320–324 (315–318).

35. Wundt, *Grundzüge der physiologischen Psychologie* (1st ed.), esp. chaps. 18, 19. For Herbart, see ibid., 796–800. Many commentators have noted Wundt's familiarity with Herbart (e.g., Danziger [1980: 75–79]), but there has been no systematic historical study of Herbart and the so-called Herbartians (e.g., Drobisch, Waitz) in relation to psychological topics in the 1850s and 1860s.

36. Wundt, *Grundzüge der physiologischen Psychologie* (5th ed.), 1: 243 (244).

37. Woodward, "Wundt's program for the new psychology," 175. On apperception, see Wundt, *Grundzüge der physiologischen Psychologie* (1st ed.), 717–725. Fearing ([1930: 207]) attributed an "inhibitory theory" of attention to Wundt.

38. Woodward, "Wundt's program for the new psychology," 183.

39. Wundt, *Grundzüge der physiologischen Psychologie* (5th ed.), 1: 323–324 (317–318).

40. Ibid., 320–327 (315–320). Wundt included a schematic picture.

41. Wundt, *Grundzüge der physiologischen Psychologie* (1st ed.), 715–725, 793–796; Ferrier, *The Functions of the Brain* (1st ed.), 284.

42. Bubnov and Heidenhain, "Ueber Erregungs- und Hemmungsvorgänge," trans. in idem, "On excitatory and inhibitory processes." The translation provided a cut and altered version, excluding the section that explained the authors' interest in hypnotism, thus portraying Bubnov and Heidenhain's work as purely experimental discovery. The translation was associated with interest in Magoun and Rhines, "An inhibitory mechanism in the bulbar reticular formation"; see below.

43. Heidenhain, *Animal Magnetism*. This included a lecture given by Heidenhain in January 1880 to the Silesian Society for Home Culture, following hypnotic performances by the well-known itinerant, Carl Hansen. The immediate translation of the small book into English indicated the international nature of the interest. The book was prefaced by G. J. Romanes, the scientist who worked up Darwin's notes on animal instinct. Heidenhain's explanation led to an account of inhibition in the *Encyclopaedia Britannica*: J. G. M'Kendrick, "Magnetism, animal," 280–281. See J. P. Williams, "Psychical research and psychiatry in late Victorian Britain," relating ideas on the suspension of the will to psychical research. Wundt (1893) also responded to the wave of interest in hypnotism in Europe and North America; see Marshall and Wendt, "Wilhelm Wundt, spiritism, and the assumptions of science." See also B. Danilevskii, "Die

Hemmungen der Reflex- und Willkürbewegungen," citing a decade of speculation linking inhibition and "nervous sleep"; Meynert, "Ueber hypnotische Erscheinungen."

44. Ellenberger, *The Discovery of the Unconscious*, 85–101, 749–784; Harrington, *Medicine, Mind, and the Double Brain*, chap. 6. For a comparison of models of hypnotism in relation to Freud, see Levin, *Freud's Early Psychology*, 64–74. For the application of inhibition to understanding hypnotism in France, see Brown-Séquard, "Recherches expérimentales et cliniques sur l'inhibition"; idem, "Le sommeil normal." For Italy, see Guarnieri, "Theatre and laboratory."

45. Heidenhain, *Animal Magnetism*, 43–44.

46. Ibid., xi–xii.

47. Ibid., 49.

48. Czermak, "Nachweis echter 'hypnotischer' Erscheinungen"; idem, "Beobachtungen und Versuche über 'hypnotische' Zustände bei Thieren"; Preyer, *Die Kataplexie und der thierische Hypnotismus*, 79–83. Preyer (ibid., 24) attributed the observation that compression of the neck induced inhibition to Lewisson, "Ueber Hemmung der Thätigkeit der motorischen Nervencentra." For Preyer's career, see Jaeger, "Origins of child psychology."

49. Kircher was a polymathic natural philosopher and writer: *D.S.B.*, "Kircher, Athanasius." I have not traced this particular phenomenon, but it appears to have been a traditional "wonder" of nature. See Preyer, *Die Kataplexie und der thierische Hypnotismus*, 3–10; Verworn, *General Physiology*, 492–496, with photographs; below. B. Danilevskii (1881: 595–596) reported that a colleague, Professor Bielskii, attempted to hypnotize a crocodile!

50. Bubnov and Heidenhain, "Ueber Erregungs- und Hemmungsvorgänge," 167, trans. in idem, "On excitatory and inhibitory processes," 191–192. (Page of translation subsequently cited in parentheses after the German.)

51. Ibid., 181 (202).

52. Ibid. H. E. Hering and Sherrington (1897) reported the strong inhibition of reflexes in mammals by direct stimulation of sensory areas in the cortex.

53. Schäfer, "The cerebral cortex," 712.

54. Meynert, "Ueber hypnotische Erscheinungen."

55. Bubnov and Heidenhain, "Ueber Erregungs- und Hemmungsvorgänge," 186 (206).

56. Munk, "Ueber Erregung und Hemmung." Munk also suggested that Bubnov and Heidenhain's results were produced by exhaustion of nerves, and this initiated a debate about the reliability of their results and interpretations. See H. E. Hering, "Die intracentralen Hemmungsvorgänge," 518–519, 525–529.

57. Bubnov and Heidenhain, "Ueber Errengungs- und Hemmungsvorgänge," 188 (207).

58. On tonicity, see Brondgeest, "Untersuchungen über den Tonus der willkürlichen Muskeln"; Vulpian, *Leçons sur la physiologie générale*, 430–434; Eckhard, "Beiträge zur Geschichte der Experimentalphysiologie des Nervensystems," 151–158. Gault (1904: 530, 547–551) claimed that the concept of tonus was introduced by J. Müller, *Handbuch der Physiologie*, 2: 29. Hall explained muscular tone by reference to his "excito-motory" system of nerves:

Hall, *Memoirs on the Nervous System*, 73, 93–94; idem, *On the Diseases and Derangements of the Nervous System*, 76–78.

59. Bubnov and Heidenhain, "Ueber Erregungs- und Hemmungsvorgänge," 191 (209).

60. Ibid., 193 (210).

61. Wundt, *Grundzüge der physiologischen Psychologie* (5th ed.), 1: 243–244 (244).

62. H. E. Hering, "Die intracentralen Hemmungsvorgänge"; Meltzer, "Inhibition"; Wundt, *Grundzüge der physiologischen Psychologie* (5th ed.), 1: 63–87 (70–93); Dodge, "Theories of inhibition"; Fearing, *Reflex Action*, 191–206; Howell, "Inhibition."

63. Hoff, "The history of vagal inhibition," 472–480; Geison, *Michael Foster and the Cambridge School of Physiology.*

64. Schiff, "Experimentelle Untersuchungen über die Nerven des Herzens"; idem, *Lehrbuch der Physiologie des Menschen*; idem, "Der modus der Herzbewegung." Hoff (1940: 474) argued that Schiff's theory was a significant but ignored anticipation of "Wedensky inhibition" (see below), though it was incorrect in relation to vagal action: "His theory of exhaustion as a cause of vagal arrest probably meant 'Wedensky inhibition.'" Of course, Schiff could not actually have "meant" something that was not to exist for over twenty years. See further: Hoff, "The history of the refractory period," 656–658.

65. Schiff, "Altes und neues Herznerven," 551–567; idem, "Recherches sur les nerfs dits arrestateurs."

66. Cf. Olmsted, *Charles-Édouard Brown-Séquard*, 161–165. For his opening course of lectures, see Brown-Séquard, "Collège de France: Cours de médecine." Brown-Séquard (1889*a*: 2) claimed to have extended the study of inhibitory processes in lectures to the Paris faculty of medicine in 1869 and 1871, but I do not know about the content of these lectures. In an encyclopedia article (1889*e*: 2–3), he claimed to have studied inhibition since 1868, but the term itself was not present in the articles he cited (1868*a*, 1868*b*). These articles noted the arrest of heart action or convulsions by peripheral stimulation.

67. See the historical summary relating Brown-Séquard's work to studies of inhibition: Richet, *Physiologie des muscles et des nerfs*, 704–711, 800–801. For psychological uses, see below.

68. Brown-Séquard, "Existence de l'excitabilité motrice," 301. Charles Rouget was professor of physiology in the medical faculty at Montpellier in the 1860s.

69. Brown-Séquard, *Course of Lectures on the Physiology and Pathology of the Nervous System.* For the significance of Brown-Séquard's work in translating "sympathy" into modern terms, see Riese, *A History of Neurology*, 133–136. Riese commented (ibid., 134) that Brown-Séquard was "little known and never cited"; his contributions to neurology appear to have been eclipsed by those of Charcot in the 1880s.

70. Brown-Séquard, "Faits nouveaux relatifs à la mise en jeu ou à l'arrêt," 494, 496. For Brown-Séquard's application of these ideas to the explanation of laterality of function and metalloscopy experiments (producing hypnotism), see Harrington, *Medicine, Mind, and the Double Brain*, 180–181.

71. Brown-Séquard, "Faits montrant que toutes les parties . . . peuvent déterminer certaines inhibitions," 323. He continued the discussion in idem, "Inhibition de certaines puissances réflexes"; idem, "Du rôle de certaines influences dynamogéniques"; idem, "De la puissance inhibitrice." For his claims to the discovery of inhibition, see his "Champ d'action de l'inhibition"; "Quelque mots sur la découverte de l'inhibition"; "De quelque règles générales relatives à l'inhibition," developing his article in *Dictionnaire encyclopédique des sciences médicales* (1889*e*).

72. A. James, "The reflex inhibitory centre theory." G. H. Lewes (1877: 288–304) discussed "discharge" and "arrest" as subspecies of more general laws of stimulation.

73. McDougall, "The nature of inhibitory processes," 169. For McDougall's work in wider perspective, see Rintoul, "Images of human nature," chaps. 6 and 7.

74. Spencer, "The social organism." See also above, chap. 2; and below.

75. McDougall, "The nature of inhibitory processes," 169. See W. James, *The Principles of Psychology*, 2: 579–592.

76. McDougall, *Physiological Psychology*, 132–133. Dodge (1926*b*) attempted to test the drainage theory in a study of the tendon reflex; cf. Fearing, *Reflex Action*, 273–274.

77. Fearing, *Reflex Action*, 194–202. This use of "interference" should be distinguished from Wundt's term, discussed above.

78. H. E. Hering, "Die intracentralen Hemmungsvorgänge," 516. For Goltz, see above.

79. Tsion, "Hemmungen und Erregungen," cols. 112–117, reprinted in idem, *Gesammelte physiologischen Arbeiten*, 96–110. Il'ya Tsion's (or Elie de Cyon's) extraordinary career is discussed in relation to Pavlov below, chap. 5. For Tsion's "reactionary" views on the heartbeat, see Geison, *Michael Foster and the Cambridge School of Physiology*, 344, 351.

80. Brunton, "Inhibition, peripheral and central," 180.

81. Ibid., 199. Cf. Simonov, "Die Hemmungsmechanismen der Säugethiere"; J. G. M'Kendrick, "On the inhibitory or restraining action," 734.

82. Brunton, "Inhibition, peripheral and central," 218.

83. Ibid.

84. Brunton, "On the nature of inhibition," 468.

85. Ibid., 421. For the significance of Romanes's research, see R. D. French, "Darwin and the physiologists."

86. Brunton, "On the nature of inhibition," 437. Brunton also noted the phenomenon, commented on by physicians since Hippocrates (see above, chap. 1), that strong irritation was an interference against pain, thus aligning his account with ancient considerations concerning sympathetic action.

87. Ibid., 487.

88. This work is now particularly associated with Bernard, and the wider research has not been studied. See Bernard's summary in *De la physiologie générale*, 25–32, 224–231; Grmek, *Raisonnement expérimental et recherches toxicologiques*, chap. 3.

89. Sedgwick, "The influence of quinine upon . . . the spinal cord."

90. E. Hering, "Zur Lehre vom Lichtsinne," 69: 182–199; "Zur Theorie der Vorgänge in der lebendigen Substanz," trans. in idem, "Theory of the functions in living matter." Hering's evidence was reviewed in A. D. Waller, "On the 'inhibition' of . . . muscular contractions." For the context of Hering's work in visual physiology (drawing on ideas of metabolic self-regulation), see E. Hering, *Outlines of a Theory of the Light Sense*, intro. and 109–113. Gaskell, "The Croonian Lecture," 1027–1029. On Gaskell, see Geison, *Michael Foster and the Cambridge School of Physiology*, esp. 314–319; Swazey, *Reflexes and Motor Integration*, 70–74.

91. Gaskell, "On the structure, distribution and function of the nerves which innervate the visceral and vascular systems," 41.

92. Ibid., 40.

93. See below, chap. 5.

94. Exner, *Entwurf zu einer physiologischen Erklärung der psychischen Erscheinungen*, 69–83. Exner apparently introduced the term "Bahnung" in 1892 in the context of a study of reaction times. See Gault, "A sketch of the history of reflex action," 540–544.

95. Exner, *Entwurf zu einer physiologischen Erklärung der psychischen Erscheinungen*, 165–167, on attention; Freud, "Project for a scientific psychology." See below, chap. 5; Amacher, *Freud's Neurological Education*, 42–54, 63–70.

96. Verworn, *Irritability*, 201–202. See also idem, "Zur Physiologie der nervösen Hemmungserscheinungen"; idem, *Die Biogenhypothese*, 105–111; Rothschuh, *History of Physiology*, 302–303.

97. Meltzer, "Inhibition," 741. The claim that inhibition was a general physiological property was reviewed and related to other views of inhibition in Howell, "Inhibition."

98. Brazier, *A History of Neurophysiology in the 19th Century*; Clarke and O'Malley, *The Human Brain and Spinal Cord*, 87–138, 209–259; Lenoir, "Models and instruments in the development of electrophysiology."

99. Schiff, *Lehrbuch der Physiologie des Menschen*, 201. Sherrington (1961: 44) attributed the first description of a "refractory phase" (in the heart) to Kronecker and Stirling, "Das charakterische Merkmal der Herzmuskelbewegung." See Hoff, "The history of the refractory period."

100. Vvedenskii, "Ueber einige Beziehungen zwischen der Reizstärke und der Tetanushöhe." On Vvedenskii's change from radicalism to insular scientist, see Todes, "From radicalism to scientific convention," 377–380.

101. The definition of Dodge, "Theories of inhibition," 169. Vvedenskii published more extensive studies in Russian in the 1880s (which I have not seen) and then made his work available in French so as to reach a wider audience: Vvedenskii, "De l'action excitatrice et inhibitoire"; idem, "Des relations entre les processus rythmiques et l'activité fonctionelle."

102. Vvedenskii, "Die Erregung, Hemmung und Narkose."

103. Koshtoyants, *Essays on the History of Physiology in Russia*, 250–256; Diamond, Balvin, and Diamond, *Inhibition and Choice*, 51–54, 201–224. A. A. Ukhtomskii was Vvdenskii's successor in directing physiological research

at the University of St. Petersburg/Leningrad: Joravsky, *Russian Psychology*, 282–286.

104. Verworn, *Irritability*, 154–234.

105. Lucas, revised by Adrian, *The Conduction of the Nervous Impulse*, 98. The "all or none" principle of conduction was supported by the experiments of the physiologist Francis Gotch: Gotch, "The submaximal electrical response of nerve." For the assimilation of Wedensky inhibition to the all or none principle, see Adrian, "Wedensky inhibition." For the precise recording of the refractory period in nerve, see Gotch and Burch, "The electrical response of nerve." Forbes (1912) criticized the metabolism theories of E. Hering and Verworn and (following Sherrington) directed attention toward the central synapses as the likely site of inhibition.

106. Brooks, "Discovery of the function of chemical mediators"; Clarke and O'Malley, *The Human Brain and Spinal Cord*, 237–240, 244–259; Diamond, Balvin, and Diamond, *Inhibition and Choice*, 88–105; Eccles, "The development of ideas on the synapse"; Granit, *Charles Scott Sherrington*, 98–141; *D.S.B.*, "Loewi, Otto." For Russian work on transmitter mechanisms, see Koshtoyants, *Essays on the History of Physiology in Russia*, 273–276.

107. Creed, Denny-Brown, Eccles, Liddell, and Sherrington, *Reflex Activity of the Spinal Cord*, 158.

108. Ash, "Psychology in twentieth-century Germany"; Ash and Geuter, eds., *Geschichte der deutschen Psychologie*; Ash and Woodward, eds., *Psychology in Twentieth-Century Thought*; Geuter, "The uses of history"; Hearnshaw, *A Short History of British Psychology*; Rose, *The Psychological Complex*.

109. Ash, "The self-presentation of a discipline"; Danziger, "The positivist repudiation of Wundt"; idem, "Wundt and the two traditions"; O'Donnell, *The Origins of Behaviorism*.

110. Breese, "On inhibition," 6. Breese (ibid., 6–10) surveyed the idea that the activity of one psychological content inhibited others.

111. Ibid., 12–13.

112. Ibid., 16–17.

113. Daston, "British responses to psycho-physiology"; Hearnshaw, *A Short History of British Psychology*; Rintoul, "Images of human nature."

114. R. J. Richards, *Darwin and the Emergence of Evolutionary Theories*; P. P. Wiener, *Evolution and the Founders of Pragmatism*; Young, "Scholarship and the history of the behavioural sciences"; idem, *Mind, Brain, and Adaptation*.

115. Especially Bain, *The Senses and the Intellect*, chaps. 1, 2.

116. Bain, *The Emotions and the Will*, 445–449.

117. Ibid., chaps. 6–10, on the will.

118. Ibid., 445–446.

119. Ibid., 447.

120. Ibid., 442.

121. Carpenter, *Principles of Mental Physiology*, 130–147, 330–336, 382–391, 413–428. This text appears to have been widely used, e.g., in teacher training, and it was taken seriously by psychologists, e.g., William James, who

adopted Carpenter's category of "ideo-motor" action: James, *The Principles of Psychology*, 2: 522–528. In his review of attention (ibid., 1: 404), James referred only casually to inhibition, to describe the state of mental vacancy opposed to the state of attention.

122. Spencer, *The Principles of Psychology*, 1: 231–233, 245–249.

123. Bain, *The Senses and the Intellect*, 557.

124. Ibid., 563. Inhibition, referring to the obstructive interference of different associations in remembering and forgetting, was used by later psychologists, e.g., Pillsbury, *The Essentials of Psychology*, 213–222.

125. Spencer, *The Principles of Psychology*, 1: 475. See Hamilton, "Philosophy of perception"; idem, "Supplementary dissertations," Note D*, 880, 886–888.

126. Spencer, *The Principles of Psychology*, 1: 496.

127. Mill, *A System of Logic*, 860–874. As young men, Bain and Spencer were both influenced by phrenology, which also linked the study of individual differences and a moral and practical ethos. See Young, *Mind, Brain, and Adaptation*, 121–133, 150–167; above, chap. 2.

128. Spencer, *The Principles of Psychology*, 1: 582.

129. Taine, *De l'intelligence*; Ribot, *La psychologie anglaise*.

130. Ribot, *The Psychology of Attention*, 46.

131. Ibid., 49–50.

132. Ribot, *Diseases of the Will*, 10, 51.

133. Ribot, *The Psychology of Attention*, 10.

134. Ibid., 50. Cf. Preyer, *Die Seele des Kindes*, 124–127, 145–148, trans. as idem, *The Mind of the Child*, 1: 188–195, 227–232; Jaeger, "Origins of child psychology"; idem, "Preyer and the German school reform movement."

135. Clouston, *Clinical Lectures on Mental Diseases*, 351. See Tuke, *Prichard and Symonds in Especial Relation to Mental Science*; R. Smith, *Trial by Medicine*, 38–40, 124–142; above, chap. 2.

136. Watson, "The moral imbecile," chap. 3.

137. Ribot, *The Diseases of the Will*, 17.

138. Nye, *Crime, Politics and Madness in Modern France*, 260–261, discussing the Chaumié circular of 1905, which required the question of responsibility to be put to medical witnesses.

139. Wolf, *Alfred Binet*, 43–64.

140. Binet and Féré, *Le magnétisme animal*, 153, trans. in Wolf, *Alfred Binet*, 68.

141. Binet, "L'inhibition dans les phénomènes de conscience."

142. Paulhan, *L'activité mentale*, 17; see also 221–314.

143. Meynert, *Psychiatrie*, 183, trans. in idem, *Psychiatry*, 196–197. (This was the first, physiological, volume of a projected two-volume study, but the second, clinical, volume was not published in this form.) In his historical review of neurology, Head (1926, 1: 54–66) referred scathingly to the "diagram makers," who included Wernicke, whose work was based on Meynert's ideas. See Jeannerod, *The Brain Machine*, 71–83.

144. Ideas about the antagonism, arrest, and inhibition of mental elements

were stressed in general textbooks, e.g., Ladd, *A Treatise . . . of Human Mental Life*, 254–259; Sully, *The Human Mind*, 2: 246–276.

145. de Watteville, "Sleep and its counterfeits," 741.

146. Ibid.

147. Nordau, *Degeneration*, 323, 324. For the European context, see Pick, *Faces of Degeneration*. These ideas were linked briefly to modern notions of "disinhibition" in Martindale, "Degeneration, disinhibition, and genius."

148. McDougall, *An Introduction to Social Psychology*, 442.

149. McDougall, "The physiological factors of the attention-process," 1902: 323, 1906: 349–355.

150. Morgan, *An Introduction to Comparative Psychology*, 213. See Boakes, *From Darwin to Behaviourism*, 35. Morgan's view of learning came between the theories of Bain and Spencer and Thorndike's "law of effect." See Postman, "Rewards and punishments."

151. Morgan, *Animal Life and Intelligence*, 385–386.

152. Ibid., 458. For behavioral choice as "disinhibition," see Diamond, Balvin, and Diamond, *Inhibition and Choice*, 133–150.

153. Morgan, *Animal Life and Intelligence*, 461. For the relations between attention, thought, and inhibition, see Diamond, Balvin, and Diamond, *Inhibition and Choice*, 151–166.

154. Morgan, *Animal Life and Intelligence*, 459.

155. Hyslop, "Inhibition and the freedom of the will," 374.

156. Ibid., 382.

157. Ibid., 386.

158. W. James, *The Principles of Psychology*, 2: 395.

159. Ibid.

160. Ibid., 583; James italicized the whole passage.

161. Ibid., 373.

162. Ibid., 584.

163. Breese, "On inhibition," 17.

164. G. E. Müller and Pilzecker, "Experimentelle Beiträge zur Lehre vom Gedächtniss." See Murray, "Research on human memory"; Scheerer, "Wilhelm Wundt's psychology of memory." For further references to early-twentieth-century discussions, see Eisler, "Hemmung," 632; Ritter, ed., *Historisches Wörterbuch der Philosophie*, col. 1056; Ebbinghaus, *Grundzüge der Psychologie*, 693–707.

165. Sechenov, "Physiologische Studien über die Hemmungsmechanismen," 171–173.

166. Exner, *Entwurf zu einer physiologischen Erklarung der psychischen Erscheinungen*.

167. Obersteiner, "Experimental researches on attention," 443.

168. Heymans, "Untersuchungen über psychische Hemmung." For the Netherlands, van Strien, "Psychology and its social legitimation."

169. Fearing, *Reflex Action*, 206–214.

170. Jacobson, "Progressive relaxation." This paper did not mention inhibition, but its ideas were founded in Jacobson's earlier research (itself based on

that of Heymans): idem, "Experiments on the inhibition of sensations"; idem, "Furthur experiments on the inhibition of sensations." See Tweney, "Programmatic research in experimental psychology," 47.

171. Dodge, "The problem of inhibition," 12.

172. Roback, *The Psychology of Character*, 543.

173. For the context of behaviorism, see Burnham, *Paths into American Culture*; O'Donnell, *The Origins of Behaviorism*. On its problematic acceptance by U.S. psychologists, see Samelson, "Organizing for the kingdom of behavior." For its methodological commitment to animal behavior studies, see Boakes, *From Darwin to Behaviourism*; Mackenzie, *Behaviourism and the Limits of Scientific Method*.

174. Hunter, "The psychological study of behavior," 24.

175. Guthrie, "Conditioning as a principle of learning," 428. For Pavlov's response, see Pavlov, "The reply of a physiologist," 91–100, reprinted in idem, *Lectures on Conditioned Reflexes*, 2: 117–145. See Gray, *Pavlov*, chap. 4; Windholz, "Pavlov's position toward American behaviorism"; Diamond, Balvin, and Diamond, *Inhibition and Choice*, 256–269. For Pavlov's use of inhibition see below, chap. 5. G. R. Wendt (1936) conducted experiments to show that inhibition was always the effect of an opposing system, thus undermining Pavlov's whole approach. For American studies of conditioning in general (incorporating Pavlov's research), see Hilgard and Marquis, *Conditioning and Learning*, 45–48, 104–134, 346. These authors subsumed inhibition under the study of "extinction" of learned responses. For a later symposium on inhibition in psychology, see *British Journal of Psychology*, "Inhibition."

176. Hull, *Principles of Behavior*, 278. For a comparison of American behaviorism and Pavlovian approaches, see Razran, "Russian physiologists' psychology."

177. B. F. Skinner, *The Behavior of Organisms*, 17; see also ibid., 160.

178. Ibid., 17. See also the application of this definition to the discussion of discriminative stimuli: ibid., 231–234.

179. Beer, *Darwin's Plots*; Burrow, *Evolution and Society*; Russett, *Sexual Science*; Stocking, *Victorian Anthropology*; Young, *Darwin's Metaphor*.

180. Spencer, *First Principles*; idem, *Principles of Psychology* (the 2d ed., completely revised from the 1st ed., 1855, and much more widely read). For Spencer's evolutionism, see Burrow, *Evolution and Society*, chap. 6; Peel, *Herbert Spencer*; R. J. Richards, *Darwin and the Emergence of Evolutionary Theories*, 343–394; Young, *Mind, Brain, and Adaptation*, 161–196.

181. Harrington, *Medicine, Mind, and the Double Brain*, esp. chap. 3. Harrington (ibid., 94–95) referred, e.g., to Jules Bernard Luys's explanation for the hyperemotionality of some left-hemiplegics in terms of a lesion in an inhibitory center in the right hemisphere.

182. See Riese, *A History of Neurology*; Star, *Regions of the Mind*; Young, *Mind, Brain, and Adaptation*, 197–210, 220–223. For Jackson's representation of the evolutionary hierarchy in bilateral terms, see Harrington, *Medicine, Mind, and the Double Brain*, 209–245.

183. Jackson, "On the anatomical and physiological localisation of movements," 46–47. See C. U. M. Smith, "Evolution and the problem of mind."

184. Jackson, "On the anatomical and physiological localisation of movements," 38.

185. Jackson, "On temporary mental disorders after epileptic paroxysms," 123 n.; idem, "On epilepsies," 146 n., 149; idem, "On affections of speech," 192; idem, "Remarks on dissolution of the nervous system," 22.

186. See Temkin, *The Falling Sickness*, 328–351.

187. Jackson, "Discussion at the Neurological Society," 477–481, discussing Mercier, "Inhibition (1888*a*)".

188. Jackson, "On post-epileptic states," 370; Jackson printed the second paragraph as a footnote to the first. B. Stilling was a German histologist and researcher on spinal cord function. His "nucleus" was a cell aggregate in the spinal cord. I am not aware that Stilling himself referred to inhibition.

189. Jackson, "On affections of speech," 192. See Anstie, *Stimulants and Narcotics*, 80; Dickson, "Matter and force," 235; idem, *The Science and Practice of Medicine*, 11–12.

190. Jackson, "On temporary mental disorders after epileptic paroxysms," 123 n.

191. Jackson, "On the anatomical and physiological localisation of movements," 50–51. See Young, *Mind, Brain, and Adaptation*, 207.

192. Collie, *Henry Maudsley*; Pick, *Faces of Degeneration*, 203–216; T. Turner, "Henry Maudsley."

193. Maudsley, *The Pathology of Mind*, 194.

194. Ibid., 136. For the psychiatric setting, see Clark, "'The data of alienism,'" 115–122.

195. Maudsley, *The Pathology of Mind*, 243.

196. Maudsley, *Body and Will*, 251.

197. Tredgold, *Mental Deficiency*, 319. See Watson, "The moral imbecile," 40–44, 75–85.

198. Maudsley, *Body and Will*, 110–111.

199. Maudsley, *The Physiology and Pathology of Mind*, 153–154. Maudsley wrote a notorious paper attacking medical education for women on the grounds of their limited energies: idem, "Sex in mind and in education." For the Victorian psychiatrists' preoccupation with Hamlet's "illness," see Bynum and Neve, "Hamlet on the couch."

200. The "analogy" between the hierarchy in the nervous system and in the army became a statement about their identical nature in Mercier, "Inhibition (1888*a*)", 376–382; idem, *Nervous System and the Mind*, 133–143.

201. Clouston, *The Hygiene of Mind*, 37.

202. Maudsley, *The Physiology and Pathology of Mind*, 94.

203. Ibid., 94–95.

204. Mercier, *The Nervous System and the Mind*, 76.

205. Ibid. Same passage also in idem, "Inhibition (1888*a*)", 370.

206. Mercier, *The Nervous System and the Mind*, 133.

207. Jackson in Mercier, "Inhibition (1888*a*)", 392 n., reprinted in Jackson, "Discussion at the Neurological Society," 481 n. Jackson quoted from his own Croonian Lecture: idem, "Evolution and dissolution of the nervous system," 58.

208. See Woodward, "Wundt's program."

209. Meynert, *Psychiatry*, 196–197. See above. Meynert's view of inhibition was linked to Freud's in Jones, *Sigmund Freud*, 1: 308–309.

210. This was the retrospective formulation of Head, "Croonian Lecture," 184. Freud (1953, esp. 86–89) was a noteworthy critic.

211. Goltz, "Der Hund ohne Grosshirn," 603–604, trans. in Clarke and O'Malley, *The Human Brain and Spinal Cord*, 563. He first expressed this view in "Ueber die Verrichtungen des Grosshirns," 39–44. The argument was summarized in W. James, *The Principles of Psychology*, 1: 67–69. For a similar view, see Brown-Séquard, "Sur l'arrêt immédiat de convulsions"; idem, "De quelques règles générales relatives à l'inhibition," 751.

212. Head, "Croonian Lecture," 184.

213. Ibid., 195.

214. Ibid., 196.

215. Ibid., 197–206. Head interpreted sensory disturbances in terms of the release of inhibition; see Riese, *A History of Neurology*, 155–157. Sherrington had analyzed the relation of central excitation and inhibition; see below, chap. 5.

216. Rivers and Head, "A human experiment in nerve division," esp. 325–326. See Miller, "The dog beneath the skin."

217. Head, "Sensation and the cerebral cortex," 650.

218. Head, "Croonian Lecture," 206.

219. Ibid., 208.

220. Maudsley, *The Pathology of Mind*, 386.

221. Bagehot, *Physics and Politics*, 105.

222. Huxley, "Evolution and ethics," 52, quoting from Tennyson's poem, "In memoriam A. H. H.," in Tennyson, *Poems*, 2: CXVIII, line 28. On Huxley's view of the dualism in human nature, see Paradis, *T. H. Huxley*, 141–163.

223. Rivers, *Instinct and the Unconscious*, 31. For the relation to theories of atavism and recapitulation, see Gould, *Ontogeny and Phylogeny*, 115–155. On the response to war neuroses, see Stone, "Shellshock and the psychologists."

224. Rivers, *Instinct and the Unconscious*, 31.

225. Ibid., 239.

226. See Berrios, "Stupor," 684–685; Ritter, ed., *Historisches Wörterbuch der Philosophie*, "Hemmung—vitale," cols. 1057–1058.

227. Kraepelin, *Manic-depressive Insanity*, 15–16. See idem, *Psychiatrie*, 3: 1295–1303.

228. Kraepelin, *Manic-depressive Insanity*, 36–40. See idem, *Psychiatrie*, 3: 1219–1224, 1299–1301.

229. Bleuler, *Textbook of Psychiatry*, 80. See ibid., 74; idem, *Psychiatrie*, 52–55; idem, *Dementia Praecox*, 34, 309–310.

230. Kretschmer, *A Text-book of Medical Psychology*, 41. Kretschmer was the president of the International Medical Society for Psychotherapy when the German section was "Nazified" in 1933, and he was dismissed as a "Jew."

231. Kretschmer, *Hysteria, Reflex and Instinct*, x; Kretschmer italicized the whole passage.

232. Magoun and Rhines, "An inhibitory mechanism in the bulbar reticular formation," 165. This research was first reported in Magoun, "Bulbar inhibi-

tion." Subsequent work on cortical arousal also focused on the functions of the reticular formation and the part played by inhibition in higher nervous activities. For the importance of inhibition to the psychology of learning, personality, and so on, see Diamond, *Personality and Temperament*, 395–426.

233. Delgado, *Physical Control of the Mind*, 176. These ideas were discussed critically in Chorover, *From Genesis to Genocide*, 173–174.

234. MacLean, "Psychosomatic disease and the 'visceral brain'"; idem, "The limbic system"; idem, "The paranoid streak in man." See Papez, "A proposed mechanism of emotion." For overviews of these theories, see Durant, "The beast in man"; idem, "The science of sentiment." Similar views have played a major part in primate studies, a field characterized by a circle of reflections about human and animal nature: Haraway, *Primate Visions*.

235. MacLean, quoted in Durant, "The beast in man," 31. The imagery of the unbridled horse has its locus classicus in Plato (1961: 246 ff.) where the human soul was portrayed as a pair of noble and ignoble horses, held together only with difficulty by the charioteer. Marcuse (1955: 99–114) sketched out the history of this theme as "the logic of domination."

5: TWENTIETH-CENTURY SCHOOLS

1. See the celebratory essay by his younger colleagues: Eccles and Gibson, *Sherrington*.

2. Sherrington's book (1961) retains its status as a classic and remains in print. His principal scientific papers were selected, abridged, and introduced, with a bibliography up to 1938, in Sherrington, *Selected Writings of Sir Charles Sherrington*. See Granit, *Charles Scott Sherrington*, 47–73; Liddell, *The Discovery of Reflexes*, chap. 4; Swazey, *Reflexes and Motor Integration*.

3. Sherrington, "Inhibition as a coordinative factor."

4. Liljestrand, "The prize in physiology or medicine," 247, also quoted in Eccles and Gibson, *Sherrington*, 70. This account should not be taken too literally. For example, it would be worth exploring whether there was also resistance to Sherrington's candidature owing to his statements in support of the Western powers in World War I, statements that some considered antithetical to the ideals of science.

5. Sherrington, *Man on His Nature*, 190. Much of the account of the mind-body relation in these lectures was introduced through the writings of the sixteenth-century French physician and humanist, Jean Fernel. See Sherrington, *The Endeavour of Jean Fernel*.

6. Sherrington, *Man on His Nature*, 163–164, quoting Morgan, *An Introduction to Comparative Psychology*, 182.

7. Swazey, *Reflexes and Motor Integration*, 168.

8. Ibid., 169. The "final common path" was Sherrington's term for the motor nerve carrying the unified result of nervous integrations to a muscle; see below.

9. Brazier, "The historical development of neurophysiology," 39.

10. Sherrington, "Inhibition as a coordinative factor," 288.

11. See above, chaps. 3, 4.

12. Sherrington, *The Integrative Action of the Nervous System*, esp. Lectures V, VI. Liddell (1960: 136–140) described the scratch reflex as "a comprehensive paradigm."

13. Liddell and Sherrington, "Responses in response to stretch." This paper was founded in Sherrington's work in the 1890s. See Granit, *Charles Scott Sherrington*, 73–78.

14. Swazey, *Reflexes and Motor Integration*, 100–101. Swazey (ibid., 124–160) provided a systematic introduction to *The Integrative Action of the Nervous System.*

15. The principal paper on reciprocal inhibition was Sherrington, "On reciprocal innervation in antagonistic muscles." See also idem, "Note on the knee-jerk"; idem, "Further experimental note on . . . antagonistic muscles"; idem, *The Integrative Action of the Nervous System*, 83–107; Swazey, *Reflexes and Motor Integration*, 68–70, 84–90, 116–118.

16. Sherrington, "Experiments in examination of the peripheral distribution of the . . . posterior roots," 178.

17. Bell and Bell, *The Anatomy and Physiology of the Human Body*, 3: 103–109. The research was solely by Charles Bell (who published this edition, which introduced the topic, after his brother's death). Even here, it was the *assumption* of the antagonism of paired muscles that guided Bell's interpretation of function. It is difficult to describe "antagonism" as an empirical discovery. There are other examples of physiologists "anticipating" the idea of reciprocal inhibition, e.g., Budge, *Untersuchungen über das Nervensystem*, 1: 62–63.

18. Descartes, *Treatise of Man*, 25–27, 29, 31–33. See Sherrington, *The Integrative Action of the Nervous System*, 286–288.

19. Meltzer, "Die Irradiationen des Schluckcentrums," 215–216, freely trans. in Sherrington, *The Integrative Action of the Nervous System*, 100–101.

20. Sherrington, *The Integrative Action of the Nervous System*, 83.

21. Ibid., 101. On Anodon, see Pavlov, "Wie die Muschel ihre Schaale öffnet." For the systematic rejection of the existence of inhibitory nerves to vertebrate skeletal muscle, see A. D. Waller, "On the 'inhibition' of . . . muscular contractions."

22. Letter to Henry Head, 1918, quoted in Eccles and Gibson, *Sherrington*, 209. See Biedermann (1887, 1888). On Gaskell, see above, chap 4.

23. Sherrington, "Reflex inhibition as a factor in the co-ordination of movements," 254.

24. Sherrington, "The correlation of reflexes"; idem, *The Integrative Action of the Nervous System*, 117–120.

25. Sherrington, "Experiments in examination of the peripheral distribution of the . . . posterior roots." See idem, *The Integrative Action of the Nervous System*, 299–302; Swazey, *Reflexes and Motor Integration*, 80–83. If one hemisphere was removed, rigidity occurred only on one side of the body.

26. Sherrington himself recognized the relation to Jackson's work, e.g., Sherrington, "Inhibition as a coordinative factor," 287.

27. Head, "Croonian Lecture."

28. Goltz and Freusberg, "Ueber die Functionen des Lendenmarks des

Hundes"; Freusberg, "Reflexbewegungen beim Hunde"; Sherrington, "Experiments in examination of the peripheral distribution of the . . . posterior roots"; idem, *The Integrative Action of the Nervous System*, 241–250; Swazey, *Reflexes and Motor Integration*, 96–100.

29. Hering and Sherrington, "Ueber Hemmung der Contraction willkürlicher Muskeln." See H. E. Hering, "Die intracentralen Hemmungsvorgänge," 519–521; Sherrington, *The Integrative Action of the Nervous System*, 289.

30. Meltzer, "Inhibition," 701.

31. Ibid., referring to Sherrington, "Experimental note on two movements of the eye." Sherrington had argued that subcortical inhibition occurred habitually in normal eye movements. He would probably have found Meltzer's extension of his argument rather speculative.

32. Nevertheless, during World War I, Sherrington became deeply involved with research on fatigue, a subject important to the occupational development of psychology.

33. Sherrington, *The Integrative Action of the Nervous System*, 299. This work involved studying the convulsive effects of strychnine and tetanus toxins.

34. Sherrington, *The Brain and Its Mechanism*, 33–34.

35. Sherrington, "Reflex inhibition as a factor in the co-ordination of movements," 308.

36. Sherrington, *The Brain and Its Mechanism*, 10. He alluded to Thomas Carlyle, *Sartor Resartus*, 108: "The end of Man is an Action, and not a Thought." See Sherrington, *Man on His Nature*, 163.

37. Sherrington, *The Integrative Action of the Nervous System*, 1947 preface, xiii–xiv.

38. Ibid., xvi. Cf. A. N. Whitehead's conception of "misplaced concreteness," used to criticize an overly physicalist metaphysics: Whitehead, *Science and the Modern World*, 64.

39. Sherrington, *The Integrative Action of the Nervous System*, 1947 preface, xvi–xvii.

40. Ibid., 353–390.

41. See Lucas, rev. Adrian, *The Conduction of the Nervous Impulse*.

42. For the theory of the neuron and the synapse, see Clarke and O'Malley, *The Human Brain and Spinal Cord*; Diamond, Balvin, and Diamond, *Inhibition and Choice*, 88–105; R. D. French, "Some concepts of nerve structure"; Liddell, *The Discovery of Reflexes*; Swazey, *Reflexes and Motor Integration*, 74–78.

43. See Sherrington, *Selected Writings of Sir Charles Sherrington*, 440–496. The argument developed in a slow and piecemeal way. Thus, in his Nobel address ([1932] 1965: 284–285), Sherrington still referred to inhibition simply as an interference with the propagation of the impulse. On synaptic transmission, see above, chap. 4.

44. Eccles and Gibson, *Sherrington*, 55; this passage was written by Eccles. Sherrington indicated in 1906 (1961: 192–200) that he favored the interface between the neurons in the spinal cord as the site for the inhibitory mechanism.

45. Sherrington, "Remarks on some aspects of reflex inhibition"; idem, "Ferrier Lecture."

46. Sherrington, "Reflex inhibition as a factor in the co-ordination of movements," 253.

47. Joravsky, *Soviet Marxism and Natural Science*; Vucinich, *Empire of Knowledge.*

48. Joravsky, *Russian Psychology*, 379–414. Other interpretations of the history of Soviet psychology include Bauer, *New Man in Soviet Psychology*; Kozulin, *Psychology in Utopia.* McLeish (1975) attempted to reconstruct the dialectical content of objective psychology. As is generally the case with the history of the USSR, there are considerable gaps in our understanding of the 1930s and 1940s.

49. Gray, *Pavlov.* The most extensive biography is by Babkin (1951), who worked with Pavlov but left after the revolution, and his account is based on personal reminiscence. For Pavlov's political views and relations with the Bolsheviks and his critics in the 1920s, see Joravsky, *Russian Psychology*, 77–83, 207–212, 286–307. Daniel Todes is writing a new biography.

50. Asratyan, *I. P. Pavlov*; Koshtoyants, *Essays on the History of Physiology in Russia*, 178–207. The continuity of Sechenov's and Pavlov's work on inhibition and recent brain research was emphasized in Asratyan, *Brain Reflexes.* Asratyan described inhibition theory as creating an earlier and alternative conception of nervous integration to that established by Sherrington. See Purpura and Waelsch, "Brain reflexes." Inhibition was a fundamental concept in post-Pavlovian Soviet textbooks: Bykov, ed., *Text-book of Physiology*, 543–544.

51. Asratyan, *I. P. Pavlov*, 153. The Russian edition of this book appeared first in 1949. Asratyan apparently added materials in the light of the 1950 decision about Pavlov's work: ibid., 161–164, on the consequences of the 1950 congress.

52. Joravsky, *Russian Psychology*, 70–76, 134–148; Todes, "From radicalism to scientific convention," 389–416. Tsion meanwhile converted to Christianity. On Pavlov's early career, see also Vucinich, *Science in Russian Culture*, 298–315.

53. Pavlov, "Wie die Muschel ihre Schaale öffnet."

54. E.g., Pavlov, *Selected Works*, 50, 52, 56, 175. See Todes, "From radicalism to scientific convention," 427–431.

55. Pavlov, *Lectures on Conditioned Reflexes*, 1: 39.

56. Todes, "From radicalism to scientific convention," 423.

57. Koshtoyants, *Essays on the History of Physiology in Russia*, 241–276. According to Jeannerod (1985: 44), Pavlov forbade his students to read Sherrington, but I do not know the source of this anecdote.

58. Gantt, "Pavlov," 178. Pavlov's approach to inhibition was explained and defended in Diamond, Balvin, and Diamond, *Inhibition and Choice*, 183–200. These authors wrote (200): "It demonstrates, over and over again, the absolute necessity of taking the inhibitory process into account whenever we wish to explain *any* response to *any* stimulus."

59. This school persisted into the 1950s: Leake, "Danilevsky, Wedensky, and Ukhtomsky."

60. Bekhterev, *General Principles of Human Reflexology*, 89. For Bekhterev's context, see Joravsky, *Russian Psychology*, 83–91, 271–281.

61. Bekhterev, *General Principles of Human Reflexology*, 272.

62. Pavlov, *Lectures on Conditioned Reflexes*, 1: 38–39.

63. Ibid., 39. For the Soviet view that Pavlov established such methods, see Anokhin, "Ivan P. Pavlov and psychology."

64. Pavlov presented a systematic theory of higher nervous activity in *Conditioned Reflexes*, which included a list of publications from his laboratories (412–427). Pavlov tightly coordinated conditioning research, and his conclusions drew together collective experimental work: Windholz, "Pavlov and the Pavlovians." For a portrayal of the Pavlov school in the 1930s, see Frolov, *Pavlov and His School*. He summarized his theory for an English-speaking audience in "Outline of the higher nervous activity," reprinted in Pavlov, *Lectures on Conditioned Reflexes*, 2: 44–59. Following convention, I refer to "conditioned" and "unconditioned" reflexes, though it has been suggested that the words "conditional" and "unconditional" might translate his meaning more accurately.

65. Pavlov, *Lectures on Conditioned Reflexes*, 1: 244.

66. Pavlov, *Conditioned Reflexes*, 29–31, 289–290; idem, *Lectures on Conditioned Reflexes*, 1: 341–342. Pavlov further analyzed external inhibition into four types.

67. As reported in Frolov, *Pavlov and His School*, 96–97.

68. Ibid., 97–98.

69. Pavlov, *Lectures on Conditioned Reflexes*, 1: 244.

70. See Pavlov, *Conditioned Reflexes*, Lecture IV.

71. Ibid., 117–151. See Gray, *Pavlov*, 48–53, 79–84.

72. See Windholz, "Pavlov's position toward American behaviorism"; above, chap. 4.

73. E.g., Pavlov's summary of his theory to the XIV International Congress of Physiology in Rome (1932): Pavlov, "Physiology of the higher nervous activity"; also in idem, *Lectures on Conditioned Reflexes*, 2: 86–94.

74. The subtitle of G. V. Anrep's translation of *Conditioned Reflexes* in 1927 was *An Investigation of the Physiological Activity of the Cerebral Cortex*. The book was published in Russian in 1926 as (in English translation) *Lectures on the Work of the Cerebral Hemispheres* or *Activity of the Cerebral Hemispheres*. For the contrast between Russian and Western views, the later Pavlovian school, and a bibliography of Soviet research, see Mecacci, *Brain and History*.

75. Gray, *Pavlov*, 92.

76. Pavlov, *Conditioned Reflexes*, Lecture XI, 188–203.

77. Frolov, *Pavlov and His School*, 140.

78. Pavlov, *Lectures on Conditioned Reflexes*, 1: 341.

79. Ibid., 348. Cf. Pavlov, *Conditioned Reflexes*, Lectures IX–XIII.

80. Pavlov, *Selected Works*, 636 n. 52.

81. Pavlov, *Lectures on Conditioned Reflexes*, 1: 349.

82. Pavlov, *Conditioned Reflexes*, 395–396.

83. Pavlov, *Lectures on Conditioned Reflexes*, 1: 245.

84. Pavlov, *Conditioned Reflexes*, Lecture XV, 250–283; idem, *Lectures on Conditioned Reflexes*, 1: 305–318. On later theories correlating sleep and decreased activity or inhibition from higher centers, see Cofer and Appley, *Motivation*, 165–167; Diamond, Balvin, and Diamond, *Inhibition and Choice*, 358–366; Jeannerod, *The Brain Machine*, 103–107.

85. Pavlov, *Lectures on Conditioned Reflexes*, 1: 294–295.

86. Ibid., 348.

87. The nature of Pavlov's influence (if any) is not clear to me. Joravsky (1989: 415–442) did not discuss Pavlov in his account of psychiatry in this period. On therapy in general, see Wortis, *Soviet Psychiatry*, 150–176. Sleep therapy or rest cures, of course, had a history that went back well beyond the nineteenth century. For the general context of military psychiatry, see Gabriel, *Soviet Military Psychiatry*.

88. Gray, *Pavlov*, 104.

89. Pavlov, *Lectures on Conditioned Reflexes*, 1: 363–378.

90. Pavlov, *Lectures on Conditioned Reflexes*, 2: 88.

91. Gray, *Pavlov*, 108–112.

92. Pavlov, *Lectures on Conditioned Reflexes*, 2: 39–43, 95–97, 102–116, 146–165.

93. Pavlov, *Conditioned Reflexes*, Lectures XVII–XVIII, 284–319, Lecture XXIII, "The experimental results obtained from animals in their application to man," 395–411; idem, *Lectures on Conditioned Reflexes*, 2; idem, *Selected Works*, Sects. X, XI.

94. Pavlov, *Conditioned Reflexes*, 313–319; idem, *Lectures on Conditioned Reflexes*, 1: 364–365; Frolov, *Pavlov and His School*, 119–120.

95. Pavlov, *Conditioned Reflexes*, 290–293; idem, *Lectures on Conditioned Reflexes*, 1: 342. See Gray, *Pavlov*, 119–120.

96. Pavlov, *Conditioned Reflexes*, 397.

97. Frolov, *Pavlov and His School*, 222. Pavlov's work therefore also provided a useful resource for criticizing Freud, whose work was under attack in the Soviet Union from the end of the 1920s. See Joravsky, *Russian Psychology*, 230–237; Kozulin, *Psychology in Utopia*, 92–94.

98. Pavlov, *Conditioned Reflexes*, 403.

99. Pavlov, *Lectures on Conditioned Reflexes*, 2: 95–97.

100. Sargant, *Battle for the Mind*, 15–54.

101. Wolpe, *Psychotherapy by Reciprocal Inhibition*. Wolpe attempted to integrate Hullian and Pavlovian learning theory. See Gantt, Pickenhain, and Zwingmann, eds., *Pavlovian Approach to Psychopathology*.

102. Eysenck, *Dimensions of Personality*, 51–58. This work became the basis for a systematic theory of personality: idem, *The Structure of Human Personality*. "Introverted" and "extraverted" were introduced in Jung, *Psychological Types*.

103. Eysenck, *The Dynamics of Anxiety and Hysteria*, 38–51, 107–113. Eysenck encouraged Gray to publish (Gray [1964]) the most important attempt to generate a Western awareness of Pavlov's typology.

104. Eysenck, *The Biological Basis of Personality*, xii.

105. Ibid., 75–83.

106. Thus, Bettelheim (1983: 108) criticized "the mistranslation of Freud's thoughts to make them fit better into a behavioristic frame of reference" by Freud's English translator, James Strachey, and canonized in the *Standard Edition*. There is even discussion of the possibility of a new English-language edition. See also Kiell, *Freud without Hindsight*, 20–24; Timms and Segal, eds., *Freud in Exile*, Pt. III. The view that Freud should indeed be regarded as a biologist was argued in Sulloway, *Freud, Biologist of the Mind*.

107. James Strachey, in the *Standard Edition of the Complete Psychological Works of Sigmund Freud*, consistently rendered *Hemmung* as inhibition. I cite from this edition.

108. Levin, *Freud's Early Psychology*. For Freud's life, see Ellenberger, *The Discovery of the Unconscious*, esp. chap. 7; Gay, *Freud*; Jones, *Sigmund Freud*.

109. Freud, *On Aphasia*; Levin, *Freud's Early Psychology*, 32–33, 74–81; Stengel, "A re-evaluation of Freud's book 'On Aphasia.'" See above, chap. 4. For the linguistic setting, see Forrester, *Language and the Origins of Psychoanalysis*.

110. Levin, *Freud's Early Psychology*, 68–74. See above, chap 4.

111. Breuer, in Breuer and Freud, *Studies on Hysteria*, 25.

112. Breuer in ibid., 192–214. As a young man, Breuer had collaborated with E. Hering in studies of the reflex inhibitory mechanism in breathing; see above, chap. 3. For Breuer's career and relations with psychoanalysis, see Hirschmüller, *Physiologie und Psychoanalyse*.

113. Freud, "Preface and footnotes to the translation of Charcot's *Tuesday Lectures*," 138.

114. Freud, "A case of successful treatment by hypnotism," 121.

115. Ibid., 122. See Levin, *Freud's Early Psychology*, 96–100.

116. Freud, "The neuro-psychoses of defence"; idem, "Further remarks on the neuro-psychoses of defence"; Breuer and Freud, *Studies on Hysteria*.

117. Rapaport, "The structure of psychoanalytic theory," 66–78, 86–97. See also Rapaport and Gill, "The points of view and assumptions of metapsychology." It seems to me that Rapaport's attempt to distinguish separate models in Freud's thought failed; rather, Freud creatively used the flexible meanings of linked metaphors. Pibram (1962) argued that Freud's modeling was suggestive for modern neuroscience. Friedman and Alexander (1983) argued that Freud was able to distance himself from contemporary neurophysiological ideas where it suited his psychological purposes.

118. Freud, *The Interpretation of Dreams*, 511.

119. Ibid., 610.

120. Ibid. Freud returned to a systematic treatment of the typographic and dynamic models in "The unconscious," and this was the basis for Rapaport's classification.

121. Freud, "Project for a scientific psychology." The natural-scientific background to Freud's work was reviewed in Amacher, *Freud's Neurological Education*; Dorer, *Historische Grundlagen der Psychoanalyse*; Jones, *Sigmund Freud*, 1: 400–444. These studies were not always historically reliable.

122. Rapaport, "The structure of psychoanalytic theory," 92. The dynamic

psychotherapy of Freud's contemporary, Pierre Janet, was equally influenced by physiological economic concepts, though Janet did not discuss inhibition specifically. See, e.g., Janet, *La force et la faiblesse psychologiques*; Ellenberger, *The Discovery of the Unconscious*, 377–386.

123. Rapaport, "The structure of psychoanalytic theory," 60.

124. Ibid., 70.

125. Levin, *Freud's Early Psychology*, 106.

126. See Griesinger, *Die Pathologie und Therapie* (2d ed., 1861); Obersteiner, "Experimental researches on attention"; Dorer, *Historisches Grundlagen der Psychoanalyse*, 103–106, 113, 165–169; Ellenberger, *The Discovery of the Unconscious*, 536. On Herbart, see above, chap. 2.

127. Freud, "Project for a scientific psychology." See Levin, *Freud's Early Psychology*, 153–183; Sulloway, *Freud, Biologist of the Mind*, 113–131.

128. Freud, "Project for a scientific psychology," 323.

129. Ibid., 327.

130. Ibid., 325.

131. Ibid., 327.

132. Ibid., 326.

133. Ibid., 323–324. See Amacher, *Freud's Neurological Education*, 69–70.

134. Freud, "Project for a scientific psychology," 357.

135. Ibid.

136. Freud, *The Interpretation of Dreams*, 599.

137. Ibid., 601.

138. Ibid., 603.

139. Freud, *Inhibitions, Symptoms and Anxiety*, 108. The immediate stimulus to this work was Freud's desire to address Theodor Rank's explanation of anxiety in *Der Trauma der Geburt* (first publ. 1924).

140. Freud, *Inhibitions, Symptoms and Anxiety*, 87.

141. Ibid., 88–89. This ambiguity was preserved in the English-language translations of the title of Freud's work: the American translation of 1927 referred to *Inhibition, Symptom and Anxiety*, while the 1936 English translation (followed by the *Standard Edition*) used *Inhibitions, Symptoms and Anxiety*. The German original was in the singular: *Hemmung, Symptom und Angst*.

142. Freud, *Inhibitions, Symptoms and Anxiety*, 90.

143. Freud, "'Civilized' sexual morality," 185.

144. Ibid., 187.

145. Ibid., 189.

146. Ibid., 190.

147. Ibid., 199.

148. Freud, *Inhibitions, Symptoms and Anxiety*, 119.

149. Ibid., 153. Freud knew of Maudsley's work (e.g., Freud [1900: 612 n.], quoting Maudsley [1867: 15]), but I do not mean that Maudsley was an "influence."

150. Freud, *Civilization and Its Discontents*, 76.

151. Ibid., 97.

152. Ibid., 102–103.
153. Ibid., 103.
154. Ibid., 119. For Freud's systematic discussion of this instinct, see Freud, *Beyond the Pleasure Principle*. On the impact of World War I, see Hoffman, "The ideological significance of Freud's social thought"; Stepansky, *Aggression in Freud*, chaps. 7, 8.
155. Freud, *Beyond the Pleasure Principle*, 36.
156. Ibid., 38, 45. For consideration of the cultural implications of Freud's dualistic theory of the instincts, see Brown, *Life Against Death*, chaps. 7, 8.
157. Freud, *Beyond the Pleasure Principle*, 49. See above, chap. 4. While noting the biological dimension, one may also note Freud's concurrent citation of poets and philosophers (notably Schopenhauer).
158. Freud, *Civilization and Its Discontents*, 108, 109.
159. Ibid., 111–112.
160. Ibid., 112. See Rieff, *Freud: The Mind of the Moralist*, 242–249, on the existence of social laws as evidence for repressed desire.
161. Freud, *Civilization and Its Discontents*, 121.
162. Ibid., 123.
163. Ibid., 123–124.
164. Ibid., 134.
165. Rapaport (1959: 68–69, 86–88) referred to this as the "genetic model" in Freud's thought. Sulloway (1979: 257–276, 393–415) particularly stressed Freud's belief that "ontogeny repeats phylogeny." See also Gould, *Ontogeny and Phylogeny*, 155–161. Rieff (1959: chap. 6) discussed recapitulation in its cultural rather than biological context.
166. For an overview, see Durant, "The beast in man."
167. B. Richards, *Images of Freud*, 22–26, 60–70.
168. Rieff, *Freud: The Mind of the Moralist*; idem, *The Triumph of the Therapeutic*.
169. Lasch, *The Culture of Narcissism*.
170. The question of the historical relations between Freudian ideas and common belief still requires attention. Writers have been more concerned to use Freudian insights than to write histories of "popular" psychology. But see Burnham, *Psychoanalysis and American Medicine*; idem, *Paths into American Culture*; Moscovici, *La psychoanalyse*; Rapp, "The reception of Freud by the British press." For reviews of Freud's published work, see Kiell, *Freud without Hindsight*. On the wider twentieth-century construction of "psychological society" in the English-speaking world, see Rose, *The Psychological Complex*; idem, *Governing the Soul*.
171. Marcuse, *Eros and Civilization*, 3.
172. See Jay, *The Dialectical Imagination*, chap. 3; Robinson, *The Freudian Left*. This critical tradition was revived in the 1950s, especially in Marcuse, *Eros and Civilization*.
173. Brown, *Life Against Death*. Brown observed (3): "There is one word which, if we only understand it, is the key to Freud's thought. That word is 'repression.'"

6: REFLECTIONS

1. Q. Skinner, "Meaning and understanding," 54, 55.

2. Bouwsma, "From history of ideas to history of meaning," 284. In a discussion of "linguistic turns" in the history of science, Jan Golinski (1990) distinguished "symbolic," "hermeneutic or semantic," and "rhetorical" approaches. I envisage my work as "hermeneutic" in his sense.

3. Baker, "On the problem of the ideological origins of the French Revolution," 198.

4. As a matter of historical information, Michel Foucault was a decisive influence on creating interest in discourse in English-language historiography, and his work was a powerful impetus to exploring language as a vehicle for the interpenetration of "science" and "politics." Whether or not he achieved a coherent notion of discourse is another matter, but it need not detain us. It should be noted, however, that the kinds of criticism raised here have been articulated by others in discussions of Foucault's work.

5. Markus, "Why is there no hermeneutics of natural science?" 43. As I hope is evident, this book is an attempt to construct such a hermeneutics—a project that Markus also accepted but broached through a systematic account of the distinctive cultural organization of the "Author-Text-Reader" relation in modern natural science. As for Markus, hermeneutics is understood here to be a cognitive and not an ontological enterprise.

6. Amacher, *Freud's Neurological Education*, 70.

7. Perry, *The Thought and Character of William James*, 2: 28, quoting from a lecture given by James in 1878.

8. Mill, *A System of Logic*, 851–852. These arguments about the sources of psychological and physiological notions deserve more attention. Graham Richards (1989) has argued that all psychological terms derive from sensory experience. On the uses of metaphor more generally in psychology, see Leary, ed., *Metaphors in the History of Psychology*.

9. Hesse, "Theory and observation"; idem, *The Structure of Scientific Inference*, chaps. 1, 2; Bloor, *Knowledge and Social Imagery*, 20–39.

10. Bloor, "Durkheim and Mauss revisited," 293.

11. Douglas, *Natural Symbols*, 112.

12. Ibid., 93.

13. Outram, *The Body and the French Revolution*, 8.

14. Elias, *The Civilizing Process: State Formation and Civilization*, 242.

15. Elias, *The Civilizing Process: The History of Manners*, 255.

16. Ibid., 258.

17. Todes, "From radicalism to scientific convention," 245.

18. Kurt Danziger, in particular, has stressed the importance of technology and its political economy in understanding what he called the "generative" quality of metaphors about control in psychology: Danziger, "Origins of the schema of stimulated motion"; idem, "Generative metaphor." See Mayr, "Adam Smith and the concept of the feedback system." Recent work by Norton Wise and Crosbie Smith (1989–1990) has pointed to the rich and multiple interactions between the mathematical and physical sciences, the political econ-

omy of profit and waste, work, and conceptions of balance in both nature and society. This suggests a route through which this study of inhibition might be opened up to broader questions (though Wise and Smith do not consider many of the forms of regulation discussed here).

19. N. McKendrick, "Josiah Wedgwood and factory discipline"; Thompson, "Time, work-discipline, and industrial capitalism." For the struggle to control leisure, see Bailey, *Leisure and Class in Victorian England.*

20. Cannon, *The Wisdom of the Body*; Cross and Albury, "Walter B. Cannon, L. J. Henderson, and the organic analogy." Cannon's work also reflected the rapid growth of an understanding of chemical regulation in the body. See, in general, Brooks and Levey, "Humorally-transported integrators of body function and the development of endocrinology"; Medvei, *A History of Endocrinology.*

21. Cannon, *The Wisdom of the Body*, 20–21, also quoted in Cross and Albury (1987: 175).

22. N. Wiener, *Cybernetics*, 41–43.

23. Maxwell, "On governors." For Watt's device, see Watt's notes to Robison, *A System of Mechanical Philosophy*, 2: 154–155; Mayr, *Feedback Control*, 109–115.

24. Bagehot, *Physics and Politics*, 136. See Babbage, *On the Economy of Machinery*, esp. 27–29; Hyman, *Charles Babbage*, 103–122.

25. These conclusions were discussed in Brooke, *Science and Religion.*

References

The date cited after the author's name is usually that of first publication, though, for recent secondary sources, the date of the version used is given. Where a substantially altered later edition has been used, the date is of that edition. Where the source is a translation, the date of translation is given. Other dates, where necessary as historical information, are given in the entry. Transliterated Russian names are standardized.

Adolph, E. F. 1961. "Early concepts of physiological regulations." *Physiological Reviews* 41: 737–770.

Adrian, E. D. 1913. "Wedensky inhibition in relation to the 'all-or-none' principle in nerve." *Journal of Physiology* 46: 384–412.

Amacher, Peter. 1964. "Thomas Laycock, I. M. Sechenov, and the reflex arc concept." *Bulletin of the History of Medicine* 38: 168–183.

———. 1965. *Freud's Neurological Education and Its Influence on Psychoanalytic Theory*. Psychological Issues, monograph 16. New York: International Universities Press.

Anokhin, Peter K. 1968. "Ivan P. Pavlov and psychology." In Benjamin B. Wolman, ed., *Historical Roots of Contemporary Psychology*, 131–159. New York: Harper & Row.

Anstie, Francis E. 1864. *Stimulants and Narcotics, Their Mutual Relations*. London: Macmillan.

Arens, Katherine. 1989. *Structures of Knowing: Psychologies of the Nineteenth Century*. Boston Studies in the Philosophy of Science 113. Dordrecht: Kluwer.

Ash, Mitchell G. 1983. "The self-presentation of a discipline: History of psychology in the United States between pedagogy and scholarship." In Loren Graham, Wolf Lepenies, and P. Weingart, eds., *Functions and Uses of Disciplinary Histories*, 143–189.

———. 1990. "Psychology in twentieth-century Germany: Science and profession." In Geoffrey Cocks and Konrad Jarausch, eds., *German Professions 1800–1950*, 289–307. New York: Oxford University Press.

Ash, Mitchell G., and Ulfried Geuter, eds. 1985. *Geschichte der deutschen Psychologie im 20. Jahrhundert: Ein Überblick*. Opladen: Westdeutscher Verlag.

Ash, Mitchell G., and William R. Woodward, eds. 1987. *Psychology in Twentieth-Century Thought and Society*. Cambridge: Cambridge University Press.

Asratyan, E. A. 1953. *I. P. Pavlov: His Life and Work*, trans. from Russian (1949). Moscow: Foreign Languages Publishing House.

———, ed. 1968. *Brain Reflexes*. Progress in Brain Research 22. Amsterdam: Elsevier.

Babbage, Charles. 1832. *On the Economy of Machinery and Manufactures*. 3d ed. London: Charles Knight, 1833.

Babkin, B. P. 1951. *Pavlov: A Biography*. London: Victor Gollancz.

Bagehot, Walter. 1872. *Physics and Politics*. In Norman St John-Stevas, ed. *The Collected Works of Walter Bagehot*, 7: 13–144. London: The Economist, 1974.

Bailey, Peter. 1978. *Leisure and Class in Victorian England: Rational Recreation and the Contest for Control, 1830–1885*. London: Routledge & Kegan Paul.

Bain, Alexander. 1868. *The Senses and the Intellect*, 3d ed. London: Longmans, Green. (First publ. 1855.)

———. 1875. *The Emotions and the Will*, 3d ed. London: Longmans, Green. (First publ. 1859.)

Baker, Keith Michael. 1982. "On the problem of the ideological origins of the French Revolution." In Dominick LaCapra and Steven L. Kaplan, eds., *Modern European Intellectual History: Reappraisals and New Perspectives*, 197–219. Ithaca: Cornell University Press.

Baldwin, James Mark, ed. 1901–1905. "Mental inhibition." In *Dictionary of Philosophy and Psychology*, 1: 546–547. Facsimile reprint. Gloucester, Mass.: Peter Smith, 1960.

Barker-Benfield, G. J. 1976. *The Horrors of the Half-known Life: Male Attitudes toward Women and Sexuality in Nineteenth-Century America*. New York: Harper & Row.

Barlow, John. 1842. *The Connection Between Physiology and Intellectual Philosophy*. London: William Pickering.

———. 1843. *On Man's Power Over Himself to Prevent or Control Insanity*. London: William Pickering.

[Barlow, William Frederick]. 1839–1840. "The influence of volition over the excito-motory function of the spinal cord." *Lancet*, pt. 1: 572–574.

Barnes, Barry. 1980. "On the conventional character of knowledge and cognition." In K. Knorr-Cetina and Michael J. Mulkay, eds., *Science Observed: Perspectives on the Social Study of Science*, 19–51. London: Sage, 1983.

Barnes, Barry, and David Edge, eds. 1982. *Science in Context: Readings in the Sociology of Science*. Milton Keynes: Open University Press.

Barnes, Barry, and Steven Shapin, eds. 1979. *Natural Order: Historical Studies of Scientific Culture*. London: Sage.

Barnes, Matthew. 1984. *Augustus Hare*. London: Allen & Unwin.

Bauer, R. A. 1952. *The New Man in Soviet Psychology*. Cambridge: Harvard University Press.

Beer, Gillian. 1985. *Darwin's Plots: Evolutionary Narrative in Darwin, George Eliot and Nineteenth-Century Fiction*. London: Ark.

Bekhterev, V. M. 1933. *General Principles of Human Reflexology: An Introduction to the Objective Study of Personality*, trans. E. Murphy and W. Murphy from 4th Russian ed. (1928, first publ. 1917). London: Jarrolds.

Bell, John, and Charles Bell. 1826. *The Anatomy and Physiology of the Human Body*, 6th ed. corrected by C. Bell. 3 vols. London: Longman, Rees, Orme, Brown and Green.

Beneke, Friedrick Eduard. 1825–1827. *Psychologische Skizzen*. 2 vols. Göttingen: Bandenhoeck und Ruprecht.

———. 1842. *Erziehungs- und Unterrichtslehre*, 2d ed. 2 vols. Berlin: E. S. Mittler und Sohn. (First publ. 1835.)

———. 1861. *Lehrbuch der Psychologie als Naturwissenschaft*, 3d ed. Ed. Johann Gottlieb Dressler. Berlin: E. S. Mittler und Sohn. (First publ. 1833.)

Bennett, John Hughes. 1851. *The Mesmeric Mania of 1851: With a Physiological Explanation of the Phenomena*. Edinburgh: Sutherland and Knox.

Beritashvili [Beritov], I. S. 1968. "Central inhibition according to I. M. Sechenov's experiments and concepts, and its modern interpretation." In E. A. Asratyan, ed., *Brain Reflexes*, 21–31.

Berman, Morris. 1978. *Social Change and Scientific Organization: The Royal Institution, 1799–1844*. London: Heinemann.

Bernard, Claude. 1851. "L'influence du grand sympathique sur la sensibilité et sur la calorification." *C.R.S.B.* 3: 163–164.

———. 1852*a*. "De l'influence du système nerveux grand sympathique sur la chaleur animale." *C.R.A.S.* 34: 472–475.

———. 1852*b*. "Expériences sur les fonctions de la portion céphalique du grand sympathique." *C.R.S.B.* 4: 155.

———. 1852*c*. "Sur les effets de la section de la portion céphalique du grand sympathique." *C.R.S.B.* 4: 168–170.

———. 1853. "Recherches expérimentales sur le grand sympathique et spécialement sur l'influence que la section de ce nerf exerce sur la chaleur animale." *C.R.S.B.* 5: 77–107.

———. 1858*a*. *Leçons sur la physiologie et la pathologie du système nerveux*. 2 vols. Paris: J.-B. Baillière.

———. 1858*b*. "Sur les variations de couleur dans le sang veineux des organes glandulaires suivant leur état de fonction ou de repos." *C.R.A.S.* 46: 159–165.

———. 1858*c*. "De l'influence de deux ordres de nerfs qui déterminent les variations de couleur du sang veineux dans les organes glandulaires." *C.R.A.S.* 47: 245–253.

———. 1864. "Du rôle des actions réflexes paralysantes dans les phénomène des sécretions." *Journal de l'anatomie et de la physiologie* 1: 507–513.

———. 1872. *De la physiologie générale*. Facsimile reprint. Bruxelles: Cultures et Civilisation, 1965.

———. 1876. *Leçons sur la chaleur animale sur les effets de la chaleur et sur la fièvre*. Paris: J.-B. Baillière.

———. 1885. *Leçons sur les phénomènes de la vie communs aux animaux et aux végétaux*, 2d ed., vol. 1. Facsimile reprint. Paris: J. Vrin, 1966. (First publ. 1878.)

———. 1927. *An Introduction to the Study of Experimental Medicine*, trans. Henry Copley Greene (1st French ed. 1865). Facsimile reprint. New York: Dover, 1957.

Berridge, Virginia, and Griffith Edwards. 1981. *Opium and the People: Opiate Use in Nineteenth-Century England*. London/New York: Allen Lane/St. Martin's Press.

Berrios, G. E. 1981. "Stupor: A conceptual history." *Psychological Medicine* 11: 677–688.

Bertalanffy, Ludwig von. 1971. *General Systems Theory: Foundations, Development, Applications*. London: Allen Lane, 1971. (First publ. 1968.)

Bettelheim, Bruno. 1983. *Freud and Man's Soul*. London: Chatto and Windus, The Hogarth Press.

Bichat, Xavier. 1962. *Recherches physiologigues sur la vie et la mort*. Paris: Masson. (First publ. 1800.)

Biedermann, Wilhelm. 1887. "Beiträge zur allgemeinen Nerven- und Muskelphysiologie. Zwanzigste Mittheilung. Über die Innervation der Krebsschere." *S.K.A.W.* 95, pt. 3: 7–46.

———. 1888. "Beiträge zur allgemeinen Nerven- und Muskelphysiologie. Einundzwanzigste Mittheilung. Über die Innervation der Krebsschere." *S.K.A.W.* 97, pt. 3: 49–82.

Binet, Alfred. 1890. "L'inhibition dans les phénomènes de conscience." *Revue philosophique* 30: 136–156.

Binet, Alfred, and C. Féré. 1887. *Le magnétisme animal*. Paris: Félix Alcan.

Blackstone, William. 1765–69. *Commentaries on the Laws of England*. Facsimile reprint. 4 vols. Chicago: University of Chicago Press, 1979.

Bleuler, E. 1916. *Lehrbuch der Psychiatrie*. Berlin: Julius Springer.

———. 1924. *Textbook of Psychiatry*, trans. A. A. Brill from 4th German ed. (1923). Facsimile reprint. New York: Arno Press, 1976.

———. 1950. *Dementia Praecox or the Group of Schizophrenias*, trans. J. Zinkin, from German (1911). New York: International Universities Press.

Bloor, David. 1976. *Knowledge and Social Imagery*. London: Routledge & Kegan Paul.

———. 1982. "Durkheim and Mauss revisited: Classification and the sociology of knowledge." *Studies in the History and Philosophy of Science* 13: 267–297.

Boakes, Robert. 1984. *From Darwin to Behaviourism: Psychology and the Mind of Animals*. Cambridge: Cambridge University Press.

Boring, Edwin G. 1950. *A History of Experimental Psychology*, 2d ed. New York: Appleton-Century-Crofts. (First publ. 1929.)

Bouwsma, William J. 1981. "From history of ideas to history of meaning." *Journal of Interdisciplinary History* 12: 279–291.

Bradley, F. H. 1876. "The vulgar notion of responsibility in connexion with the theories of freewill and necessity." In *Ethical Studies*, 2d ed., 1–57. Oxford: Clarendon Press, 1927.

Braid, James. 1843. *Neurypnology; Or, the Rationale of Nervous Sleep, Considered in Relation with Animal Magnetism.* London: John Churchill.

Brandt, Francis Burke. 1865. *Friedrick Eduard Beneke, The Man and His Philosophy: An Introductory Study.* New York/Berlin: Macmillan/Mayer and Müller.

Brazier, Mary A. B. 1959. "The historical development of neurophysiology." In John Field, ed., *Handbook of Physiology* 1: 1–58. Washington: American Physiological Society.

———. 1984. *A History of Neurophysiology in the 17th and 18th Centuries.* New York: Raven Press.

———. 1988. *A History of Neurophysiology in the 19th Century.* New York: Raven Press.

Breese, B. B. 1899. "On inhibition." *Psychological Review, Series of Monograph Supplements* 3, no. 1.

Breuer, Josef. 1868. "Die Selbstseuerung der Athmung durch den *Nervus vagus.*" *S.K.A.W.* 58, pt. 2: 909–937.

Breuer, Josef, and Sigmund Freud. 1893–1895. *Studies on Hysteria. S.E.* 2.

British and Foreign Medico-chirurgical Review [Review of physiology: nervous system] 24 (1859): 235–239.

British Journal of Psychology ["Symposium on inhibition"] 51 (1960): 193–236.

Brodie, Benjamin Collins. 1854. *Psychological Inquiries: In a Series of Essays, Intended to Illustrate the Mutual Relations of the Physical Organisation and the Mental Faculties.* London: Longman, Brown, Green and Longmans.

Brondgeest, P. J. 1860. "Untersuchungen über den Tonus der willkürlickhen Muskeln" [Report of Academisch Proefschrift, Utrecht, 1860]. *Archiv für Anatomie, Physiologie* n.v.: 703–704.

Brooke, John Hedley. 1991. *Science and Religion: Some Historical Perspectives.* New York: Cambridge University Press.

Brooks, Chandler McC. 1959. "Discovery of the function of chemical mediators in the transmission of excitation and inhibition to effector tissues." In Chandler McC. Brooks and Paul F. Cranefield, eds., *The Historical Development of Physiological Thought*, 169–181. New York: Hafner.

Brooks, Chandler McC., and Harold A. Levey. 1959. "Humorally-transported integrators of body function and the development of endocrinology." In Chandler McC. Brooks and Paul F. Cranefield, eds., *The Historical Development of Physiological Thought*, 183–238. New York: Hafner.

Brown, Norman O. 1970. *Life Against Death: The Psychoanalytical Meaning of History.* Middletown: Wesleyan University Press. (First publ. 1959.)

Browne, J. Crichton. 1863. "Notes on homicidal insanity." *Journal of Mental Science* 9: 197–210.

Brown-Séquard, C.-É. 1860. *Course of Lectures on the Physiology and Pathology of the Central Nervous System.* Philadelphia: Collins.

———. 1868*a*. "Sur l'arrêt immediat de convulsions violentes par l'influence de l'irritation de quelques nerfs sensitifs." *Archives de physiologie normale et pathologique* 1: 157–160.

———. 1868*b*. "Note sur l'avortement d'attaques d'épilepsie par l'irritation de nerfs à action centripète." *Archives de physiologie normale et pathologique* 1: 317–318.

———. 1879*a*. "Faits nouveaux relatifs à la mise en jeu ou à l'arrêt (inhibition) des propriétés motrices ou sensitives de diverses parties du centre cérébro-rachidien." *Archives de physiologie normale et pathologique*, 2d ser., 6: 494–499.

[Brown-Séquard, C.-É.] 1879*b*. "Collège de France. Cours de médecine par. M. Brown-Séquard." *Gazette hebdomadaire de médecine et de chirurgie*, 2d ser., 16: 771.

Brown-Séquard, C.-É. 1882. "Recherches expérimentales et cliniques sur l'inhibition et la dynamogénie.—Application des connaissances fournies par ces recherches aux phénomènes principaux de l'hypnotisme, de l'extase et du transfert." *Gazette hebdomadaire de médecine et de chirurgie*, 2d ser., 19: 35–36, 53–55, 75–77, 105–107, 136–138.

———. 1884*a*. "Existence de l'excitabilité motrice et de l'excitabilité inhibitoire dans les régions occipitales et sphenoidales de l'écorce cérébrale." *C.R.S.B.*, 8th ser., 1: 301–303.

———. 1884*b*. "Faits montrant que toutes les parties de l'encéphale, chez l'homme, peuvent déterminer certaines inhibitions." *C.R.S.B.*, 8th ser., 1: 320–324.

———. 1884*c*. "Inhibition de certaines puissances réflexes du bulbe rachidien et de la moelle épinière, sous l'influence d'irritations de diverse parties de l'encéphale." *C.R.S.B.*, 8th ser., 1: 350–352.

———. 1884*d*. "Du rôle de certaines influences dynamogéniques réflexes dans des cas de suture de nerfs récemment publiés." *C.R.S.B.*, 8th ser., 1: 423–425.

———. 1884*e*. "De la puissance inhibitrice et de la puissance convulsivante de l'acide carbonique." *C.R.S.B.*, 8th ser., 1: 556–559.

———. 1889*a*. "Champ d'action de l'inhibition en physiologie, en pathogénie et en thérapeutique." *Archives de physiologie normale et pathologique*, 5th ser., 1: 1–23.

———. 1889*b*. "Le sommeil normal, comme le sommeil hypnotique, est le résultat d'une inhibition de l'activité intellectuelle." *Archives de physiologie normale et pathologique*, 5th ser., 1: 333–335.

———. 1889*c*. "Quelque mots sur la découverte de l'inhibition." *Archives de physiologie normale et pathologique*, 5th ser., 1: 337–339.

———. 1889*d*. "De quelques règles générales relatives à l'inhibition." *Archives de physiologie normale et pathologique*, 5th ser., 1: 751–761.

———. 1889*e*. "Inhibition." In *Dictionnaire encyclopédique des sciences médicales*, 4th ser., vol. 16: 1–19. Paris: Asselin et Houzeau/G. Masson.

Brožek, Josef. 1971. "The psychology and physiology of behaviour: Some recent Soviet writings on their history." *History of Science* 10: 56–87.

———. 1973–74. "Soviet historiography of psychology." *Journal of the His-*

tory of the Behavioral Sciences 9 (1973): 152–161, 213–216; 10 (1974): 195–201, 348–351.

Brunton, T. Lauder. 1874. "Inhibition, peripheral and central." *West Riding Lunatic Asylum Medical Reports* 4: 179–222.

———. 1883. "On the nature of inhibition, and the action of drugs upon it." *Nature* 27: 419–422, 436–439, 467–468, 485–487.

Bubnov, N., and R. Heidenhain. 1881. "Ueber Erregungs- und Hemmungsvorgänge innerhalb der motorischen Hirncentren." *Archiv für die gesammte Physiologie* 26: 137–200.

———. 1944. "On excitatory and inhibitory processes within the motor centers of the brain," trans. G. von Bonin and W. S. McCulloch from German (1881). *Illinois Monographs in Medical Science* 4: 173–210.

Bucknill, John Charles, and Daniel Hack Tuke. 1858. *A Manual of Psychological Medicine.* London: John Churchill.

Budge, Julius. 1841–42. *Untersuchungen über das Nervensystem.* 2 vols. Frankfurt am Main: Jäger.

Budge, Julius, and Augustus V. Waller. 1851. *Neue Untersuchungen über das Nervensystem.* N.p.

Burnham, John Chynoweth. 1967. *Psychoanalysis and American Medicine, 1894–1918: Medicine, Science and Culture.* Psychological Issues, monograph 20. New York: International Universities Press.

———. 1988. *Paths into American Culture: Psychology, Medicine and Morals.* Philadelphia: Temple University Press.

Burrow, J. W. 1970. *Evolution and Society: A Study in Victorian Social Theory.* Cambridge: Cambridge University Press.

Burstyn, Joan N. 1980. *Victorian Education and the Ideal of Womanhood.* London: Croom Helm.

Bykov, K. M., ed. 1960. *Text-book of Physiology*, trans. S. Belsky and O. Myshne from Russian. Moscow: Foreign Languages Publishing House.

Bynum, William F. 1974. "Rationales for therapy in British psychiatry: 1780–1835." *Medical History* 18: 317–334.

Bynum, William F., and Michael Neve. 1985. "Hamlet on the couch." In W. F. Bynum, Roy Porter, and Michael Shepherd, eds., *The Anatomy of Madness: Essays in the History of Psychiatry* 1: 289–304. London: Tavistock.

Bynum, William F., and Roy Porter, eds. 1988. *Brunonianism in Britain and Europe.* Medical History, suppl. no. 8. London: Wellcome Institute for the History of Medicine.

Canguilhem, Georges. 1955. *La formation du concept de réflexe aux XVIIe et XVIIIe siècles.* Paris: Presses Universitaires de France.

———. 1964. "Le concept de réflexe au XIXe siècle." In *Études d'histoire et de philosophie des sciences*, 295–304. Paris: J. Vrin, 1968.

———. 1978. *The Normal and the Pathological*, trans. Carolyn R. Fawcett, in collaboration with Robert S. Cohen, from French (1972, first publ. 1966). New York: Zone Books, 1989.

———. 1988*a*. "John Brown's system: An example of medical ideology," trans. Arthur Goldhammer from French (1974). In *Ideology and Rationality in the History of the Life Sciences*, 41–50. Cambridge: MIT Press.

———. 1988*b*. "The development of the concept of biological regulation in the eighteenth and nineteenth centuries," trans. Arthur Goldhammer from French (1977). In *Ideology and Rationality in the History of the Life Sciences*, 81–102. Cambridge: MIT Press.

Cannon, Walter B. 1932. *The Wisdom of the Body*. London: Kegan Paul, Trench, Trübner.

Carlyle, Thomas. 1833–34. *Sartor Resartus: The Life and Opinions of Herr Teufelsdröckh*. London: Chapman and Hall, 1885.

Caron, Joseph A. 1988. "'Biology' in the life sciences: A historiographical contribution." *History of Science* 26: 223–268.

Carpenter, W. B. 1842. *Principles of Human Physiology*. London: John Churchill.

———. 1850. *On the Use and Abuse of Alcoholic Liquors, in Health and Disease*. London: Charles Gilpin, John Churchill.

———. 1852. "On the influence of suggestion in modifying and directing muscular movements, independently of volition." *Proceedings of the Royal Institution* 1: 147–153.

———. 1853*a*. *Principles of Human Physiology*, 4th ed. London: John Churchill.

———. 1853*b*. "Electrobiology and mesmerism." *Quarterly Review* 93: 501–557.

———. 1874. *Principles of Mental Physiology*, 7th ed. London: Kegan Paul, Trench, Trübner, 1896.

Carr, Edward Hallett. 1961. *The Romantic Exiles: A Nineteenth-Century Portrait Gallery*. Boston: Beacon Press. (First publ. 1933.)

Carter, Robert Brudenell. 1853. *On the Pathology and Treatment of Hysteria*. London: John Churchill.

Casper, Johann Ludwig. 1861–1865. *A Handbook of the Practice of Forensic Medicine*, trans. G. W. Balfour from 3d German ed. (1860). 4 vols. London: The New Sydenham Society.

Chorover, Stephen L. 1980. *From Genesis to Genocide: The Meaning of Human Nature and the Power of Behavior Control*. Cambridge: MIT Press, 1980.

Clark, Michael J. 1981. "The rejection of psychological approaches to mental disorder in late nineteenth-century British psychiatry." In Andrew Scull, ed., *Madhouses, Mad-doctors, and Madmen: The Social History of Psychiatry in the Victorian Era*, 271–312. Philadelphia: University of Pennsylvania Press.

———. 1982. "'The data of alienism': Evolutionary neurology, physiological psychology, and the reconstruction of British psychiatric theory, c. 1850–c. 1900." D. Phil. diss., University of Oxford.

———. 1988. "Morbid introspection, unsoundness of mind, and British psychological medicine, c. 1830–c. 1900." In W. F. Bynum, Roy Porter, and Michael Shepherd, eds., *The Anatomy of Madness: Essays in the History of Psychiatry*, 3: 71–101. London: Routledge.

Clarke, Edwin, and L. S. Jacyna. 1987. *Nineteenth-Century Origins of Neuroscientific Concepts*. Berkeley, Los Angeles, London: University of California Press.

Clarke, Edwin, and C. D. O'Malley. 1968. *The Human Brain and Spinal Cord: A Historical Study Illustrated by Writings from Antiquity to the Twentieth Century*. Berkeley, Los Angeles, London: University of California Press.

Clouston, T. S. 1883. *Clinical Lectures on Mental Diseases*, 2d ed. London: J. & A. Churchill, 1887.

———. 1906. *The Hygiene of Mind*. London: Methuen.

Cofer, C. N., and M. H. Appley. 1964. *Motivation: Theory and Research*. New York: John Wiley.

Cohen, Stanley, and Andrew Scull, eds. 1983. *Social Control and the State: Historical and Comparative Essays*. Oxford: Martin Robertson.

Coleman, William. 1985. "The cognitive basis of the discipline: Claude Bernard on physiology." *Isis* 76: 49–70.

Coleman, William, and Frederic L. Holmes, eds. 1988. *The Investigative Enterprise: Experimental Physiology in Nineteenth-Century Medicine*. Berkeley, Los Angeles, London: University of California Press.

Collie, Michael. 1988. *Henry Maudsley, Victorian Psychiatrist: A Bibliographic Study*. Winchester: St. Paul's Bibliographies.

Collins, H. M. 1985. *Changing Order: Replication and Induction in Scientific Practice*. London: Sage.

Combe, George. 1828. *The Constitution of Man Considered in Relation to External Objects*, 8th ed. (1847). Facsimile reprint. Westmead, Farnborough: Gregg International, 1970.

Cooter, Roger. 1976. "Phrenology and British alienists, ca. 1825–1845." In Andrew Scull, ed., *Madhouses, Mad-doctors, and Madmen: The Social History of Psychiatry in the Victorian Era*, 58–104. Philadelphia: University of Pennsylvania Press.

———. 1979. "The power of the body: The early nineteenth century." In Barry Barnes and Steven Shapin, eds., *Natural Order*, 73–92.

———. 1984. *The Cultural Meaning of Popular Science: Phrenology and the Organization of Consent in Nineteenth-Century Britain*. Cambridge: Cambridge University Press.

Cortelazzo, Menlio, and Paolo Zolli. 1983. *Dizionario etimologico della lingua italiana*, vol. 3. Bologna: Zanichelli.

Cranefield, Paul F. 1957. "The organic physics of 1847 and the biophysics of today." *Journal of the History of Medicine* 12: 407–423.

———. 1974. *The Way In and the Way Out: François Magendie, Charles Bell and the Roots of the Spinal Nerves*. Mount Kisco, N.Y.: Futura.

Creed, R. S., D. Denny-Brown, J. C. Eccles, E. G. T. Liddell, and C. S. Sherrington. 1932. *Reflex Activity of the Spinal Cord*. Oxford: Clarendon Press.

Cross, Stephen J., and William R. Albury. 1987. "Walter B. Cannon, L. J. Henderson, and the organic analogy." *Osiris*, 2d ser., 3: 165–192.

Czermak, J. 1872. "Nachweis echter 'hypnotischer' Erscheinungen bei Thieren." *S.K.A.W.* 66, pt. 3: 364–381.

———. 1873. "Beobachtungen und Versuche über 'hypnotische' Zustände bei Thieren." *Archiv für die gesammte Physiologie* 7: 107–121.

Danilevskii, A. 1866. "Untersuchungen zur Physiologie des Centralnervensystems." *Archiv für Anatomie, Physiologie* n.v.: 677–691.

Danilevskii, B. 1881. "Die Hemmungen der Reflex- und Willkürbewegungen

Beiträge zur Lehre vom thierischen Hypnotismus." *Archiv für die gesammte Physiologie* 24: 489–525, 595–596.

Danziger, Kurt. 1979. "The positivist repudiation of Wundt." *Journal of the History of the Behavioral Sciences* 15: 205–230.

———. 1980*a*. "Wundt and the two traditions of psychology." In R. W. Rieber, ed., *Wilhelm Wundt and the Making of a Scientific Psychology*, 73–87. New York: Plenum Press.

———. 1980*b*. "Wundt's theory of behavior and volition." In R. W. Rieber, ed., *Wilhelm Wundt and the Making of a Scientific Psychology*, 89–115. New York: Plenum Press.

———. 1982. "Mid-nineteenth-century British psycho-physiology: A neglected chapter in the history of psychology." In William R. Woodward and Mitchell G. Ash, eds., *The Problematic Science*, 119–146.

———. 1983. "Origins of the schema of stimulated motion: Towards a prehistory of modern psychology." *History of Science* 21: 182–210.

———. 1984. "Toward a conceptual framework for a critical history of psychology." In H. Carpintero and J. M. Peiró, eds., *Psychology in Its Historical Context*, 99–107. Valencia: Monografiás de la Rivista de Historia de la Psicología, Universidad de Valencia.

———. 1990. "Generative metaphor and the history of psychological discourse." In David E. Leary, ed., *Metaphors in the History of Psychology*, 331–356.

Darwin, Erasmus. 1794–96. *Zoonomia; Or, the Laws of Organic Life*. 2 vols. London: J. Johnson.

Daston, Lorraine J. 1978. "British responses to psycho-physiology, 1860–1900." *Isis* 69: 192–208.

Delgado, José M. R. 1969. *Physical Control of the Mind: Toward a Psychocivilized Society*. New York: Harper & Row.

Descartes, René. 1972. *Treatise of Man*, French text (1664) and trans. Thomas Steele Hall. Cambridge: Harvard University Press. (Latin ed., *De homine*, publ. 1662.)

Desmond, Adrian. 1989. *The Politics of Evolution: Morphology, Medicine, and Reform in Radical London*. Chicago: University of Chicago Press.

Diamond, Solomon. 1957. *Personality and Temperament*. New York: Harper & Brothers.

———. 1980. "Wundt before Leipzig." In R. W. Rieber, ed., *Wilhelm Wundt and the Making of a Scientific Psychology*, 3–70. New York: Plenum Press.

Diamond, Solomon, Richard S. Balvin, and Florence Rand Diamond. 1963. *Inhibition and Choice: A Neurobehavioral Approach to Problems of Plasticity in Behavior*. New York: Harper & Row.

Dickson, J. Thompson. 1869. "Matter and force considered in relation to mental and cerebral phenomena." *Journal of Mental Science* 15: 217–239.

———. 1874. *The Science and Practice of Medicine in Relation to Mind, the Pathology of Nerve Centres and the Jurisprudence of Insanity*. London: H. K. Lewis.

Dodge, Raymond. 1926*a*. "The problem of inhibition." *Psychological Review* 33: 1–12.

———. 1926*b*. "Theories of inhibition." *Psychological Review* 33: 106–122, 167–187.

Doerner, Klaus. 1981. *Madmen and the Bourgeoisie: A Social History of Insanity and Psychiatry*, trans. Joachim Neugroschel and Jean Steinberg from German (1969). Oxford: Basil Blackwell.

Donnelly, Michael. 1983. *Managing the Mind: A Study of Medical Psychology in Early Nineteenth-Century Britain*. London: Tavistock.

Dorer, M. 1932. *Historische Grundlagen der Psychoanalyse*. Leipzig: Felix Meiner.

Douglas, Mary. 1970. *Natural Symbols: Explorations in Cosmology*, 2d ed. London: Barrie and Jenkins, 1973.

Drobisch, Moritz Wilhelm. 1842. *Empirische Psychologie nach naturwissenschaftlicher Methode*. Leipzig: Leopold Voss.

———. 1850. *Erste Grundlehren der mathematischen Psychologie*. Leipzig: Leopold Voss.

Dunkel, Harold B. 1970. *Herbart and Herbartianism: An Educational Ghost Story*. Chicago: University of Chicago Press.

Durant, John R. 1981. "The beast in man: An historical perspective on the biology of human aggression." In Paul F. Brain and David Benton, eds., *The Biology of Aggression*, 17–46. Alphen an den Rijn: Sijthoff and Noordhoff.

———. 1985. "The science of sentiment: The problem of the cerebral localization of emotion." In P. P. G. Bateson and Peter H. Klopfer, eds., *Perspectives in Ethology*, 6: 1–31. New York: Plenum Press.

Ebbinghaus, Hermann. 1905. *Grundzüge der Psychologie*, vol. 1, 2d ed. Leipzig: Veit.

Eccles, John C. 1959. "The development of ideas on the synapse." In Chandler McC. Brooks and Paul F. Cranefield, eds., *The Historical Development of Physiological Thought*, 39–66. New York: Hafner.

Eccles, John C., and William C. Gibson. 1979. *Sherrington: His Life and Thought*. Berlin: Springer.

Eckhard, C. 1862. "Über die Erection des Penis." *S.K.A.W.* 45, pt. 2: 542–543.

———. 1863. "Untersuchungen über die Erection des Penis beim Hunde." In *Beiträge zur Anatomie und Physiologie*, 3: 123–166. Giessen: Ferber'sche Universitäts-Buchandlung.

———. 1881. "Beiträge zur Geschichte der Experimentalphysiologie des Nervensystems. Geschichte der Lehre von dem Reflexerscheinungen." In *Beiträge zur Anatomie und Physiologie*, 9: 29–192. Giessen: Emil Roth.

Eisler, Rudolf. 1927. "Hemmung." In *Wörterbuch der philosophischen Begriffe: Historisch- quellenmassig Bearbeitet*, 1: 630–633. 4th ed. Berlin: E. S. Mittler und Sohn.

Elias, Norbert. 1978. *The Civilizing Process: The History of Manners*, trans. Edmund Jephcott from German (1939). Oxford: Basil Blackwell.

———. 1982. *The Civilizing Process: State Formation and Civilization*, trans. Edmund Jephcott from German (1939). Oxford: Basil Blackwell.

Ellenberger, Henri F. 1970. *The Discovery of the Unconscious: The History and Evolution of Dynamic Psychiatry*. London: Allen Lane, Penguin Press.

Eulenburg, A., and L. Landois. 1866. "Die Hemmungsneurose." *Wiener Medi-*

zinische Wochenschrift 16: cols. 521–525, 537–540, 553–555, 569–571, 585–589.

Exner, Sigmund. 1894. *Entwurf zu einer physiologischen Erklarung der psychischen Erscheinungen.* Leipzig: Franz Deuticke.

Eysenck, H. J. 1947. *Dimensions of Personality.* London: Routledge & Kegan Paul.

———. 1953. *The Structure of Human Personality.* London: Methuen.

———. 1957. *The Dynamics of Anxiety and Hysteria: An Experimental Application of Modern Learning Theory to Psychiatry.* London: Routledge & Kegan Paul.

———. 1967. *The Biological Basis of Personality.* Springfield, Ill.: Charles C. Thomas.

Fearing, Franklin. 1930. *Reflex Action: A Study in the History of Physiological Psychology.* Facsimile reprint. New York: Hafner, 1964.

Ferrier, David. 1873. "Experimental researches in cerebral physiology and pathology." *West Riding Lunatic Asylum Medical Reports* 3: 30–96.

———. 1876. *The Functions of the Brain.* London: Smith, Elder.

———. 1886. *The Functions of the Brain,* 2d ed. London: Smith, Elder.

Figlio, Karl M. 1975. "Theories of perception and the physiology of mind in the late eighteenth century." *History of Science* 12: 177–212.

———. 1976. "The metaphor of organization: An historiographical perspective on the bio-medical sciences of the early nineteenth century." *History of Science* 14: 17–53.

Flourens, P.-J. 1842*a*. *Recherches expérimentales sur les propriétés et les fonctions du système nerveux dans les animaux vertébrés,* 2d ed. Paris: J.-B. Baillière. (First publ. 1824, based on memoirs of 1822 and 1823.)

———. 1842*b*. *Examen de la Phrenologie,* 2d ed. Paris: Paulin, 1845.

Forbes, Alexander. 1912. "Reflex inhibition of skeletal muscle." *Quarterly Journal of Experimental Physiology* 5: 149–187.

Forrester, John. 1980. *Language and the Origins of Psychoanalysis.* London: Macmillan.

Foster, Michael. 1877. *A Text Book of Physiology.* London: Macmillan.

Foucault, Michel. 1981. *The History of Sexuality.* Vol. 1: *An Introduction,* trans. Robert Harley from French (1976). Harmondsworth: Penguin Books.

French, Richard D. 1970*a*. "Darwin and the physiologists, or the medusa and modern cardiology." *Journal of the History of Biology* 3: 253–274.

———. 1970*b*. "Some concepts of nerve structure and function in Britain, 1875–1885: Background to Sir Charles Sherrington and the synapse concept." *Medical History* 14: 154–165.

———. 1971. "Some problems and sources in the foundations of modern physiology in Great Britain." *History of Science* 10: 28–55.

French, Roger K. 1969. *Robert Whytt, the Soul and Medicine.* London: Wellcome Institute for the History of Medicine.

Freud, Sigmund. 1892–1893. "A case of successful treatment by hypnotism." *S.E.* 1, 115–128.

———. 1892–1894. "Preface and footnotes to the translation of Charcot's *Tuesday Lectures.*" *S.E.* 1, 129–143.

———. 1894. "The neuro-psychoses of defence." *S.E.* 3, 41–68.

———. 1895. "Project for a scientific psychology." *S.E.* 1, 281–397.

———. 1896. "Further remarks on the neuro-psychoses of defence." *S.E.* 3, 157–185.

———. 1900. *The Interpretation of Dreams. S.E.* 4, 5.

———. 1908. "'Civilized' sexual morality and modern nervous illness." *S.E.* 9, 177–204.

———. 1915. "The unconscious." *S.E.* 14, 159–215.

———. 1920. *Beyond the Pleasure Principle. S.E.* 18, 1–64.

———. 1926. *Inhibitions, Symptoms and Anxiety. S.E.* 20, 77–175.

———. 1930. *Civilization and Its Discontents. S.E.* 21, 57–145.

———. 1953. *On Aphasia: A Critical Study*, trans. E. Stengel from German (1891). London: Imago.

Freusberg, A. 1874. "Reflexbewegungen beim Hunde." *Archiv für die gesammte Physiologie* 9: 358–389.

———. 1875. "Ueber die Erregung und Hemmung der Thätigkeit der nervösen Centralorgane." *Archiv für die gesammte Physiologie* 10: 174–208.

Frieden, Nancy Mandelker. 1981. *Russian Physicians in an Era of Reform and Revolution, 1856–1905.* Princeton: Princeton University Press.

Friedman, John, and James Alexander. 1983. "Psychoanalysis and natural science: Freud's 1895 *Project* revisited." *International Review of Psychoanalysis* 10: 303–318.

Fritsch, G., and E. Hitzig. 1870. "Ueber die elektrische Erregbarkeit des Grosshirns." *Archiv für Anatomie, Physiologie* n.v.: 300–332.

———. 1960. "On the electrical excitability of the cerebrum," trans. and ed. G. von Bonin. In G. von Bonin, ed., *Some Papers on the Cerebral Cortex*, 73–96. Springfield, Ill.: Charles C. Thomas.

Frolov, Iu. P. 1937. *Pavlov and His School: The Theory of Conditional Reflexes*, trans. D. P. Dutt from Russian. London: Kegan Paul, Trench, Trubner.

Gabbay, John. 1982. "Asthma attacked? Tactics for the reconstruction of a disease concept." In Peter Wright and Andrew Treacher, eds., *The Problem of Medical Knowledge: Examining the Social Construction of Medicine*, 23–48. Edinburgh: Edinburgh University Press.

Gabriel, Richard A. 1986. *Soviet Military Psychiatry: The Theory and Practice of Coping with Battle Stress.* New York: Greenwood.

Gallagher, Catherine, and Thomas Laqueur, eds. 1987. *The Making of the Modern Body: Sexuality and Society in the Nineteenth Century.* Berkeley, Los Angeles, London: University of California Press.

Gantt, W. Horsley. 1959. "Pavlov." In Mary A. B. Brazier, ed., *The Central Nervous System and Behavior: Transactions of the First Conference*, 163–186. New York: Josiah Macy, Jr., Foundation.

Gantt, W. H., L. Pickenhain, and C. Zwingmann, eds. 1970. *Pavlovian Approach to Psychopathology: History and Perspectives.* Oxford: Pergamon.

Gaskell, W. H. 1882. "The Croonian Lecture—On the rhythm of the heart of the frog, and on the nature of the action of the vagus nerve." *Philosophical Transactions of the Royal Society of London* 173: 993–1033.

———. 1886. "On the structure, distribution and function of the nerves which innervate the visceral and vascular systems." *Journal of Physiology* 7: 1–80.

———. 1900. "The contraction of cardiac muscle." In E. A. Schäfer, ed., *Text-book of Physiology*, 2: 169–227. Edinburgh: Young J. Pentland.

Gault, Robert H. 1904. "A sketch of the history of reflex action in the latter half of the nineteenth century." *American Journal of Psychology* 15: 526–568.

Gay, Peter. 1985. *The Bourgeois Experience Victoria to Freud*. Vol. 1: *Education of the Senses*. New York: Oxford University Press.

———. 1988. *Freud: A Life for Our Time*. London: J. M. Dent.

Geison, Gerald L. 1978. *Michael Foster and the Cambridge School of Physiology: The Scientific Enterprise in Late Victorian Society*. Princeton: Princeton University Press.

Geuter, Ulfried. 1983. "The uses of history for the shaping of a field: Observations on German psychology." In Loren Graham, Wolf Lepenies, and P. Weingart, eds., *Functions and Uses of Disciplinary Histories*, 191–228.

Gillispie, Charles Coulston. 1960. *The Edge of Objectivity: An Essay in the History of Scientific Ideas*. Princeton: Princeton University Press.

Godlee, Rickman John. 1917. *Lord Lister*. London: Macmillan.

Goldstein, Jan. 1987. *Console and Classify: The French Psychiatric Profession in the Nineteenth Century*. Cambridge: Cambridge University Press.

Golinski, Jan. 1990. "Language, discourse and science." In R. C. Olby, G. N. Cantor, J. R. R. Christie, and M. J. S. Hodge, eds., *Companion to the History of Modern Science*, 110–123. London: Routledge.

Goltz, Friedrich. 1863. "Vagus und Herz." *Archiv für pathologische Anatomie und Physiologie* 26: 1–33.

———. 1869. *Beiträge zur Lehre von den Functionen der Nervencentren des Frosches*. Berlin: August Hirschwald.

———. 1892. "Der Hund ohne Grosshirn. Siebente Abhandlung über die Verrichtungen des Grosshirns." *Archiv für die gesammte Physiologie* 51: 570–614.

Goltz, Friedrich, and A. Freusberg. 1874. "Ueber die Functionen des Lendenmarks des Hundes." *Archiv für die gesammte Physiologie* 8: 460–498.

Goltz, Friedrich, and E. Gergens. 1876. "Ueber die Verrichtungen des Grosshirns." *Archiv für die gesammte Physiologie* 13: 1–44.

Gotch, Francis. 1903. "The submaximal electrical response of nerve to a single stimulus." *Journal of Physiology* 28: 395–416.

Gotch, Francis, and G. J. Burch. 1899. "The electrical response of nerve to two stimuli." *Journal of Physiology* 24: 410–426.

Gould, Stephen Jay. 1977. *Ontogeny and Phylogeny*. Cambridge: Belknap Press of Harvard University Press.

Graham, Loren, Wolf Lepenies, and P. Weingart, eds. 1983. *Functions and Uses of Disciplinary Histories*. Sociology of the Sciences Yearbook, vol. 7. Dordrecht: D. Reidel.

Granit, Ragnar. 1966. *Charles Scott Sherrington: An Appraisal*. London: Nelson.

Gray, J. A., ed. and trans. 1964. *Pavlov's Typology: Recent Theoretical and Experimental Developments from the Laboratory of B. M. Teplov*. Oxford: Pergamon.

Gray, J. A. 1979. *Pavlov*. Brighton: Harvester Press.

Gregory, Frederick. 1977. *Scientific Materialism in Nineteenth Century Germany*. Dordrecht: D. Reidel.

Griesinger, Wilhelm. 1843. "Ueber psychische Reflexactionen. Mit einem Blick auf das Wesen der psychischen Krankheiten." *Archiv für physiologische Heilkunde* 2: 76–113.

———. 1844. "Neue Beiträge zur Physiologie und Pathologie des Gehirns." *Archiv für physiologische Heilkunde* 3: 69–98.

———. 1845. *Die Pathologie und Therapie der psychishen Krankheiten*. Stuttgart: Adolph Krabbe.

———. 1867. *Mental Pathology and Therapeutics*, trans. C. L. Robertson and J. Rutherford from 2d German ed. (1861). Facsimile reprint. New York: Hafner, 1965.

Grimm, Jacob, and Wilhelm Grimm. 1877. *Deutsches Wörterbuch*, vol. 4, 2d ed. Leipzig: S. Hirzel.

Grmek, Mirko Drazen. 1967. "Évolution des conceptions de Claude Bernard sur le milieu intérieur." In Étienne Wolff et al., *Philosophie et méthodologique scientifiques de Claude Bernard*, 117–150. Paris: Masson.

———. 1973. *Raisonnement expérimental et recherches toxicologiques chez Claude Bernard*. Geneva: Droz.

Guarnieri, Patrizia. 1987. "Moritz Schiff (1823–96): Experimental physiology and noble sentiment in Florence." In Nicholaas A. Rupke, ed., *Vivisection in Historical Perspective*, 105–124.

———. 1988. "Theatre and laboratory: Medical attitudes to animal magnetism in late-nineteenth-century Italy." In Roger Cooter, ed., *Studies in the History of Alternative Medicine*, 118–139. London: Macmillan.

Gundlach, Horst. 1976. *Reiz - Zur Verwendung: Eines Begriffes in der Psychologie*. Bern: Hans Huber.

Guthrie, Edwin R. 1930. "Conditioning as a principle of learning." *Psychological Review* 37: 412–428.

Haines, Barbara. 1978. "The inter-relations between social, biological, and medical thought, 1750–1850: Saint-Simon and Comte." *British Journal for the History of Science* 11: 19–35.

Hall, Marshall. 1837. *Memoirs on the Nervous System*. London: Sherwood, Gilbert and Piper.

———. 1839. "Memoirs on some principles of pathology in the nervous system." *Medico-chirurgical Transactions* 22: 191–217.

———. 1841. *On the Diseases and Derangements of the Nervous System*. London: H. Baillière.

———. 1850. *Synopsis of the Diastaltic Nervous System*. London: privately printed.

Haller, John S., and Robin M. Haller. 1974. *The Physician and Sexuality in Victorian America*. Urbana: University of Illinois Press.

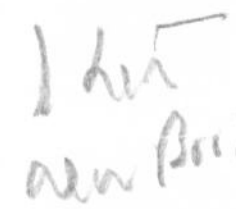

Hamilton, William. 1830. "Philosophy of perception." In *Discussions on Philosophy and Literature, Education and University Reform*, 38–97. London: Longman, Brown, Green and Longman, 1852.

———. 1846. "Supplementary dissertations; or excursive notes, critical and historical." In W. Hamilton, ed., *The Works of Thomas Reid D.D.*, 3d ed., 741–914. Edinburgh: Maclachlan and Stewart, 1852.

Haraway, Donna. 1990. *Primate Visions: Gender, Race, and Nature in the World of Modern Science*. New York: Routledge.

Harrington, Anne. 1987. *Medicine, Mind, and the Double Brain: A Study in Nineteenth-Century Thought*. Princeton: Princeton University Press.

Harrison, Brian. 1971. *Drink and the Victorians: The Temperance Question in England, 1815–1872*. London: Faber and Faber.

———. 1982. *Peaceable Kingdom: Stability and Change in Modern Britain*. Oxford: Clarendon Press.

Haymaker, Webb, and Francis Schiller, eds. 1970. *The Founders of Neurology: One Hundred and Forty-six Biographical Sketches by Eighty-eight Authors*, 2d ed. Springfield, Ill.: Charles C. Thomas.

Head, Henry. 1918. "Sensation and the cerebral cortex." In *Studies in Neurology* 2: 639–800. London: Henry Frowde, Hodder & Stoughton, 1920.

———. 1921. "Croonian Lecture: Release of function in the nervous system." *Proceedings of the Royal Society of London* 92B: 184–209.

———. 1926. *Aphasia and Kindred Disorders of Speech*. 2 vols. Cambridge: Cambridge University Press.

Hearnshaw, L. S. 1964. *A Short History of British Psychology, 1840–1940*. London: Methuen.

Heidenhain, Rudolf. 1880. *Animal Magnetism: Physiological Observations*, trans. I. C. Woolridge from 4th German ed. (1880, first publ. 1880). London: C. Kegan Paul.

Heinroth, J. C. A. 1818. *Lehrbuch der Störungen des Seelenlebens oder der Seelenstörungen und inhrer Behandlung*. 2 vols. Leipzig: F. C. W. Vogel.

———. 1975. *Textbook of Disturbances of Mental Life or Disturbances of the Soul and Their Treatment*, trans. and intro. George Mora. 2 vols. Baltimore: Johns Hopkins University Press.

Herbart, J. F. 1821. "Ueber einige Beziehungen zwischen Psychologie und Staatswissenschaft." In *Sämtliche Werke*, 5: 25–40. Langensalza: Hermann Beyer und Söhne, 1890.

———. 1824–25. *Psychologie als Wissenschaft neu gegründet auf Erfahrung, Metaphysik und Mathematik*. In *Sämtliche Werke*, 5: 177–434; 6: 1–340. Langensalza: Hermann Beyer und Söhne, 1890–1892.

———. 1834. *Lehrbuch zur Psychologie*, 2d ed. (first publ. 1816). In *Sämtliche Werke*, 4: 295–436. Langensalza: Hermann Beyer und Söhne, 1891.

———. 1891. *A Text-book in Psychology: An Attempt to Found the Science of Psychology on Experience, Metaphysics, and Mathematics*, trans. Margaret K. Smith from German. New York: D. Appleton.

Hering, Ewald. 1868. "Die Selbstseuerung der Athmung durch den *Nervus vagus*." *S.K.A.W.* 57, pt. 2: 672–677.

———. 1872–1874. "Zur Lehre vom Lichtsinne." *S.K.A.W.* 66, pt. 3 (1872):

5–24; 68, pt. 3 (1873): 185–201, 229–244; 69, pt. 3 (1874): 85–104, 179–217; 70, pt. 3 (1874): 169–204.

———. 1889. "Zur Theorie der Vorgänge in der lebendigen Substanz." *Lotos. Jahrbuch für Naturwissenschaft*, n.s., 9: 35–70.

———. 1897. "Theory of the functions in living matter," trans. F. A. Welby from German (1889). *Brain* 20: 232–258.

———. 1964. *Outlines of a Theory of the Light Sense*, trans. Leo M. Hurvich and Dorothea Jameson from German (1920). Cambridge: Harvard University Press.

Hering, H. E. 1902. "Die intracentralen Hemmungsvorgänge in ihrer Beziehung zur Skelettmuskulatur." *Ergebnisse der Physiologie* 1, pt. 2: 503–533.

Hering, H. E., and C. S. Sherrington. 1897. "Ueber Hemmung der Contraction willkürlicher Muskeln bei elecktrischer Reizung der Grosshirnrinde." *Archiv für die gesammte Physiologie* 68: 222–228.

Herzen, Alexandre A. 1864. *Expériences sur les centres modérateurs de l'action réflexe*. Turin: H. Loescher.

Hesse, Mary. 1970. "Theory and observation." In *Revolutions and Reconstructions in the Philosophy of Science*, 63–110. Brighton: Harvester Press, 1980.

———. 1974. *The Structure of Scientific Inference*. Berkeley, Los Angeles, London: University of California Press.

Heymans, G. 1899–1909. "Untersuchungen über psychische Hemmung." *Zeitschrift für Psychologie und Physiologie der Sinnesorgane* 21 (1899): 321–359; 26 (1901): 305–382; 34 (1904): 15–28; 41 (1906): 28–37, 89–116; 53 (1909): 401–415.

Hilgard, Ernest R., and Donald G. Marquis. 1940. *Conditioning and Learning*. New York: Appleton-Century-Crofts.

Hirschmüller, Albrecht. 1978. *Physiologie und Psychoanalyse in Leben und Werk Josef Breuers*. Bern: Hans Huber.

Hoff, Hebbel E. 1940. "The history of vagal inhibition." *Bulletin of the History of Medicine* 8: 461–496.

———. 1942. "The history of the refractory period: A neglected contribution of Felice Fontana." *Yale Journal of Biological Medicine* 14: 635–672.

Hoffman, Louise E. 1987. "The ideological significance of Freud's social thought." In Mitchell G. Ash and William R. Woodward, eds., *Psychology in Twentieth-Century Thought and Society*, 253–269.

Holland, H. 1852. *Chapters on Mental Physiology*. London: Longman, Brown, Green and Longmans.

Houghton, Walter E. 1957. *The Victorian Frame of Mind 1830–1870*. New Haven: Yale University Press.

Howell, W. H. 1925. "Inhibition." *Physiological Review* 5: 161–181.

Hull, Clark L. 1943. *Principles of Behavior: An Introduction to Behavior Theory*. New York: D. Appleton-Century.

Hunter, Walter S. 1932. "The psychological study of behavior." *Psychological Review* 39: 1–24.

Huxley, Thomas Henry. 1871. "Administrative nihilism." In Huxley, *Method and Results* (*Collected Essays*, vol. 1), 251–289. London: Macmillan, 1893.

———. 1893. "Evolution and ethics." In Huxley, *Evolution and Ethics and Other Essays* (*Collected Essays*, vol. 9), 46–116. London: Macmillan, 1894.

Hyman, Anthony. 1984. *Charles Babbage: Pioneer of the Computer*. Oxford: Oxford University Press.

Hyslop, James H. 1892. "Inhibition and the freedom of the will." *Philosophical Review* 1: 369–388.

Iaroshevskii, Mikhail G. 1968. "I. M. Sechenov—the founder of objective psychology," trans. Basil Haigh from Russian. In Benjamin B. Wolman, ed., *Historical Roots of Contemporary Psychology*, 77–110. New York: Harper & Row.

———. 1974. *Psychologie im 20. Jahrhundert: Theoretische Entwicklungsprobleme der psychologischen Wissenschaft*, trans. Ruth Kossert from Russian. Berlin: Volk und Wissen Volkseigner Verlag, 1975.

———. 1982. "The logic of scientific development and the scientific school: The example of Ivan Mikhailovich Sechenov," trans. from Russian. In William R. Woodward and Mitchell G. Ash, eds., *The Problematic Science*, 231–254.

———. 1986. *Ivan Sechenov*, trans. Michael Burov from Russian. Moscow: Mir.

Jackson, John Hughlings. 1866. "Notes on the physiology and pathology of language." *S.W.* 2: 121–128.

———. 1874. "On the nature of duality of the brain." *S.W.* 2: 129–145.

———. 1875*a*. "On the anatomical and physiological localisation of movements in the brain." *S.W.* 1: 37–76.

———. 1875*b*. "On temporary mental disorders after epileptic paroxysms." *S.W.* 1: 119–134.

———. 1876. "On epilepsies and on the after-effects of epileptic discharges (Todd and Robertson's hypothesis)." *S.W.* 1: 135–161.

———. 1878–1880. "On affections of speech from disease of the brain." *S.W.* 2: 155–204.

———. 1881. "Remarks on dissolution of the nervous system as exemplified by certain post-epileptic conditions." *S.W.* 2: 3–28.

———. 1884. "Evolution and dissolution of the nervous system." *S.W.* 2: 45–75.

———. 1888. "Discussion at the Neurological Society on Dr. Mercier's paper on 'Inhibition.'" *S.W.* 2: 476–481.

———. 1888–89. "On post-epileptic states: A contribution to the comparative study of insanities." *S.W.* 1: 366–384.

Jacob, François. 1974. *The Logic of Living Systems: A History of Heredity*, trans. Betty E. Spillman from French (1970). London: Allen Lane.

Jacobson, Edmund. 1911. "Experiments on the inhibition of sensations." *Psychological Review* 18: 24–53.

———. 1912. "Further experiments on the inhibition of sensations." *American Journal of Psychology* 23: 345–369.

———. 1925. "Progressive relaxation." *American Journal of Psychology* 36: 73–87.

Jacyna, L. S. 1981. "The physiology of mind, the unity of nature, and the moral order in Victorian thought." *British Journal for the History of Science* 14: 109–132.

———. 1982. "Somatic theories of mind and the interests of medicine in Britain, 1850–1879." *Medical History* 26: 233–258.

Jaeger, Siegfried. 1982. "Origins of child psychology: William Preyer." In William R. Woodward and Mitchell G. Ash, eds., *The Problematic Science*, 300–321.

———. 1985. "Preyer and the German school reform movement." In Georg Eckardt, ed., *Contributions to a History of Developmental Psychology: International William T. Preyer Symposium*, 231–243. Berlin: Mouton.

Jaeger, Siegfried, and Irmingard Staeuble. 1978. *Die Gesellschaftliche Genese der Psychologie*. Frankfurt/Main: Campus Verlag.

James, Alexander. 1881. "The reflex inhibitory centre theory." *Brain* 4: 287–302.

James, William. 1890. *The Principles of Psychology*. 2 vols. Facsimile reprint. New York: Dover, 1950.

Janet, Pierre. 1932. *La force et la faiblesse psychologiques*. Paris: Norbert Maloine.

Jay, Martin. 1973. *The Dialectical Imagination: A History of the Frankfurt School and the Institute of Social Research, 1923–1950*. London: Heinemann.

Jeannerod, Marc. 1985. *The Brain Machine: The Development of Neurophysiological Thought*, trans. David Union from French (1983). Cambridge: Harvard University Press.

Jones, Ernest. 1953–1957. *Sigmund Freud: Life and Work*. 3 vols. London: Hogarth Press.

Joravsky, David. 1961. *Soviet Marxism and Natural Science 1917–1932*. London: Routledge & Kegan Paul.

———. 1989. *Russian Psychology: A Critical History*. Oxford: Basil Blackwell.

Jordanova, Ludmilla, ed. 1986. *Languages of Nature: Critical Essays on Science and Literature*. London: Free Association Books.

Jordanova, Ludmilla. 1989. *Sexual Visions: Images of Gender in Science and Medicine between the Eighteenth and Twentieth Centuries*. New York: Harvester Wheatsheaf.

Jung, C. G. 1923. *Psychological Types*, trans. H. G. Baynes, rev. R. F. C. Hull, from German (1921) (*The Collected Works of C. G. Jung*, vol. 6). London: Routledge & Kegan Paul, 1971.

Käbin, Ilo. 1986. *Die medizinische Forschung und Lehre an der Universität Dorpat/Tartu 1802–1940: Ergebnisse und Bedeutung für die Entwicklung der Medizin*. Sydsvenska medicinhistoriska sällskapets Årsskrift, suppl. 6. Lüneburg: Verlag Nordostdeutches Kulturwerk.

Kane, Alison, and Eric T. Carlson. 1982. "A different drummer: Robert Carter and nineteenth century hysteria." *Bulletin of the New York Academy of Medicine* 58: 519–534.

Kant, Immanuel. 1798. *Anthropologie in pragmatischer Hinsicht*. In *Kant's gesammelte Schriften*, 7: 117–333. Berlin: Georg Reimer, 1917.

———. 1974. *Anthropology from a Pragmatic Point of View*, trans. Mary J. Gregor from 2d German ed. (1800). The Hague: Martinus Nijhoff.

Kelly, Alfred. 1981. *Descent of Darwin: The Popularization of Darwinism in Germany, 1860–1914*. Chapel Hill: University of North Carolina Press.

Kiell, Norman. 1988. *Freud Without Hindsight: Reviews of His Work (1893–1939)*. Madison, Conn.: International Universities Press.

Koblitz, Ann Hibner. 1988. "Science, women, and the Russian intelligentsia: The generation of the 1860s." *Isis* 79: 208–226.

Kohn, David, ed. 1985. *The Darwinian Heritage*. Princeton: Princeton University Press.

Koshtoyants, K. S. 1960. "I. Sechenov (1829–1905)." In I. M. Sechenov, *Selected Physiological and Psychological Works*, 7–27.

———. 1964. *Essays on the History of Physiology in Russia*, trans. David P. Boder, Kristan Hanes, and Natalie O'Brien from Russian (1946), ed. Donald B. Lindsley. Washington: American Institute of Biological Sciences.

Kozulin, Alex. 1984. *Psychology in Utopia: Toward a Social History of Soviet Psychology*. Cambridge: MIT Press.

Kraepelin, Emil. 1909–1915. *Psychiatrie: Ein Lehrbuch für Studierende und Ärzte*, 8th ed. 4 vols. Leipzig: Johann Ambrosius Barth.

———. 1921. *Manic-depressive Insanity and Paranoia*, trans. R. Mary Barclay from *Psychiatrie*, 8th German ed., vols. 3 and 4. Facsimile reprint. New York: Arno Press, 1976.

Kretschmer, Ernst. 1934. *A Text-book of Medical Psychology*, trans. E. B. Strauss from 4th German ed. (1930). London: Oxford University Press.

———. 1961. *Hysteria, Reflex and Instinct*, trans. Vlasta Baskin and Wade Baskin from 6th German ed. (1958). London: Peter Owen.

Kronecker, Hugo, and S. Meltzer. 1883. "Der Schluckmechanismus, seine Erregung und seine Hemmung." *Archiv für Anatomie und Physiologie* suppl. vol.: 328–360.

Kronecker, Hugo, and W. Stirling. 1874. "Das charakterische Merkmal der Herzmuskelbewegung." In *Beitraege zur Anatomie und Physiologie als Festgabe Carl Ludwig*, 173–204. Leipzig: F. C. W. Vogel.

Ladd, George Trumbull. 1894. *A Treatise of the Phenomena, Laws, and Development of Human Mental Life*. London: Longmans, Green.

La Mettrie, J. O. de. 1912. *Man A Machine*, trans. Gertrude C. Bussey from French (1747). La Salle: Open Court, 1961.

Langendorff, Oscar. 1877. "Ueber Reflexhemmung." *Archiv für Physiologie* n.v.: 96–115.

Lasch, Christopher. 1980. *The Culture of Narcissism: American Life in an Age of Diminishing Expectations*. London: Abacus.

Lawrence, Christopher. 1979. "The nervous system and society in the Scottish Enlightenment." In Barry Barnes and Steven Shapin, eds., *Natural Order*, 19–40.

Laycock, Thomas. 1845. "On the reflex functions of the brain." *British and Foreign Medical Review* 19: 298–311.

Leake, Chauncey D. 1959. "Danilevsky, Wedensky, and Ukhtomsky." In Mary A. B. Brazier, ed., *The Central Nervous System and Behavior: Transactions of the First Conference*, 151–162. New York: Josiah Macy, Jr., Foundation.

Leary, David E. 1978. "The philosophical development of the conception of psychology in Germany, 1780–1850." *Journal of the History of the Behavioral Sciences* 14: 113–121.

———. 1980. "The historical foundations of Herbart's mathematization of psychology." *Journal of the History of the Behavioral Sciences* 16: 150–163.

Leary, David E., ed. 1990. *Metaphors in the History of Psychology*. Cambridge: Cambridge University Press.

Legallois, J. C. C. 1812. *Expériences sur le principe de la vie, notamment sur celui des mouvements du coeur, et sur le siége de ce principe*. Paris: D'Hautel.

Lemaine, G., R. MacLeod, M. Mulkay, and P. Weingart, eds. 1976. *Perspectives on the Emergence of Scientific Disciplines*. The Hague: Mouton.

Lenoir, Timothy. 1986. "Models and instruments in the development of electrophysiology, 1845–1912." *Historical Studies in the Physical and Biological Sciences* 17: 1–54.

Lesch, John E. 1984. *Science and Medicine in France: The Emergence of Experimental Physiology, 1790–1855*. Cambridge: Harvard University Press.

Levin, Kenneth. 1978. *Freud's Early Psychology of the Neuroses: A Historical Perspective*. Hassocks, Sussex: Harvester Press.

Lewes, George Henry. 1877. *The Physical Basis of Mind: Being the Second Series of Problems of Life and Mind*. London: Trübner.

Lewisson, M. 1869. "Ueber Hemmung der Thätigkeit der motorischen Nervencentra durch Reizung sensibler Nerven." *Archiv für Anatomie, Physiologie* n.v.: 255–266.

Leys, Ruth. 1980. "Background to the reflex controversy: William Alison and the doctrine of sympathy before Hall." *Studies in History of Biology* 4: 1–66.

Liddell, E. G. T. 1960. *The Discovery of Reflexes*. Oxford: Clarendon Press.

Liddell, E. G. T., and C. S. Sherrington. 1924. "Responses in response to stretch (myotactic reflexes)." *Proceedings of the Royal Society of London* 96B: 212–242.

Liljestrand, Göran. 1950. "The prize in physiology or medicine." In The Nobel Foundation and W. Odelberg, eds., *Nobel: The Man & His Prizes*, 3d ed., 139–278. New York: American Elsevier, 1972.

Lister, Joseph. 1858. "Preliminary account of an inquiry into the functions of the visceral nerves, with special reference to the so-called 'inhibitory system.'" *Proceedings of the Royal Society of London* 9: 367–380.

———. 1909. *The Collected Papers of Joseph, Baron Lister*. 2 vols. Oxford: Clarendon Press.

Littré, Émil. 1863–1872. *Dictionnaire de la langue français*, vol. 4. Facsimile reprint. Paris: Gallimard/Hachette, 1962.

Lloyd, G. E. R., ed. 1978. *Hippocratic Writings*. Harmondsworth: Penguin Books.

Lotze, Hermann. 1885. *Microcosmus: An Essay Concerning Man and His Relations to the World*, trans. Elizabeth Hamilton and E. E. Constance Jones from 3d German ed. (1876). 2 vols. Edinburgh: T. & T. Clark.

Lucas, Keith. 1917. *The Conduction of the Nervous Impulse*, rev. E. D. Adrian. London: Longmans, Green.

McDougall, William. 1902–1906. "The physiological factors of the attention-process." *Mind*, n.s., 11 (1902): 316–351; 12 (1903): 289–302, 473–488; 15 (1906): 329–359.

———. 1903. "The nature of inhibitory processes within the nervous system." *Brain* 26: 153–191.

———. 1905. *Physiological Psychology*. London: J. M. Dent, 1918.

———. 1908. *An Introduction to Social Psychology*, 23d ed. London: Methuen, 1936.

M'Kendrick, John G. 1874. "On the inhibitory or restraining action which the encephalon exerts on the reflex centres of the spinal cord." *Edinburgh Medical Journal* 19: 733–737.

———. 1883. "Magnetism, animal." In *Encyclopaedia Britannica*, 9th ed., 15: 277–283. Edinburgh: Adam and Charles Black.

McKendrick, Neil. 1961. "Josiah Wedgwood and factory discipline." *Historical Journal* 4: 30–55.

Mackenzie, Brian D. 1977. *Behaviourism and the Limits of Scientific Method*. London: Routledge & Kegan Paul.

MacLean, Paul D. 1949. "Psychosomatic disease and the 'visceral brain': Recent developments bearing on the Papez theory of emotion." *Psychosomatic Medicine* 11: 338–353.

———. 1959. "The limbic system with respect to two basic life principles." In Mary A. B. Brazier, ed., *The Central Nervous System and Behavior*, 31–118. Transactions of the Second Conference on the Central Nervous System and Behavior. New York: Josiah Macy, Jr., Foundation.

———. 1971. "The paranoid streak in man." In Arthur Koestler and J. R. Smythies, eds., *Beyond Reductionism: New Perspectives in the Life Sciences*, 258–278. Boston: Beacon Press.

McLeish, John. 1975. *Soviet Psychology: History, Theory, Content*. London: Methuen.

Magendie, François. 1822. "Expériences sur les fonctions des racines des nerfs rachidiens." Facsimile reprint. In Paul F. Cranefield, *The Way In and the Way Out*.

———. 1822. "Expériences sur les fonctions des racines des nerfs qui naissent de la moelle épinière." Facsimile reprint. In Paul F. Cranefield, *The Way In and The Way Out*.

———. 1839. *Leçons sur les fonctions et les maladies du système nerveux*. 2 vols. Paris: Ébrard.

Magoun, H. W. 1944. "Bulbar inhibition and facilitation of motor activity." *Science* 100: 549–550.

Magoun, H. W., and Ruth Rhines. 1946. "An inhibitory mechanism in the bulbar reticular formation." *Journal of Neurophysiology* 9: 165–171.

Marcuse, Herbert. 1962. *Eros and Civilization: A Philosophical Inquiry into Freud*. New York: Vintage Books. (First publ. 1955.)

Markus, G. 1987. "Why is there no hermeneutics of natural science? Some preliminary theses." *Science in Context* 1: 5–51.

Marshall, Marilyn E., and Russel A. Wendt. 1980. "Wilhelm Wundt, spiritism, and the assumptions of science." In Wolfgang G. Bringmann and Ryan D. Tweney, eds., *Wundt Studies: A Centennial Collection*, 158–175. Toronto: C. J. Hogrefe.

Martindale, Colin. 1971. "Degeneration, disinhibition and genius." *Journal of the History of the Behavioral Sciences* 7: 177–182.

Marx, Otto M. 1965. "A re-evaluation of the mentalists in early 19th century German psychiatry." *American Journal of Psychiatry* 121: 752–760.

———. 1968. "J. C. A. Heinroth (1773–1843) on psychiatry and law." *Journal of the History of the Behavioral Sciences* 4: 163–179.

———. 1972. "Wilhelm Griesinger and the history of psychiatry: A reassessment." *Bulletin of the History of Medicine* 46: 519–544.

Matkevich, F. 1864. "Ueber die Wirkung des Alkohols, Strychnins und Opiums auf die reflexhemmenden Mechanismen des Frosches." *Zeitschrift für rationelle Medicin*, n.s., 21: 230–268.

Maudsley, Henry. 1867. *The Physiology and Pathology of Mind*, 2d ed. London: Macmillan, 1868.

———. 1874. "Sex in mind and in education." *Fortnightly Review*, n.s., 15: 466–483.

———. 1883. *Body and Will: Being an Essay Concerning Will in Its Metaphysical, Physiological, and Pathological Aspects.* London: Kegan Paul, Trench.

———. 1895. *The Pathology of Mind: A Study of Its Distempers, Deformities and Disorders.* Facsimile reprint. London: Julian Friedmann, 1979.

Maxwell, J. C. 1868. "On governors." *Proceedings of the Royal Society of London* 16: 270–283.

Mayo, Thomas. 1854. *Medical Testimony and Evidence in Cases of Lunacy.* London: John W. Parker.

Mayr, Otto. 1970. *The Origins of Feedback Control*, trans. from German (1969). Cambridge: MIT Press.

———. 1971. "Adam Smith and the concept of the feedback system."*Technology and Culture* 12: 1–22.

Mecacci, Luciano. 1979. *Brain and History: The Relationship between Neurophysiology and Psychology in Soviet Research*, trans. Henry A. Buchtel from Italian. New York: Brunner/Mazel.

Medvei, Victor Cornelius. 1982. *A History of Endocrinology*. Lancaster: MTP Press.

Meijer, Onno G. 1988. *The Hierarchy Debate: Perspectives for a Theory and History of Movement Science* (Academisch Proefschrift). Amsterdam: Free University Press.

Meltzer, S. J. 1883. "Die Irradiationen des Schluckcentrums und ihre allgemeine Bedeuting." *Archiv für Physiologie* n.v.: 209–238.

———. 1899. "Inhibition." *New York Medical Journal* 69: 661–666, 699–703, 739–743.

Mercier, Charles. 1888*a*. "Inhibition." *Brain* 11: 361–386, and disc. 386–405.

———. 1888*b*. *The Nervous System and the Mind: A Treatise on the Dynamics of the Human Organism.* London: Macmillan.

———. 1892. "Inhibition." In Daniel Hack Tuke, ed., *A Dictionary of Psychological Medicine*, 2: 691–692. London: J. & A. Churchill.

Meynert, Theodor. 1884. *Psychiatrie. Klinik der Erkrankungen des Vorderhirns begründet auf dessen Bau, Leistungen und Ernährung*. Wien: Wilhelm Braumüller.

———. 1885. *Psychiatry: A Clinical Treatise on Diseases of the Fore-brain Based upon a Study of Its Structure, Functions and Nutrition*, trans. B. Sachs from German (1884). Facsimile reprint. New York: Hafner, 1968.

———. 1888. "Ueber hypnotische Erscheinungen." *Wiener klinische Wochenschrift* 1: 451–453, 473–476, 495–498.

———. 1960. "On the collaboration of parts of the brain," trans. Gerhardt von Bonin from German (1891). In Gerhardt von Bonin, ed., *Some Papers on the Cerebral Cortex*, 159–180. Springfield, Ill.: Charles C. Thomas.

Micale, Mark S. 1990. "Hysteria and its historiography: The future prospect." *History of Psychiatry* 1: 33–124.

Mill, John Stuart. 1973–74. *A System of Logic Ratiocinative and Inductive* (*Collected Works of John Stuart Mill*, vols. 7, 8). Toronto: University of Toronto Press. (First publ. 1843.)

Miller, Jonathan. 1972. "The dog beneath the skin." *The Listener* 88 (20 July): 74–76.

Milne Edwards, H. 1859. *Leçons sur la physiologie et l'anatomie comparée de l'homme et des animaux*, vol. 4. Paris: Victor Masson.

Morgan, C. Lloyd. 1890–91. *Animal Life and Intelligence*. London: Edward Arnold.

———. 1894. *An Introduction to Comparative Psychology*. London: Walter Scott.

Mort, Frank. 1987. *Dangerous Sexualities: Medico-moral Politics in England since 1830*. London: Routledge & Kegan Paul.

Moscovici, Serge. 1976. *La psychoanalyse: Son image et son public*, 2d ed. Paris: Presses Universitaires de France. (First publ. 1961.)

Mulkay, Michael. 1979. *Science and the Sociology of Knowledge*. London: George Allen & Unwin.

Müller, G. E., and A. Pilzecker. 1900. "Experimentelle Beiträge zur Lehre vom Gedächtniss." *Zeitschrift für Psychologie und Physiologie der Sinnesorgane*, Ergänungsband 1. Leipzig: Johann Ambrosius Barth.

Müller, Johannes. 1834–40. *Handbuch der Physiologie des Menschen für Vorlesungen*, 2d ed., vol. 1; 3d ed., vol. 2. Coblenz: J. Hölscher.

———. 1839–42. *Elements of Physiology*, trans. William Baly from German. 2 vols. London: Taylor and Walton.

Munk, Hermann. 1881. "Ueber Erregung und Hemmung." *Archiv für Physiologie* n.v.: 553–559.

Murray, D. J. 1976. "Research on human memory in the nineteenth century." *Canadian Journal of Psychology* 30: 201–220.

Neuburger, Max. 1981. *The Historical Development of Experimental Brain and Spinal Cord Physiology before Flourens*, trans. and ed. E. Clarke from German (1897). Baltimore: Johns Hopkins University Press.

Nordau, Max. 1895. *Degeneration*, trans. from 2d German ed. (1893). Facsimile reprint. New York: Howard Fertig, 1968.

Nothnagel, H. 1869. "Bewegungshemmende Mechanismen im Rückenmark des

Frosches." *Centralblatt für die medicinischen Wissenschaften*, no. 14: 211–212.

———. 1875–76. "Beobachtungen über Reflexhemmung." *Archiv für Psychiatrie und Nervenkrankheiten* 6: 332–343.

Nye, Robert. 1984. *Crime, Politics and Madness in Modern France: The Medical Concept of National Decline*. Princeton: Princeton University Press.

Obersteiner, H. 1879. "Experimental researches on attention." *Brain* 1: 439–453.

O'Donnell, John M. 1979. "The crisis of experimentalism in the 1920's: E. G. Boring and his uses of history." *American Psychologist* 34: 289–295.

———. 1986. *The Origins of Behaviorism: American Psychology, 1870–1920*. New York: New York University Press.

Olmsted, J. M. D. 1946. *Charles-Édouard Brown-Séquard: A Nineteenth Century Neurologist and Endocrinologist*. Baltimore: Johns Hopkins University Press.

Olmsted, J. M. D., and E. Harris Olmsted. 1952. *Claude Bernard & the Experimental Method in Medicine*. London: Abelard-Schuman.

Outram, Dorinda. 1989. *The Body and the French Revolution: Sex, Class, and Political Culture*. New Haven: Yale University Press.

Papez, James W. 1937. "A proposed mechanism of emotion." *Archives of Neurology and Psychiatry* 38: 725–743.

Paradis, James G. 1978. *T. H. Huxley: Man's Place in Nature*. Lincoln: University of Nebraska Press.

Paulhan, F. 1889. *L'activité mentale et les éléments de l'esprit*. Paris: Félix Alcan.

Pavlov, Ivan Petrovich. 1885. "Wie die Muschel ihre Schaale öffnet. Versuche und Fragen zur allgemeinen Muskel- und Nervenphysiologie." *Archiv für die gesammte Physiologie* 37: 6–31.

———. 1927. *Conditioned Reflexes: An Investigation of the Physiological Activity of the Cerebral Cortex*, trans. from Russian and ed. G. V. Anrep. Facsimile reprint. New York: Dover, 1960.

———. 1928. *Lectures on Conditioned Reflexes: Twenty-five Years of Objective Study of the Higher Nervous Activity (Behaviour) of Animals. Volume 1*, trans. from Russian and ed. W. Horsley Gantt. New York: International Publishers.

———. 1930. "A brief outline of the higher nervous activity," trans. D. L. Zyre from Russian. In Carl Murchison, ed., *Psychologies of 1930*, 207–220. Facsimile reprint. New York: Arno Press, 1973.

———. 1932. "The reply of a physiologist to psychologists." *Psychological Review* 39: 91–127.

———. 1941. *Lectures on Conditioned Reflexes. Volume Two: Conditioned Reflexes and Psychiatry*, trans. from Russian and ed. W. Horsley Gantt. New York: International Publishers.

———. 1955. *Selected Works*, ed. K. S. Koshtoyants, trans. S. Belsky from Russian and ed. J. Gibbons. Moscow: Foreign Languages Publishing House.

———. 1955. "Physiology of the higher nervous activity." In *Selected Works*, 271–286.

Peel, J. D. Y. 1971. *Herbert Spencer: The Evolution of a Sociologist*. London: Heinemann.

Perry, Ralph Barton. 1935. *The Thought and Character of William James as Revealed in Unpublished Correspondence and Notes, Together with His Published Writings*. 2 vols. Boston: Little, Brown.

Pflüger, Eduard. 1857. *Ueber das Hemmungs-Nervensystem für die peristaltischen Bewegungen der Gedärme*. Berlin: August Hirschwald.

———. 1859. "Experimentalbeitrag zur Theorie der Hemmungnerven." *Archiv für Anatomie, Physiologie* n.v.: 13–29.

Phillips, D. C. 1977. *Holistic Thought in Social Science*. London: Macmillan.

Pick, Daniel. 1989. *Faces of Degeneration: A European Disorder, c. 1848–1918*. Cambridge: Cambridge University Press.

Pillsbury, W. B. 1911. *The Essentials of Psychology*, 2d ed. New York: Macmillan, 1925.

Pinel, Philippe. 1806. *A Treatise on Insanity*, trans. D. D. Davis from French (1801). London: Cadell and Davies.

Plato. 1961. "Phaedrus," trans. R. Hackforth (1952). In Edith Hamilton and Huntington Cairns, eds., *The Collected Dialogues of Plato, Including the Letters*, 475–525. Bollingen Series 71. New York: Pantheon Books.

Pope, Alexander. 1963. *The Poems of Alexander Pope*, ed. John Butt. London: Methuen.

Postman, Leo. 1962. "Rewards and punishments in human learning." In L. Postman, ed., *Psychology in the Making: Histories of Selected Research Problems*, 331–401. New York: Knopf.

Preyer, William T. 1878. *Die Kataplexie und der thierische Hypnotismus*. Jena: Gustav Fischer.

———. 1888. *The Mind of the Child*, trans. H. W. Brown from 2d German ed. (1884). 2 vols. New York: D. Appleton, 1893.

———. 1905. *Die Seele des Kindes: Beobachtungen über die geistige Entwicklung des Menschen in den ersten Lebensjahren*, 6th ed. Leipzig: Th. Grieben's Verlag. (First publ. 1881.)

Pribram, Karl H. 1962. "The neuropsychology of Sigmund Freud." In Arthur J. Bachrach, ed., *Experimental Foundations of Clinical Psychology*, 442–468. New York: Basic Books.

Prichard, James Cowles. 1842. *On the Different Forms of Insanity, in Relation to Jurisprudence*. London: H. Baillière.

Purpura, D. P., and H. Waelsch. 1964. "Brain reflexes." *Science* 143: 598–604.

Rapaport, David. 1959. "The structure of psychoanalytic theory: A systematizing attempt." In Sigmund Koch, ed., *Psychology: A Study of a Science. Study 1. Conceptual and Systematic.* Volume 3: *Formulations of the Person and the Social Context*, 55–183. New York: McGraw-Hill.

Rapaport, David, and Merton M. Gill. 1959. "The points of view and assumptions of metapsychology." In Merton M. Gill, ed., *The Collected Papers of David Rapaport*, 795–811. New York: Basic Books, 1967.

Rapp, Dean A. 1988. "The reception of Freud by the British press: General interest and literary magazines, 1920–1925." *Journal of the History of the Behavioral Sciences* 24: 191–201.

Ravetz, Jerome R. 1973. *Scientific Knowledge and Its Social Problems*. Harmondsworth: Penguin Books.

Razran, Gregory. 1965. "Russian physiologists' psychology and American experimental psychology: A historical and systematic collation and a look into the future." *Psychological Bulletin* 63: 42–64.

Ribot, Théodule. 1870. *La psychologie anglaise contemporaine*. (*École expérimentale*). Paris: Ladrange.

———. 1886. *German Psychology of To-day: The Empirical School*, trans. J. M. Baldwin from 2d French ed. (1885). New York: Charles Scribner's Sons.

———. 1890. *The Psychology of Attention*, trans. from French (1889). Chicago: Open Court.

———. 1894. *Diseases of the Will*, trans. Merwin-Marie Snell from 8th French ed. Chicago: Open Court.

Richards, Barry. 1989. *Images of Freud: Cultural Responses to Psychoanalysis*. London: J. M. Dent.

Richards, Graham. 1987. "Of what is the history of psychology a history?" *British Journal for the History of Science* 20: 201–211.

———. 1989. *On Psychological Language and the Physiomorphic Basis of Human Nature*. London: Routledge.

Richards, Robert J. 1987. *Darwin and the Emergence of Evolutionary Theories of Mind and Behavior*. Chicago: University of Chicago Press.

Richet, Charles. 1882. *Physiologie des muscles et des nerfs*. Paris: Germer Baillière.

Rieff, Philip. 1961. *Freud: The Mind of the Moralist*. New York: Anchor Books.

———. 1973. *The Triumph of the Therapeutic: Uses of Faith after Freud*. Harmondsworth: Penguin Books.

Riese, Walther. 1942. "The principle of integration: Its history and its nature." *Journal of Nervous and Mental Diseases* 96: 296–312.

———. 1959. *A History of Neurology*. New York: M.D. Publications.

Riese, Walther, and Hebbel E. Hoff. 1950–51. "A history of the doctrine of cerebral localization." *Journal of the History of Medicine* 5(1950): 50–71; 6(1951): 439–470.

Ringer, Fritz K. 1969. *The Decline of the German Mandarins: The German Academic Community, 1890–1933*. Cambridge: Harvard University Press.

Rintoul, Gordon C. 1984. "Images of human nature: Experimental psychology in Victorian Britain." Ph.D. diss., University of Manchester.

Risse, Günter B. 1970. "The Brownian system of medicine: Its theoretical and practical implications." *Clio Medica* 5: 45–51.

Ritter, Joachim, ed. 1974. *Historisches Wörterbuch der Philosophie*, vol. 3. Basel/Stuttgart: Schwabe.

Rivers, W. H. R. 1920. *Instinct and the Unconscious: A Contribution to a Biological Theory of the Psycho-neuroses*, 2d ed. Cambridge: Cambridge University Press, 1922.

Rivers, W. H. R., and Henry Head. 1908. "A human experiment in nerve division." In Henry Head, *Studies in Neurology*, 1: 225–329. London: Henry Frowde, Hodder & Stoughton, 1920.

Roback, A. A. 1927. *The Psychology of Character: With a Survey of Temperament.* London: Kegan Paul, Trench, Trubner.

Robert, Paul. 1963. *Dictionnaire alphabêtique et analogique de la langue français*, vol. 4. Paris: Société du Nouveau Littré.

Robinson, Paul A. 1969. *The Freudian Left: Wilhelm Reich, Geza Roheim, Herbert Marcuse.* New York: Harper & Row.

Robison, John. 1822. *A System of Mechanical Philosophy.* 4 vols. Edinburgh: John Murray.

Romberg, Moritz Heinrich. 1853. *A Manual of the Nervous Diseases of Man*, trans. and ed. Eduard H. Seiveking from 2d German ed. (1851). 2 vols. London: Sydenham Society.

Rose, Nikolas. 1985. *The Psychological Complex: Social Regulation and the Psychology of the Individual.* London: Routledge & Kegan Paul.

———. 1990. *Governing the Soul: The Shaping of the Private Self.* London: Routledge.

Rosenbleuth, Arturo, Norbert Wiener, and Julian Bigelow. 1943. "Behavior, purpose and teleology." *Philosophy of Science* 10: 18–24.

Rosenthal, J. 1861. "De l'influence du nerf pneumogastrique et du nerf laryngé supérieur sur les mouvements du diaphragme." *C.R.A.S.* 52: 754–756.

———. 1862. *Die Athembewegungen und ihre Beziehungen zum Nerven Vagus.* Berlin: August Hirschwald.

Rothschuh, K. E., ed. 1964. *Von Boerhaave bis Berger: Die Entwicklung der kontinentalen Physiologie im 18. und 19. Jahrhundert mit besonderer Berücksichtigung der Neurophysiologie.* Stuttgart: Gustav Fischer.

Rothschuh, K. E. 1973. *History of Physiology*, trans. Günter B. Risse from German (1953). Huntington, N.Y.: Robert E. Krieger.

Rudwick, Martin J. S. 1985. *The Great Devonian Controversy: The Shaping of Scientific Knowledge among Gentlemanly Specialists.* Chicago: University of Chicago Press.

Rupke, Nicolaas A., ed. 1987. *Vivisection in Historical Perspective.* London: Croom Helm.

Russell, Colin A. 1983. *Science and Social Change 1700–1900.* London: Macmillan.

Russett, C. E. 1989. *Sexual Science: The Victorian Construction of Womanhood.* Cambridge: Harvard University Press.

Rutherford, William. 1871–72. "Lectures on experimental physiology." *Lancet* 1 (1871): 1–3, 75–78, 183–185, 295–298, 437–439, 563–567, 705–707; 2 (1871): 665–669, 739–742, 841–844; 1 (1872): 69–72, 211–215, 673–677.

Sackler, Arthur M., Mortimer D. Sackler, Raymond R. Sackler, and Felix Marti-Ibanez, eds. 1956. *The Great Physiodynamic Therapies in Psychiatry: An Historical Reappraisal.* New York: Hoeber-Harper.

Salter, Henry G. 1860. *On Asthma: Its Pathology and Treatment.* London: John Churchill.

Samelson, Franz. 1985. "Organizing for the kingdom of behavior: Academic battles and organizational policies in the Twenties." *Journal of the History of the Behavioral Sciences* 21: 33–47.

Sargant, William. 1959. *Battle for the Mind: A Physiology of Conversion and Brain-washing.* London: Pan Books. (First publ. 1957.)

Schäfer, E. A. 1900. "The cerebral cortex." In E. A. Schäfer, ed., *Text-book of Physiology,* 2: 697–782. Edinburgh: Young J. Pentland.

Scheerer, Eckart. 1980. "Wilhelm Wundt's psychology of memory." *Psychological Research* 42: 135–155.

Schiff, Moritz. 1849. "Experimentelle Untersuchungen über die Nerven des Herzens." *Archiv für physiologische Heilkunde* 8: 166–234, 442–488.

———. 1858–59. *Lehrbuch der Physiologie des Menschen. I. Muskel- und Nervenphysiologie.* Lahr: M. Schauenburg.

———. 1859. "Zur Physiologie der sogenannten 'Hemmungsnerven.' Eine Erwiederung an Dr. Eduard Pflüger in Berlin." In *Gesammelte Beiträge zur Physiologie,* 2: 344–374. Lausanne: B. Benda, 1894.

———. 1866. "Kritisch und Polemisches zur Physiologie des Nervensystems." In *Gesammelte Beiträge zur Physiologie,* 2: 476–512. Lausanne: B. Benda, 1894.

———. 1868. *Leçons sur la physiologie de la digestion, faites au Muséum d'Histoire Naturelle de Florence.* 2 vols. Florence and Turin: Hermann Loescher.

———. 1873. "Altes und neues Herznerven." In *Gesammelte Beiträge zur Physiologie,* 2: 551–633. Lausanne: B. Benda, 1894.

———. 1877–78. "Recherches sur les nerfs dits arrestateurs." In *Gesammelte Beiträge zur Physiologie,* 1: 619–659. Lausanne: B. Benda, 1894.

———. 1894. "Der Modus der Herzbewegung." In *Gesammelte Beiträge zur Physiologie,* 2: 236–343. Lausanne: B. Benda.

Schiller, Joseph. 1967. *Claude Bernard et les problèmes scientifiques de son temps.* Paris: Les éditions du cèdre.

———. 1978. *La notion d'organisation dans l'histoire de la biologie.* Paris: Maloine.

Schröer, Heinz. 1967. *Carl Ludwig: Begrunder der messenden Experimentalphysiologie 1816–1895.* Stuttgart: Wissenschaftliche Verlagsgesellschaft.

Scull, Andrew T. 1979. *Museums of Madness: The Social Organization of Insanity in Nineteenth-Century England.* London: Allen Lane.

———. 1981. "Moral treatment reconsidered: Some sociological comments on an episode in the history of British psychiatry." In Andrew Scull, ed., *Madness, Mad-doctors, and Madmen: The Social History of Psychiatry in the Victorian Era,* 105–118. Philadelphia: University of Pennsylvania Press.

Sechenov, Ivan Mikhailovich. 1863*a*. "Sous les modérateurs des mouvements réflexes dans le cerveau de la grenouille." *C.R.A.S.* 56: 50–53, 185–187.

———. 1863*b*. "Études physiologiques sur les centres modérateurs des mouvements réflexes dans le cerveau de la grenouille." *Annales des sciences naturelles,* 4th ser., 19: 109–134.

———. 1863*c*. "Physiologische Studien über die Hemmungsmechanismen für die Reflexthätigkeit des Rückenmarks im Gehirne des Frosches." In *Selected*

Works (1935), 153–176. Facsimile reprint. Amsterdam: E. J. Bonset, 1968.

———. 1865. "Weiteres über die Reflexhemmungen beim Frosche." *Zeitschrift für rationelle Medicin*, 3d ser., 23: 6–15.

———. 1868. "Über die elektrische und chemische Reizung der sensiblen Rückenmarksnerven des Frosches." In *Selected Works* (1935), 177–211. Facsimile reprint. Amsterdam: E. J. Bonset, 1968.

———. 1875*a*. "Notiz die reflexhemmenden Mechanismen betreffend." *Bulletin de l'Académie Impériale des Sciences de St-Pétersbourg* 20: cols. 322–323.

———. 1875*b*. "Notiz, die reflexhemmenden Mechanismen betreffend." *Archiv für die gesammte Physiologie* 10: 163–164.

———. 1875*c*. "Zur Frage über die Reflexhemmungen." *Bulletin de l'Académie Impériale des Sciences de St-Pétersbourg* 20: cols. 337–342.

———. 1882. "Galvanische Erscheinungen an dem Verlängerten Marke des Frosches." In *Selected Works* (1935), 212–242. Facsimile reprint. Amsterdam: E. J. Bonset, 1968.

———. 1884. *Études psychologiques*, trans. Victor Derély from Russian, intro. M. G. Vyrubov. Paris: C. Reinwald.

———. 1935*a*. "Reflexes of the brain," trans. A. A. Subkov from Russian (1863, rev. 1866). In *Selected Works*, 263–336. Facsimile reprint. Amsterdam: E. J. Bonset, 1968.

———. 1935*b*. "Who must investigate the problems of psychology, and how," trans. A. A. Subkov from Russian (1873). In *Selected Works*, 337–391. Facsimile reprint. Amsterdam: E. J. Bonset, 1968.

———. 1935*c*. "The elements of thought," trans. A. A. Subkov from Russian (1878, rev. 1903). In *Selected Works*, 403–489. Facsimile reprint. Amsterdam: E. J. Bonset, 1968.

———. 1960*a*. *Selected Physiological and Psychological Works*, ed. K. Koshtoyants, trans. S. Belsky from Russian and ed. G. Gibbons. Moscow: Foreign Languages Publishing House.

———. 1960*b*. "Observations on Mr. Kavelin's book 'The Tasks of Psychology.'" In *Selected Physiological and Psychological Works*, 140–178.

———. 1965*a*. *Autobiographical Notes*, trans. Kristan Hanes from Russian (1952; written about 1904) and ed. Donald B. Lindsley. Washington: American Institute of Biological Sciences.

———. 1965*b*. *Reflexes of the Brain*, trans. S. Belsky from Russian (1863, rev. 1866) and ed. G. Gibbons. Cambridge: MIT Press.

Sechenov, I. M., and B. Pashutin. 1865. *Neue Versuche am Hirn und Rückenmark des Frosches*. Berlin: August Hirschwald.

Sedgwick, William T. 1880–82. "The influence of quinine upon the reflex-excitability of the spinal cord." *Journal of Physiology* 3: 22–36.

Shapin, Steven. 1979. "Homo phrenologicus: Anthropological perspectives on an historical problem." In Barry Barnes and Steven Shapin, eds., *Natural Order*, 41–71.

———. 1982. "History of science and its sociological reconstructions." *History of Science* 20: 157–211.

Shapin, Steven, and Barry Barnes. 1976. "Head and hand: Rhetorical resources in British pedagogical writing, 1770–1850." *Oxford Review of Education* 2: 231–254.

———. 1977. "Science, nature and control: Interpreting Mechanics' Institutes." *Social Studies of Science* 7: 31–74.

Shaternikov, M. N. 1935. "The life of I. M. Sechenov." In I. M. Sechenov, *Selected Works*, vii–xxxvi. Facsimile reprint. Amsterdam: E. J. Bonset, 1968.

Sherrington, Charles Scott. 1893*a*. "Note on the knee-jerk and the correlation of action of antagonistic muscles." *Proceedings of the Royal Society of London* 52: 556–564.

———. 1893*b*. "Further experimental note on the correlation of action of antagonistic muscles." *Proceedings of the Royal Society of London* 53: 407–420.

———. 1894. "Experimental note on two movements of the eye." *Journal of Physiology* 17: 27–29.

———. 1897. "On reciprocal innervation in antagonistic muscles. Third note." *Proceedings of the Royal Society of London* 60: 414–417.

———. 1898. "Experiments in examination of the peripheral distribution of the fibres of the posterior roots of some spinal nerves. Part II." *Philosophical Transactions of the Royal Society of London* 190B: 45–186.

———. 1900. "The spinal cord." In E. A. Schäfer, ed., *Text-book of Physiology*, 2: 783–883. Edinburgh: Young J. Pentland.

———. 1904. "The correlation of reflexes and the principle of the common path." *British Association Reports* 74: 728–741.

———. 1913. "Reflex inhibition as a factor in the co-ordination of movements and postures." *Quarterly Journal of Experimental Physiology* 6: 251–310.

———. 1925. "Remarks on some aspects of reflex inhibition." *Proceedings of the Royal Society of London* 97B: 519–545.

———. 1929. "Ferrier Lecture—Some functional problems attaching to convergence." *Proceedings of the Royal Society of London* 105B: 332–362.

———. 1933. *The Brain and Its Mechanism*. Cambridge: Cambridge University Press.

———. 1939. *Selected Writings of Sir Charles Sherrington*, ed. D. Denny-Brown. Facsimile reprint. Oxford: Oxford University Press, 1979.

———. 1940. *Man on His Nature*, 2d ed. London: Cambridge University Press, 1951.

———. 1946. *The Endeavour of Jean Fernel*. Cambridge: Cambridge University Press.

———. 1961. *The Integrative Action of the Nervous System*, 2d ed. New Haven: Yale University Press. (First publ. 1906.)

———. 1965. "Inhibition as a coordinative factor. Nobel Lecture, December 12, 1932." In *Nobel Lectures, Including Presentation Speeches and Laureates' Biographies. Physiology or Medicine 1922–1941*, 278–289. Amsterdam: Elsevier, for the Nobel Foundation.

Shortt, S. E. D. 1986. *Victorian Lunacy: Richard M. Bucke and the Practice of Late Nineteenth-Century Psychiatry*. Cambridge: Cambridge University Press.

Showalter, Elaine. 1987. *The Female Malady: Women, Madness and English Culture, 1830–1980.* London: Virago.

Shuttleworth, Sally. 1984. *George Eliot and Nineteenth-Century Science: The Make-believe of a Beginning.* Cambridge: Cambridge University Press.

———. 1990. "Female circulation: Medical discourse and popular advertising in the mid-Victorian era." In Mary Jacobus, Evelyn Fox Keller, and Sally Shuttleworth, eds., *Body Politics: Women and the Discourse of Science*, 47–68. London: Routledge.

Simonov, L. N. 1866. "Die Hemmungsmechanismen der Säugethiere experimentell bewiesen." *Archiv für Anatomie, Physiologie* n.v.: 545–564.

Skinner, B. F. 1938. *The Behavior of Organisms: An Experimental Analysis.* New York: Appleton-Century-Crofts.

Skinner, Quentin. 1969. "Meaning and understanding in the history of ideas." In James Tully, ed., *Meaning and Context: Quentin Skinner and His Critics*, 29–67. Oxford: Polity Press, 1988.

Smith, C. U. M. 1982. "Evolution and the problem of mind." *Journal of the History of Biology* 15: 55–88, 241–262.

Smith, Roger. 1973. "The background of physiological psychology in natural philosophy." *History of Science* 11: 75–123.

———. 1977. "The human significance of biology: Carpenter, Darwin, and the *vera causa.*" In U. C. Knoepflmacher and G. B. Tennyson, eds., *Nature and the Victorian Imagination*, 216–230. Berkeley, Los Angeles, London: University of California Press.

———. 1981. *Trial by Medicine: Insanity and Responsibility in Victorian Trials.* Edinburgh: Edinburgh University Press.

———. 1983. "Defining murder and madness: An introduction to medicolegal belief in the case of Mary Ann Brough, 1854." In Robert Alun Jones and Henrika Kuklick, eds., *Knowledge and Society: Studies in the Sociology of Culture Past and Present. Current Perspectives on the History of the Social Sciences* 4: 173–225. Greenwich, Conn.: JAI Press.

———. 1988. "Does the history of psychology have a subject?" *History of the Human Sciences* 1: 147–177.

Smith-Rosenberg, Carroll. 1985. *Disorderly Conduct: Visions of Gender in Victorian America.* New York: Oxford University Press.

Sonntag, Michael. 1986. "'Zeitlose Dokumente der Seele'—Von der Abschaffung der Geschichte in der Geschichtsschreibung der Psychologie." In Gero Jütterman, ed., *Die Geschichtlichkeit des Seelischen: Der historischen Zugang zum Gegenstand der Psychologie*, 116–142. Weinheim: Beltz.

Spencer, Herbert. 1852. "A theory of population, deduced from the general law of animal fertility." *Westminster Review*, n.s., 1: 468–501.

———. 1860. "The social organism." In *Essays: Scientific, Political and Speculative*, 1: 384–428. London: Williams and Norgate, 1868.

——— 1862. *First Principles.* London: Williams and Norgate.

———. 1870–72. *The Principles of Psychology*, 2d ed. 2 vols. London: Williams and Norgate. (First publ. 1855.)

———. 1871. "Specialized administration." In *Essays: Scientific, Political and Speculative*, 3d ed. 3: 125–170. London: Williams and Norgate, 1878.

Spillane, John D. 1981. *The Doctrine of the Nerves: Chapters in the History of Neurology*. Oxford: Oxford University Press.

Star, Susan Leigh. 1989. *Regions of the Mind: Brain Research and the Quest for Scientific Certainty*. Stanford: Stanford University Press.

Starling, E. H. 1900*a*. "The nervous and muscular mechanism of the respiratory movements." In E. A. Schäfer, ed., *Text-book of Physiology*, 2: 274–312. Edinburgh: Young J. Pentland.

———. 1900*b*. "The nervous and muscular mechanisms of the digestive tract." In E. A. Schäfer, ed., *Text-book of Physiology*, 2: 313–337. Edinburgh: Young J. Pentland.

Stengel, E. A. 1954. "A re-evaluation of Freud's book 'On Aphasia': Its significance for psycho-analysis." *International Journal of Psycho-analysis* 35: 85–89.

Stepansky, Paul E. 1977. *A History of Aggression in Freud*. Psychological Issues, monograph 39. New York: International Universities Press.

Stephen, James Fitzjames. 1863. *A General View of the Criminal Law of England*. London: Macmillan.

Stirling, William. 1876. "On the reflex function of the spinal cord." *Edinburgh Medical Journal* 21: 914–919, 1092–1107.

Stocking, George W., Jr. 1987. *Victorian Anthropology*. New York: Free Press.

Stone, Martin. 1985. "Shellshock and the psychologists." In W. F. Bynum, Roy Porter, and Michael Shepherd, eds., *The Anatomy of Madness: Essays in the History of Psychiatry*, 2: 242–271. London: Tavistock.

Stout, G. F. 1888. "The Herbartian psychology." *Mind* 13: 321–338, 473–498.

———. 1889*a*. "Herbart compared with English psychologists and with Beneke." *Mind* 14: 1–26.

———. 1889*b*. "The psychological work of Herbart's disciples." *Mind* 14: 353–368.

Sturdy, Steve. 1988. "Biology as social theory: John Scott Haldane and physiological regulation." *British Journal for the History of Science* 21: 315–340.

Sulloway, Frank J. 1979. *Freud, Biologist of the Mind: Beyond the Psychoanalytic Legend*. London: Burnett Books, Andre Deutsch.

Sully, James. 1892. *The Human Mind: A Text-book of Psychology*. 2 vols. London: Longmans, Green.

Suslova, Nadeshda P. 1868. "Beiträge zur Physiologie der Lymphherzen." *Zeitschrift für rationelle Medicin* 31: 224–233.

Swazey, Judith P. 1969. *Reflexes and Motor Integration: Sherrington's Concept of Integrative Action*. Cambridge: Harvard University Press.

Taine, H. 1870. *De l'intelligence*. 2 vols. Paris: Librairie Hachette.

Taylor, D. W. 1971. "The life and teaching of William Sharpey (1802–1880): 'Father of modern physiology' in Britain." *Medical History* 15: 126–153, 241–259.

Temkin, Owsei. 1946. *The Falling Sickness: A History of Epilepsy from the Greeks to the Beginnings of Modern Neurology*, 2d ed. Baltimore: Johns Hopkins University Press, 1971.

Tennyson, Alfred. 1969. *The Poems of Tennyson*, ed. Christopher Ricks, 2d ed. 3 vols. Harlow: Longman, 1987.

Thompson, E. P. 1967. "Time, work-discipline, and industrial capitalism." *Past & Present*, no. 38: 56–97.

Timms, Edward, and Naomi Segal, eds. 1988. *Freud in Exile: Psychoanalysis and Its Vicissitudes*. New Haven: Yale University Press.

Todd, Robert B. 1847. "Nervous system" and "Physiology of the nervous system." In Robert B. Todd, ed., *The Cyclopaedia of Anatomy and Physiology*, 3: 585–723G. London: Longman, Brown, Green, Longmans, and Roberts.

Todd, Robert B., and William Bowman. 1845. *The Physiological Anatomy and Physiology of Man*. 2 vols. London: John W. Parker.

Todes, Daniel Philip. 1981. "From radicalism to scientific convention: Biological psychology in Russia from Sechenov to Pavlov." Ph.D. diss., University of Pennsylvania.

———. 1984. "Biological psychology and the tsarist censor: The dilemma of scientific development." *Bulletin of the History of Medicine* 58: 529–544.

Traube, J. 1848. "Entgegnung auf die Einwürfe gegen meine Theorie über die Ursachen der nach Durchschneidung der Nn. vagi eintretenden Lungenaffection." *Archiv für physiologische Heilkunde* 7: 454–471.

Tredgold, A. F. 1914. *Mental Deficiency (Amentia)*, 2d ed. London: Baillière, Tindall and Cox. (First publ. 1908.)

Tsion, I. [Cyon, E.] 1871. "Hemmungen und Erregungen im Central-System der Gefässnerven." *Bulletin de l'Académie Impériale des Sciences de St-Pétersbourg* 16: cols. 97–117.

———. 1874. "Über die Fortpflanzungsgeschwindigkeit der Erregung im Rückenmarke." *Bulletin de l'Académie Impériale des Sciences de St-Pétersbourg* 19: cols. 394–399.

———. 1888. *Gesammelte physiologischen Arbeiten*. Berlin: August Hirschwald.

Tsion, I., and C. Ludwig. 1866. "Die Reflexe eines der sensiblen Nerven des Herzens auf die motorischen der Blutgefässe." In *Arbeiten aus der physiologischen Anstalt zu Leipzig vom Jahre 1866 mitgetheilt durch C. Ludwig*, 128–149. Leipzig: S. Hirzel, 1867.

Tuke, D. H. 1891. *Prichard and Symonds in Especial Relation to Mental Science: With Chapters on Moral Insanity*. London: J. & A. Churchill.

Türck, Ludwig. 1851. "Ueber den Zustand der Sensibilität nach theilweiser Trennung des Rückenmarkes." *Zeitschrift der k. k. [kaiserlich-königlich] Gesellschaft der Aerzte zu Wien* 7th year, Heft 3: 189–201.

Turgenev, Ivan Sergeivich. 1960. *Fathers and Sons*. In *The Vintage Turgenev*, trans. Harry Stevens (1950) from Russian (first publ. 1861), 1: 165–352. New York: Vintage Books.

Turner, R. Steven. 1971. "The growth of professorial research in Prussia, 1818 to 1848—Causes and context." *Historical Studies in the Physical Sciences* 3: 137–182.

———. 1987. "Paradigms and productivity: The case of physiological optics, 1840–94." *Social Studies of Science* 17: 35–68.

Turner, R. Steven, Edward Kerwin, and David Woolwine. 1984. "Careers and creativity in nineteenth-century physiology: Zloczower *redux*." *Isis* 75: 523–529.

Turner, Trevor. 1988. "Henry Maudsley: Psychiatrist, philosopher, and entrepreneur." In W. F. Bynum, Roy Porter, and Michael Shepherd, eds., *The Anatomy of Madness: Essays in the History of Psychiatry*, 3: 151–189. London: Routledge.

Tweney, Ryan D. 1987. "Programmatic research in experimental psychology: E. B. Titchener's laboratory investigations, 1891–1927." In Mitchell G. Ash and William R. Woodward, eds., *Psychology in Twentieth-Century Thought and Society*, 35–57.

van Hoorn, Willem, and Thom Verhave. 1980. "Wundt's changing conceptions of a general and theoretical psychology." In Wolfgang G. Bringmann and Ryan D. Tweney, eds., *Wundt Studies: A Centennial Collection*, 71–113. Toronto: C. J. Hogrefe.

van Strien, P. J. 1984. "Psychology and its social legitimation: The case of the Netherlands." In Sacha Bem, Hans Rappard, and Willem van Hoorn, eds., *Studies in the History of Psychology and the Social Sciences* 2, 80–98. Proceedings of the Second Meeting of Cheiron: European Society for the History of the Behavioral and Social Sciences. Leiden: Psychologisch Instituut van de Rijksuniversiteit Leiden.

Verwey, Gerlof. 1984. *Psychiatry in an Anthropological and Biomedical Context: Philosophical Presuppositions and Implications of German Psychiatry, 1820–1870*. Dordrecht: D. Reidel.

Verworn, Max. 1899. *General Physiology: An Outline of the Science of Life*, trans. and ed. Frederic S. Lee from 2d German ed. (1897). London: Macmillan.

———. 1900. "Zur Physiologie der nervösen Hemmungserscheinungen." *Archiv für Physiologie* suppl. vol.: 105–123.

———. 1903. *Die Biogenhypothese: Eine kritisch-experimentelle Studie über die Vorgänge in der lebendigen Substanz*. Jena: Gustav Fischer.

———. 1913. *Irritability: A Physiological Analysis of the General Effect of Stimuli in Living Substance*. New Haven: Yale University Press.

Volkmann, A. W. 1838*a*. "Ueber Reflexbewegungen." *Archiv für Anatomie, Physiologie* n.v.: 15–43.

———. 1838*b*. "Von dem Baue und den Verrichtungen der Kopfnerven des Frosches." *Archiv für Anatomie, Physiologie* n.v.: 70–89.

———. 1842. "Ueber die Beweiskraft derjenigen Experimente, durch welche man einen directien Einfluss der Centralorgane auf die Eingeweide zu erweisen suchte." *Archiv für Anatomie, Physiologie* n.v.: 372–377.

———. 1844. "Nervenphysiologie." In Rudolph Wagner, ed., *Handwörterbuch der Physiologie mit Rücksicht auf physiologische Pathologie*, 2: 476–627. Braunschweig: Friedrich Vieweg und Sohn.

———. 1845. "Beitrag zur nähern Kenntniss der motorischen Nervenwirkungen." *Archiv für Anatomie, Physiologie*, n.v.: 407–429.

Volkmann, Wilhelm. 1875–76. *Lehrbuch der Psychologie vom Standpunkte des Realismus und nach genetischer Methode*. 2 vols. Cöthen: Otto Schulze.

Voltaire, François-Marie Arouet de. 1817. *Oeuvres complètes de Voltaire. Poésie*, vol. 3, pt. 2. Paris: Th. Desoer.

Vucinich, Alexander. 1970. *Science in Russian Culture 1861–1917*. Stanford: Stanford University Press.

———. 1984. *Empire of Knowledge: The Academy of Sciences of the USSR (1917–1970)*. Berkeley, Los Angeles, London: University of California Press.

Vulpian, A. 1866. *Leçons sur la physiologie générale et comparée du système nerveux*. Paris: Germer Baillière.

———. 1874. "Moelle épinière (physiologie)." In *Dictionnaire encyclopédique des sciences médicales*, 2d ser., 8: 343–604. Paris: P. Asselin and G. Masson.

Vvedenskii, N. E. 1885. "Ueber einige Beziehungen zwischen der Reizstärke und der Tetanushöhe bei indirecter Reizung." *Archiv für die gesammte Physiologie* 37: 69–72.

———. 1891. "De l'action excitatrice et inhibitoire du courant électrique sur l'appareil neuro-musculaire." *Archives de physiologie normale et pathologique*, 5th ser., 3: 687–696.

———. 1892. "Des relations entre les processus rythmiques et l'activité fonctionelle de l'appareil neuro-musculaire excité." *Archives de physiologie normale et pathologique*, 5th ser., 4: 50–59.

———. 1903. "Die Erregung, Hemmung und Narkose." *Archiv für die gesammte Physiologie* 100: 1–144.

Waitz, Theodor. 1849. *Lehrbuch der Psychologie als Naturwissenschaft*. Braunschweig: Friedrich Vieweg und Sohn.

Waller, Augustus V. 1892. "On the 'inhibition' of voluntarily and of electrically excited muscular contractions by peripheral excitations." *Brain* 15: 35–64.

Ward, James. 1886. "Psychology." In *Encyclopaedia Britannica*, 9th ed., 20: 37–85. Edinburgh: Adam and Charles Black.

Warren, Howard C. 1912. *A History of the Association Psychology*. London: Constable.

Watson, Stephen. 1988. "The moral imbecile: A study of the relations between penal practice and psychiatric knowledge of the habitual offender." Ph.D. diss., University of Lancaster.

Watteville, A. de. 1887. "Sleep and its counterfeits." *Fortnightly Review* 41: 732–742.

Weber, Eduard F. W. 1846. "Muskelbewegung." In Rudolf Wagner, ed., *Handwörterbuch der Physiologie mit Rücksicht auf physiologische Pathologie*, 3, pt. 2: 1–122. Braunschweig: Friedrich Vieweg und Sohn.

Weber, Eduard F. W., and E. H. Weber. 1846. "Expériences physiologiques faites dans le musée anatomique de Leipsik." *Archives générales de médecine*, 4th ser., 21, suppl. vol.: 9–17.

Weeks, Jeffrey. 1981. *Sex, Politics and Society: The Regulation of Sexuality Since 1800*. London: Longman.

Weindling, Paul. 1981. "Theories of the cell state in Imperial Germany." In Charles Webster, ed., *Biology, Medicine and Society 1840–1940*, 99–155. Cambridge: Cambridge University Press.

Wendt, G. R. 1936. "An interpretation of inhibition of conditional reflexes as competition between reaction systems." *Psychological Review* 43: 258–281.

Whitehead, A. N. 1926. *Science and the Modern World.* Cambridge: Cambridge University Press, 1953.

Whytt, Robert. 1768. *The Works*, published by his son. Edinburgh: T. Becket.

Wiener, Norbert. 1948. *Cybernetics: Or Control and Communication in the Animal and the Machine*, 2d ed. Cambridge: MIT Press, 1965.

Wiener, Philip Paul. 1949. *Evolution and the Founders of Pragmatism.* New York: Harper Torchbooks, 1965.

Williams, J. P. 1985. "Psychical research and psychiatry in late Victorian Britain: Trance as ecstasy or trance as insanity." In W. F. Bynum, Roy Porter, and Michael Shepherd, eds., *The Anatomy of Madness: Essays in the History of Psychiatry*, 1: 233–254. London: Tavistock.

Williams, Raymond. 1976. *Keywords: A Vocabulary of Culture and Society.* London: Fontana/Croom Helm.

Windholz, George. 1983. "Pavlov's position toward American behaviorism." *Journal of the History of the Behavioral Sciences* 19: 394–407.

———. 1990. "Pavlov and the Pavlovians in the laboratory." *Journal of the History of the Behavioral Sciences* 26: 64–74.

Wise, M. Norton, in collaboration with Crosbie Smith. 1989–90. "Work and waste: Political economy and natural philosophy in nineteenth century Britain." *History of Science* 27 (1989): 263–301, 391–449; 28 (1990): 221–261.

Wolf, Theta H. 1973. *Alfred Binet.* Chicago: University of Chicago Press.

Wolpe, Joseph. 1958. *Psychotherapy by Reciprocal Inhibition.* Stanford: Stanford University Press.

Wood, Alexander. 1851. *What Is Mesmerism? An Attempt to Explain Its Phenomena on the Admitted Principles of Physiological and Psychical Science.* Edinburgh: Sutherland and Knox.

Woodward, William R. 1982. "Wundt's program for the new psychology: Vicissitudes of experiment, theory and system." In William R. Woodward and Mitchell G. Ash, eds., *The Problematic Science*, 167–197.

Woodward, William R., and Mitchell G. Ash, eds. 1982. *The Problematic Science: Psychology in Nineteenth-Century Thought.* New York: Praeger.

Wortis, Joseph. 1950. *Soviet Psychiatry.* Baltimore: Williams & Wilkins.

Wundt, Wilhelm. 1871–1876. *Untersuchungen zur Mechanik der Nerven und Nervencentren.* Vol. 1, Erlangen: Ferdinand Enke; vol. 2, Stuttgart: Ferdinand Enke.

———. 1874. *Grundzüge der physiologischen Psychologie.* Leipzig: Wilhelm Engelmann.

———. 1893. "Hypnotismus und Suggestion." *Philosophische Studien* 8: 1–85.

———. 1902. *Grundzüge der physiologischen Psychologie*, 5th ed. 3 vols. Leipzig: Wilhelm Engelmann.

———. 1910. *Principles of Physiological Psychology. Vol. 1*, trans. Edward Bradford Titchener from 5th German ed. (1902). Facsimile reprint of 2d ed. New York: Kraus Reprint, 1969.

Young, Robert M. 1966. "Scholarship and the history of the behavioural sciences." *History of Science* 5: 1–51.

———. 1970. *Mind, Brain, and Adaptation in the Nineteenth Century: Cerebral Localization and Its Biological Context from Gall to Ferrier*. Oxford: Clarendon Press.

———. 1973*a*. "The role of psychology in the nineteenth-century evolutionary debate." In Robert M. Young, *Darwin's Metaphor*, 56–78.

———. 1973*b*. "The historiographic and ideological contexts of the nineteenth-century debate on man's place in nature." In Robert M. Young, *Darwin's Metaphor*, 164–247.

———. 1985. *Darwin's Metaphor: Nature's Place in Victorian Culture*. Cambridge: Cambridge University Press.

Zloczower, A. 1981. *Career Opportunities and the Growth of Scientific Discovery in 19th Century Germany* [Ph.D. diss., Hebrew University, Jerusalem, 1960]. New York: Arno Press.

Index

Printed in the United States
47656LVS00002B/290

9 780520 0758

(1) step 1 think – Alternative – Moving
2 thinking

Sherrington, Gaulov, Freud – 20th Ce.